Strategies for Student Success on the

NEXT GENERATION
NCLEX® (NGN)
TEST ITEMS

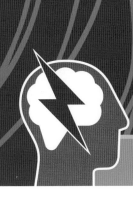

Strategies for Student Success on the

NEXT GENERATION NCLEX® (NGN) TEST ITEMS

Linda Anne Silvestri, PhD, RN, FAAN

Nursing Instructor
University of Nevada, Las Vegas
Las Vegas, Nevada;
President
Nursing Reviews, Inc. and Professional Nursing Seminars, Inc.
Henderson, Nevada;
Next Generation NCLEX® (NGN) Consultant and Subject Matter Expert
Elsevier Inc.

Angela Elizabeth Silvestri, PhD, APRN, FNP-BC, CNE

Associate Professor and BSN Program Director
University of Nevada, Las Vegas
Las Vegas, Nevada;
President
Nurse Prep, LLC
Henderson, Nevada;
Next Generation NCLEX® (NGN) Subject Matter Expert
Elsevier Inc.

Donna D. Ignatavicius, MS, RN, CNE, CNEcl, ANEF, FAADN

Speaker and Curriculum Consultant for Academic Nursing Programs
Founder
Boot Camp for Nurse Educators;
President
DI Associates, Inc.
Littleton, Colorado;
Next Generation NCLEX® (NGN) Consultant and Subject Matter Expert
Elsevier Inc.

ELSEVIER

Elsevier
3251 Riverport Lane
St. Louis, Missouri 63043

STRATEGIES FOR STUDENT SUCCESS ON THE NEXT GENERATION
NCLEX® (NGN) TEST ITEMS   ISBN: 978-0-323-87229-4
Copyright © 2023 by Elsevier Inc. All rights reserved.

Notice

International Standard Book Number: 978-0-323-87229-4

Content Strategist: Heather D. Bays-Petrovic
Content Development Manager: Ellen M. Wurm-Cutter
Content Development Specialist: Laura Klein; Meredith Madeira
Publishing Services Manager: Julie Eddy
Senior Project Manager: Jodi Willard
Design Direction: Amy Buxton

Printed in India

Last digit is the print number: 9 8 7 6 5 4

Working together
to grow libraries in
developing countries

www.elsevier.com • www.bookaid.org

In loving memory of my parents and Angela's grandparents,
Arnold Lawrence and Frances Mary, who opened my door of opportunity
to this amazing profession of nursing. My memories of their love, support,
and words of encouragement will remain in my heart forever!
And, to my husband, Larry, for being my rock of support
through all of my life's journeys.
Linda Anne Silvestri

To my husband, Brent, who has supported my work since the day we met.
I will always remember how he anticipated what I would need
to be successful in this journey.
To nursing students, you have chosen a wonderful profession that will
give back to you what you are putting in now. You can do this!
Angela Elizabeth Silvestri

To my family, who has supported my work as an author and consultant
for many decades.
To nursing students, who have chosen the caring profession that can
change the lives of so many, and to nurse educators, whose passion and
role modeling continues to shape the future of the nursing profession.
Donna D. Ignatavicius

About the Authors

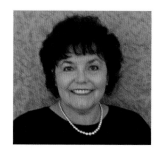

Linda Anne Silvestri, PhD, RN, FAAN

Linda is a well-known nurse educator, entrepreneur, and philanthropist whose professional aspirations focus on assisting nursing students to become successful. She has been teaching nursing students at all levels of nursing education for many years. Dr. Silvestri is currently a nursing instructor at the University of Nevada, Las Vegas (UNLV). She earned her PhD in Nursing from UNLV and conducted research on self-efficacy and the predictors of NCLEX® success. Her research findings are published in the *Journal of Nursing Education and Practice.* Dr. Silvestri has received several awards and honors. In 2019 she was inducted as a Fellow in the American Academy of Nursing. In 2012 she received the UNLV School of Nursing Alumna of the Year Award. In 2010 she received the School of Nursing Certificate of Recognition for the Outstanding PhD Student. Dr. Silvestri is a member of several national nursing organizations, some of which include the Honor Society of Nursing, Sigma Theta Tau International, the National League for Nursing, the American Nurses Association, and the American Academy of Nursing. Dr. Silvestri is a successful Elsevier author of numerous best-selling NCLEX® preparation resources on national and international levels. She also serves as an Elsevier Consultant and Subject Matter Expert for the Next Generation NCLEX® (NGN) and has presented numerous webinars on NCLEX® preparation and success. Dr. Silvestri is the President and Owner of Nursing Reviews, Inc. and Professional Nursing Seminars, Inc. Both companies are dedicated to helping nursing graduates achieve their goals of becoming licensed nurses.

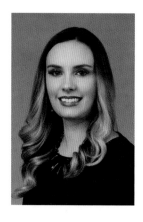

Angela E. Silvestri, PhD, APRN, FNP-BC, CNE

Angela Silvestri is a well-known nurse educator, researcher, and author. She has been teaching and working in university administrative roles for the last 10 years at all levels of nursing education. She has experience teaching across the program and in both classroom and clinical settings and working with graduate students on their culminating projects and research dissertations. She is currently serving in a leadership role as the Program Director for the undergraduate BSN program at the University of Nevada, Las Vegas (UNLV). Angela earned a bachelor's in Nursing and in Sociology from Salve Regina University in Newport, RI, and her master's—with a focus in nursing education—and PhD from the University of Nevada, Las Vegas. She also has a post-master's graduate certificate in Advanced Practice and is a board-certified Family Nurse Practitioner. She is a Scholar in Sigma Theta Tau's New Academic Leadership Academy. Angela is passionate about college student success. She works as a Family Nurse Practitioner with faculty, staff, and students on managing primary and episodic health care needs at UNLV's Student Wellness Center and Faculty and Staff Treatment Center. Dr. Silvestri is a successful Elsevier author of numerous best-selling NCLEX® preparation resources on national and international levels. She also serves as an Elsevier Subject Matter Expert for the Next Generation NCLEX® (NGN). This passion also comes through in her work at the School of Nursing teaching leadership and licensure exam preparation, as well as in publishing research and best-selling licensure exam review resources on national and international levels.

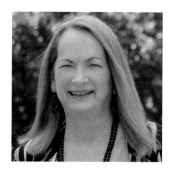

Donna D. Ignatavicius, MS, RN, CNE, CNEcl, ANEF, FAADN

Nationally recognized as an expert in nursing education and medical-surgical nursing, Donna, better known as "Iggy," has a wealth of experience in education, clinical nursing, and administration. Through her company, DI Associates, Inc., Iggy speaks at national and state conferences and provides consultation on such topics as curriculum transformation and NGN preparation. In addition, she is the author of a number of articles, chapters, and books, including the tenth edition of her leading textbook, *Medical-Surgical Nursing: Concepts for Interprofessional Collaborative Care.* In 2007 Iggy was inducted as a fellow into the very prestigious Academy of Nursing Education for her national contributions to nursing education. In 2021 she was also inducted as a fellow into the Academy of Associate Degree Nursing for her national influence and contributions to programs preparing students for nursing practice. Iggy obtained her Certified Nurse Educator® credential in 2016 and her Certified Academic Clinical Educator® credential in 2020.

Acknowledgments

We want to acknowledge the many people from Elsevier who were such a significant part of our journey as we prepared this resource for nursing students. First and foremost, we extend our deepest appreciation to Heather Bays-Petrovic, Content Strategist, for accepting our proposal and promoting our vision for this project and for supporting us every step of the way from start to finish. Thank you, Heather! Jodi Willard, Senior Project Manager, has been instrumental in moving this publication forward. Jodi's work and attention to detail has been significant in the design and final product. Thank you, Jodi! We also extend our sincere gratitude to Laura Klein, Senior Content Development Specialist; Amy Buxton, Senior Book Designer; and Julie Eddy, Publishing Services Manager. We thank all of you for your willingness and flexibility to design this resource ensuring that our ideas and vision were executed and for your consistent attention to the many details in our manuscript. Finally, we want to thank Bruce Seibert, Senior Digital Media Producer, and Bala Cherukumilli, Digital Media Producer, for all of your patience and assistance in implementing our requests for the electronic platform that accompanies this resource. A very grateful and appreciative "Thank You" from us to all of you— we could not have achieved our aspirations for this resource without you!

Preface

Welcome to the *Strategies for Student Success on the Next Generation NCLEX® (NGN) Test Items!*

This book is focused on providing you with information about the Next Generation NCLEX® (NGN) and practice questions to prepare you to successfully answer the new test item types expected on the NGN.[a] This book highlights general NGN Tips and unique test-taking strategies. Chapter 1 introduces the clinical judgment (CJ) cognitive skills upon which the new test items will be based. Chapter 2 presents examples of the new NGN test item types. Chapters 3 through 8 describe the CJ cognitive skills and present unique test-taking strategies on how to answer practice items that measure each skill. Chapter 9 demonstrates how Stand-alone items and Unfolding Case Studies will be presented on the NGN, and Chapter 10 provides an NGN Practice Test to apply what was learned throughout the book. The answers, rationales, test-taking strategies, content area, and CJ cognitive skill(s) for each practice question throughout the book are presented at the end of the book. In addition, the priority concept is identified. The specific focus of each chapter is summarized below.

Organization of the Book

- Chapter 1, *Introduction to the Cognitive Skills of Clinical Judgment*, describes how clinical judgment builds on the nursing process and introduces you to the six essential cognitive skills of the NCSBN Clinical Judgment Measurement Model (NCJMM). These cognitive skills are the basis for the new NGN test item types.
- Chapter 2, *Introduction to the NGN and the New NGN Item Types*, explains the purpose and design of the NGN and presents the new test item types. An example of each item type is presented, and the correct responses are provided with brief rationales.
- Chapter 3, *Strategies for Answering NGN Questions: Recognize Cues*, describes the CJ cognitive skill, *Recognize Cues*, which requires you to identify relevant clinical findings and decide which findings are of *immediate* concern and *most* important based on the clinical scenario. This chapter also identifies test items and enhanced test-taking strategies that you can use when answering items that measure this skill. Examples of these test items allow you the opportunity to practice applying these strategies within the chapter and in the practice test at the end of the chapter.

- Chapter 4, *Strategies for Answering NGN Questions: Analyze Cues*, describes the CJ cognitive skill, *Analyze Cues*, which requires you to connect or link relevant cues to the clinical scenario, interpret these cues, and establish their significance. This chapter also identifies test items and enhanced test-taking strategies that you can use when answering items that measure this skill. Examples of these test items allow you the opportunity to practice applying these strategies within the chapter and in the practice test at the end of the chapter.
- Chapter 5, *Strategies for Answering NGN Questions: Prioritize Hypotheses*, describes the CJ cognitive skill, *Prioritize Hypotheses*, which requires you to establish and rank client needs or hypotheses in order of priority. This chapter also identifies test items and enhanced test-taking strategies that you can use when answering items that measure this skill. Examples of these test items allow you the opportunity to practice applying these strategies within the chapter and in the practice test at the end of the chapter.
- Chapter 6, *Strategies for Answering NGN Questions: Generate Solutions*, describes the CJ cognitive skill, *Generate Solutions*, which requires you to use knowledge of evidence-based solutions about treatments and interventions that would address identified client needs and modify them to meet priorities of care. This chapter also identifies test items and enhanced test-taking strategies that you can use when answering items that measure this skill. Examples of these test items allow you the opportunity to practice applying these strategies within the chapter and in the practice test at the end of the chapter.
- Chapter 7, *Strategies for Answering NGN Questions: Take Action*, describes the CJ cognitive skill, *Take Action*, which requires that you perform appropriate and necessary interventions based on the client's situation and generated solutions. This chapter also identifies test items and enhanced test-taking strategies that you can use when answering items that measure this skill. Examples of these test items allow you the opportunity to practice applying these strategies within the chapter and in the practice test at the end of the chapter.
- Chapter 8, *Strategies for Answering NGN Questions: Evaluate Outcomes*, describes the CJ cognitive skill, *Evaluate Outcomes*, which requires that you examine outcomes and measure client progress towards meeting those outcomes in the plan of care. This chapter also identifies test items and enhanced test-taking strategies that you can use when answering items that measure this skill. Examples of these test items allow you the opportunity to practice applying these strategies within the chapter and in the practice test at the end of the chapter.

---

[a] **Please note:** The NGN content provided in this book and on the Evolve site reflects the information available at the time of production of this resource. The NCSBN research about NGN is ongoing, and changes in the items to measure each cognitive skill may be forthcoming. The NCSBN website at www.ncsbn.org provides you with the latest updates.

- Chapter 9, *Strategies for Answering NGN Stand-alone Items and Unfolding Case Studies*, describes the differences between Stand-alone items and Unfolding Case Studies. Samples of Stand-alone items (including the bow-tie and trend) are illustrated, as well as Unfolding Case Studies. This chapter also identifies test items and enhanced test-taking strategies that you can use when answering questions accompanying each type of case study. Examples of these test items allow you the opportunity to practice applying these strategies within the chapter. This chapter also points out external factors to consider in NGN cases, such as the environmental and individual factors.
- Chapter 10, *NGN Practice Test: Putting It All Together*, provides you with the opportunity to practice all of the new types of test items expected on the NGN, starting with Unfolding Cases Studies and ending with Stand-alone Bow-tie and Trend items.

Special Features of the Book

- *NGN tips within each chapter.* These unique tips provide the student with key points to remember, such as the NGN item type or cognitive skill (CS) features.
- *In-chapter sample questions* are presented within Chapters 3 through 9 to provide examples of the new NGN test item types that best measure the clinical judgment cognitive skill presented in the chapter. Each question within the chapter specifies the priority concept and content area being tested. The answer, rationale, enhanced test-taking strategy, and references are also presented to help students learn the thinking process needed to select the correct test item response.
- *End-of-chapter practice* questions are presented at the end of Chapters 3 through 8 to provide the opportunity for students to apply what they learned in each chapter and experience answering selected test items that measure each of the NCSBN's clinical judgment cognitive skills. Chapter 9 presents Stand-alone items, both Bow-tie and Trend items, and Unfolding Case Studies.
- *A comprehensive practice test* is presented in Chapter 10 to allow students to apply what they learned in Chapters 1 through 9. Students have the opportunity to answer multiple Unfolding Case Studies and Stand-alone items representing all clinical specialty areas. The priority concept, content area, answer, rationale, enhanced test-taking strategy, and reference for each test item are provided at the end of the book.
- *Enhanced test-taking strategies for the NGN.* This unique feature walks students through the thinking process needed to navigate complex NGN cases. Each strategy explains how to apply the cognitive skill when considering the information presented in the clinical scenario. Each question is accompanied by test-taking strategies that are presented both narratively and in a table format to guide the student through a logical thinking process and to suit multiple learning styles. This thinking process with test-taking strategies will also help on current NCLEX-style (Stand-alone) items and nursing course exams.

- *Thinking Space.* The Thinking Spaces located in the margins of the book is a place for personal note-taking. The student can use these spaces to write down new and important information they want to remember. To become most familiar with the cognitive skills and to build clinical judgment skills, using the Thinking Space to make important linkages between clinical scenario information and the cognitive skill will reinforce the aspects of the NCJMM model as the student is studying and preparing for the NGN.

Special Features Found on Evolve

The Evolve site accompanying this resource provides the student with all of the case studies and practice test questions in the book plus an additional 30 unfolding case studies, each with 6 NGN items. The book includes 60 single cases (each with 1 NGN item), 10 Stand-alone items (5 Bow-tie and 5 Trend), and 5 Unfolding Case Studies (items with 6 NGN items). This equals a total of 100 NGN items. Then there are an additional 30 unfolding cases, each with 6 NGN items, and 4 additional Stand-alone items (2 Bow-tie and 2 Trend) totaling 184 NGN items. Altogether, there are a total of 284 NGN items on Evolve.

The Evolve site lists various category selections. You can select by type of question—either single case, Stand-alone items (either bow-tie or trend), or Unfolding Case Study. You can also select by the specific cognitive skill, content area, or priority concept. The table below illustrates the various categories for selection.

Type	Cognitive Skill	Content Area	Priority Concept
Single	Recognize Cues	Foundations	Clotting
Stand-	Analyze Cues	of Nursing	Cognition
alone	Prioritize	Maternal-	Elimination
Unfolding	Hypotheses	Newborn	Fluid and
	Generate	Nursing	Electrolyte
	Solutions	Medical-	Balance
	Take Action	Surgical	Gas
	Evaluate	Nursing	Exchange
	Outcomes	Mental Health	Glucose
		Nursing	Regulation
		Pediatric	Immunity
		Nursing	Mobility
		Pharmacology	Mood and
			Affect
			Perfusion
			Stress and
			Coping
			Tissue
			Integrity

How to Use This Book

For Students

As implied in the title, this book was written to help you be successful when taking the new test item types that will be part of the Next Generation NCLEX® (NGN). The first two book chapters present a review of clinical judgment and the NGN item types. All new item types are based on the six cognitive (thinking) skills needed for safe, appropriate clinical judgment. Be sure that you are very familiar with this information before beginning to practice answering the test questions later in the book.

Chapters 3 through 8 describe each clinical judgment cognitive skill and provide general NGN Tips on how to answer test items that measure each skill. Sample NGN test items are then presented with the Rationale and Test-Taking Strategy for the correct and incorrect responses, followed by six end-of-chapter practice questions for you to answer. The practice questions in each chapter represent all content specialties. The rationale and test-taking strategy that you can use for each question to determine the correct answers are described in detail, with tables to help organize the information in each question. In addition, each test item is labeled by priority nursing concept and content specialty. References are also provided to help you review the content associated with each test item if needed.

When working through Chapters 3 through 8, start with Chapters 3 and 4 early in your program so that you can learn how to determine the most important client findings in a clinical scenario and what they mean (Recognize Cues and Analyze Cues). When you feel you have mastered these cognitive skills, work through Chapter 5, which will help you learn to prioritize client needs and the care required to meet them. Chapters 6 and 7 are focused on helping you learn to plan and implement nursing actions to meet the client's needs. Finally, Chapter 8 will assist you in determining whether the client's condition has improved after care has been implemented.

After working through Chapters 3 through 8 and when you feel ready to put all the cognitive skills together, Chapter 9 provides examples for NGN Unfolding Case Studies and Stand-alone items. Chapter 10 presents a comprehensive practice test that simulates what you can expect on the NGN. The rationale and test-taking strategy for each practice test item in these chapters are described in detail. Many additional practice NGN test items are available on the Evolve site with rationale, test-taking strategy, content specialty, priority nursing concept, and reference for each Unfolding Case Study or Stand-alone item.

For Faculty

This book is designed for you to use as it is organized, beginning with helping students learn what CJ is and gain an understanding of each of the essential CJ cognitive skills as described in Chapter 1. Students in their first nursing course should learn how to use these skills to make safe, appropriate clinical judgments to ensure client safety. If students are already making clinical judgments using these skills, Chapter 1 could be used for review. Then students should become familiar with the NGN test design and new item types as presented in Chapter 2. Finally, by the end of the first semester (or other term), students should learn how to Recognize Cues and Analyze Cues (Chapters 3 and 4). These cognitive skills

focus on assessing the client, discerning how to determine which client findings are the most important, and deciding what those findings mean. End-of-chapter practice questions can be used during class, online, simulation pre- or post-briefing, or clinical post-conference. The test items can be assigned to students as individuals or in groups to answer. Regardless of where or how practice test items are used, such as in the classroom, online, lab sessions, or clinical setting, be sure to review the answers, rationales, and strategies for arriving at the correct response(s) to identify and improve students' thinking process as needed.

As students progress to the next course, they should begin to learn how to prioritize care to determine what nursing actions they would plan and implement. Part of this thinking process includes an assessment to decide if the actions were effective and the client's condition has improved. Therefore students in this semester would focus on Chapters 5 through 8. Again, you can assign the practice items to students as individuals or in groups and review the items to help students improve their thinking as needed.

Chapters 9 and 10 puts together all the cognitive skill steps and new NGN test item types—both Stand-alone items and Unfolding Case Studies. These chapters can be used whenever students are applying the individual CJ cognitive skills to successfully answer the new test items in preparation for the NGN. Assign these practice Unfolding Case Studies and Stand-alone items as individual student practice to determine any skill areas where improvement is needed. Students needing improvement can then review any of the six earlier chapters (Chapters 3 through 8) to hone their thinking skills.

Faculty Tool Kit

The Faculty Tool Kit was created to guide faculty in using this book with their students at any stage in the program to prepare them for the NGN.

The Tool Kit:

- Furnishes a guide for how to use this book, *Strategies for Student Success on the Next Generation NCLEX® (NGN) Test Items,* to prepare students for the NGN
- Provides chapter-to-chapter strategic points to emphasize to students and ways to prepare students for answering NGN items
- Provides suggestions for using the Evolve site accompanying this book
- Presents step-by-step guides for writing Stand-alone items and Unfolding Case Studies
- Presents step-by-step guides for writing NGN items
- Specifies NCSBN resources that focus on NGN for students and faculty
- Provides Elsevier resources and references for preparing students for the NGN

Additional Resources for Students

- Ignatavicius, D.D. (2021). *Developing Clinical Judgment for Professional Nursing and the Next-Generation NCLEX-RN® Examination.* St. Louis: Elsevier.

This workbook helps students preparing to become RNs learn how to develop NCSBN's six clinical judgment cognitive skills through practice in answering new NGN test item types embedded in unfolding and single-episode cases throughout the entire curriculum. Clinical scenarios are presented from more basic care to complex, multisystem care of clients in multiple specialty areas.

- Ignatavicius, D.D. (2022). *Developing Clinical Judgment for Practical-Vocational Nursing and the Next-Generation NCLEX-PN® Examination.* St. Louis: Elsevier.

This workbook helps students preparing to become LPNs or LVNs learn how to develop NCSBN's six clinical judgment cognitive skills through practice in answering new NGN test item types embedded in unfolding and single-episode cases. Clinical scenarios in multiple specialty areas are included, with a primary emphasis on the care of older adults in a variety of health care settings, and can be used throughout the entire curriculum.

- Silvestri, L., & Silvestri, A. (2023). *Saunders Comprehensive Review for the NCLEX-RN® Examination* (9th ed.). St. Louis: Elsevier.

This is an excellent resource to use both while you are in nursing school and in preparation for the NCLEX® examination. This book contains 20 units with 70 chapters, and each chapter is designed to identify specific components of nursing content. The book and accompanying software contain more than 5200 practice questions and include alternate item format questions. The software also contains a 75-question preassessment test that generates an individualized study calendar. A postassessment test is included, as well as case studies and accompanying NGN item type practice questions.

- Silvestri, L., & Silvestri, A. (2021). *Saunders Q&A Review for the NCLEX-RN® Examination* (8th ed.). St. Louis: Elsevier.

This book and accompanying Evolve site provide you with more than 6000 practice questions based on the NCLEX-RN® test plan. Each practice question includes a priority nursing tip that provides you with a piece of important information to remember that will help you answer questions on nursing exams and on the NCLEX® examination. The chapters in this book are uniquely designed and are based on the NCLEX-RN® examination test plan framework, including Client Needs and Integrated Processes. Alternate item format questions and accompanying NGN item type practice questions are included. With practice questions focused on the Client Needs, Integrated Processes, and Clinical Judgment/Cognitive Skills, you can assess your level of competence.

- Silvestri, L., & Silvestri, A. (2020). *HESI/Saunders Online Review Course for the NCLEX-RN® Examination.* (3rd ed.) St. Louis: Elsevier.

The online NCLEX-RN® review course provides a systematic and individualized approach and addresses all areas of the test plan identified by the National Council of State Boards of Nursing, Inc. This self-paced online review contains 10 interactive, multimedia-rich modules featuring animations and videos, practice questions, end-of-lesson case studies, and much more! A diagnostic pretest generates a study calendar to guide your review. NCLEX®-style questions—including every type of alternate item format question—are provided, concluding with a comprehensive examination that will sharpen your test-taking skills. In addition, case studies and accompanying NGN practice questions are included. Unique videos that simulate a live review course focus on difficult subjects such as dysrhythmias and make them easier to understand.

- Silvestri, L., & Silvestri, A. (2021). *Saunders 2022-2023 Clinical Judgment and Test-Taking Strategies* (7th ed.) St. Louis: Elsevier.

This book is designed for both RN and PN nursing students and provides a foundation for understanding and unpacking the complexities of NCLEX® exam questions, including alternate item formats. *Saunders 2022-2023 Clinical Judgment and Test-Taking Strategies* takes a detailed look at all the test-taking strategies you will need to know in order to pass any nursing examination, including the NCLEX® examination. Special nursing content tips are integrated along with other tips, such as clinical preparation tips and life-planning tips. There are 1200 practice questions included so you can apply the testing strategies. NGN items and practice test questions are also included on the Evolve site accompanying this resource.

- Silvestri, L., & Silvestri, A. (2022). *Saunders Comprehensive Review for the NCLEX-PN® Examination* (8th ed.). St. Louis: Elsevier.

This is an excellent resource to use both while you are in nursing school and in preparation for the NCLEX® examination. This book contains 19 units and 65 chapters, and each chapter is designed to identify specific components of nursing content. The book and accompanying Evolve site contain more than 4500 practice questions and include alternate item format questions. The software also contains a 75-question preassessment test that generates an individualized study calendar. A post-assessment test is also included, as well as case studies and accompanying NGN item type practice questions.

- Silvestri, L., & Silvestri, A. (2020). *Saunders Q&A Review for the NCLEX-PN® Examination* (6th ed.). St. Louis: Elsevier.

This book and accompanying Evolve site provide you with more than 5900 practice questions based on the NCLEX-PN test plan. Each practice question includes a priority nursing tip that provides you with a piece of important information to remember that will help you answer questions on nursing exams and on the NCLEX® examination. The chapters in this book are uniquely designed and are based on the NCLEX-PN® examination test plan framework, including Client Needs and Integrated Processes. Alternate item format questions and accompanying NGN item type practice questions are included. With practice questions focused on the Client Needs, Integrated Processes, and Clinical Judgment/Cognitive Skills, you can assess your level of competence.

- Silvestri, L., & Silvestri, A. (2020). *HESI/Saunders Online Review Course for the NCLEX-PN® Examination.* (3rd ed.) St. Louis: Elsevier.

  This online NCLEX-PN® review course provides a systematic and individualized approach and addresses all areas of the test plan identified by the National Council of State Boards of Nursing, Inc. This self-paced online review contains 10 interactive, multimedia-rich modules featuring animations and videos, practice questions, end-of-lesson case studies, and much more! A diagnostic pretest generates a study calendar to guide your review. NCLEX®-style questions—including every type of alternate item format question—are provided, concluding with a comprehensive examination that will sharpen your test-taking skills. In addition, case studies and accompanying NGN practice questions are included. Unique videos that simulate a live review course focus on difficult subjects such as dysrhythmias and make them easier to understand.

Contents

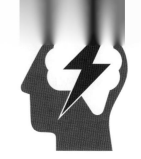

CHAPTER 1

Introduction to the Cognitive Skills of Clinical Judgment

This chapter will help you understand the need for change in the NCLEX® and the six clinical judgment cognitive (thinking) skills that serve as the basis for new test item types on the NGN. After a brief review of the *current* NCLEX® design, thinking skills needed to make safe, evidence-based clinical judgment are introduced. General NGN Tips are provided to help you relate each thinking skill with the new exam.

The new NGN item types will be included on the NCLEX® no sooner than 2023 and are described in Chapter 2 of this book. Specific Test-Taking Strategies that will help you correctly answer these new items are provided throughout other chapters of this book and accompany all practice questions in the book and on the Evolve site. Be sure to review this chapter *before* reading the rest of this book or practicing NGN questions!

What Are the Purpose and Design of the Current NCLEX®?

As you know, prelicensure nursing education programs like the one you're currently in prepare students for eligibility to take either the NCLEX-RN® or the NCLEX-PN® after graduation. These national licensure examinations are developed and updated under the direction of the NCSBN. This organization also oversees the administration of the NCLEX® in the United States, Canada, and a number of other countries.

The primary purpose of the NCSBN is to *protect the public* by providing competency assessments, such as the NCLEX®, that are sound and secure. The NCLEX® is comprehensive and reflects current nursing practice. To ensure examination currency, the NCSBN collects and analyzes nursing practice data every 3 years from thousands of graduates to determine what knowledge and activities are required in their jobs as new nurses. This information is used to develop the content of the NCLEX® and is organized in a new licensure test plan every 3 years (https://www.ncsbn.org/testplans.htm). The test plan is organized by four major Client Needs Categories, some of which have subcategories. In addition, five Integrated Processes are defined and included throughout the NCLEX® Test Plan as shown in Box 1.1.

The NCLEX® currently measures the new graduate's minimum competence in safety to ensure public protection through a variety of test items. Most of the test items (about 95%) are either Multiple Choice or Multiple Response, also known as Select All That Apply (SATA) questions. For each of these item types, client information is presented in a short clinical scenario followed by a question about the nurse's role in client care. Examples of these test item types are presented in Box 1.2.

As you'll notice in the aforementioned test items, each question focuses on what the nurse would do or say in response to specific client data. Only the client information that is the most important, relevant, or, in some cases, of immediate concern to the nurse is presented in the clinical situation. The answer is then selected from a list of choices provided. The narrow focus of these test items does not represent the scope of actual nursing practice and does not allow measurement of clinical judgment. Rather, these types of items reflect whether the candidate can distinguish between right and wrong. At this point in your education, you likely are very familiar with these item types on your course exams.

THINKING SPACE

BOX 1.1   NCLEX-RN® Test Plan Organizing Concepts

Integrated Processes	Client Needs Categories/Subcategories
Nursing Process[a] Teaching and Learning Communication and Documentation Caring Culture and Spirituality	Safe and Effective Care Environment • Management of Care[b] • Safety and Infection Control Health Promotion and Maintenance Psychosocial Integrity Physiological Integrity • Basic Care and Comfort • Pharmacological and Parenteral Therapies[c] • Reduction of Risk Potential • Physiological Adaptation

[a]This Integrated Process on the NCLEX-PN® Test Plan is the Problem-Solving Process.
[b]This Client Needs subcategory on the NCLEX-PN® Test Plan is Coordinated Care.
[c]This Client Needs subcategory on the NCLEX-PN® Test Plan is Pharmacological Therapies.

BOX 1.2   Examples of Current Multiple Choice and Multiple Response NCLEX® Test Items

Example 1: Multiple Choice Single Response

The nurse is planning care for a client admitted to the hospital with a diagnosis of acute pancreatitis and controlled hypertension. What is the nurse's **priority** for the client's care at this time?

☐ Administer an antiemetic medication.

☐ Manage the client's acute pain. ⚡

☐ Monitor the client's blood pressure.

☐ Administer supplemental oxygen.

Example 2: Multiple Response (Select All That Apply)

The nurse is assessing an adolescent who was taken to the ED for threatening to commit suicide. What is (are) the **most appropriate** question(s) for the nurse to ask the client at this time? **Select all that apply.**

☐ "What made you want to kill yourself?"

☐ "Do you have a plan for killing yourself?" ⚡

☐ "Do you plan to kill yourself with anyone else?" ⚡

☐ "Is this the first time you've threatened to kill yourself?"

☐ "Did you write a suicide note to explain why you are doing this?"

Note: ⚡ Indicates correct response(s).

Why Is There a Need for NCLEX® Change?

Although national NCLEX® first-time pass rates for both RN and PN graduates have been above 80% for many years, health care employers continue to report increasing errors in client care and lack of appropriate clinical judgment skills among new nursing graduates. A recent literature review conducted by the NCSBN found that 50% of all nurses have been involved in at least one client error. Sixty percent of those errors were the result of poor clinical judgment. Over 80% of nursing employers are *not* satisfied with the ability of new nursing graduates to make accurate or appropriate clinical decisions regarding client care. In response to these data, the NCSBN began to question if the NCLEX® was measuring "the best thing" to protect the public.

The 2013–2014 Strategic Practice Analysis of activities performed by practicing RNs and RN role experts confirmed the importance of sound clinical judgment skills for many tasks and activities performed by entry-level nurses. This analysis also highlighted that nurses today make more complex decisions to provide safe care for clients with higher acuity and advanced age.

The NCSBN literature review also found that the nurse's primary practice activity is the ability to problem solve and critically think—thinking processes needed for making appropriate clinical judgments. *Problem solving* is the process of developing and evaluating nursing solutions or approaches to client problems. *Critical thinking* can be described as a process requiring the use of logic and clinical reasoning to identify the strengths and weaknesses of nursing solutions or approaches to client problems. The NCBSN built on these process descriptions to create a definition and model of clinical judgment to be used as a basis for developing new NCLEX® test item types.

What Is the NCSBN'S Definition and Model of Clinical Judgment?

As a result of the literature review, Strategic Practice Analysis, and input from a variety of nurse clinicians and educators, the NCSBN developed this definition of clinical judgment:

Clinical judgment is defined as the observed outcome of critical thinking and decision making. It is an iterative process that uses nursing knowledge to observe and assess presenting situations, identify a prioritized client concern, and generate the best possible evidence-based solutions in order to deliver safe client care.

So, what does this definition mean for you as a nursing student and future professional nurse? Think about each of these key points in the clinical judgment definition:

- Recognize that clinical judgment is the result or *outcome of thinking* to make decisions about client care when potential or actual health problems occur. The same process of thinking to make clinical decisions occurs repeatedly as you manage client problems *(iterative process).*
- Acquire and recall *nursing knowledge* to make appropriate clinical judgments. (However, having knowledge does not guarantee that an accurate or appropriate clinical judgment will be made.)
- Learn how to *prioritize* a client's need for care based on the data presented about a clinical situation.
- Be familiar with the *best current evidence* regarding a presented client situation so you can come up with possible solutions or approaches for care to keep the client *safe.*

You will want to acquire these skills and a strong knowledge base during your nursing program to be ready for a dynamic, complex health care system and the NGN.

After the NCSBN developed its definition of clinical judgment, the organization created a model of clinical judgment, called the NCSBN Clinical Judgment Measurement Model (NCJMM). As the name implies, this model was created to measure the nursing graduate's ability to make clinical judgments. Although it is not important for you to be familiar with the entire model, it is essential that you master the thinking skills associated with clinical judgment. The NCJMM identifies six cognitive (thinking) skills that are needed for effective professional nursing practice and serve as the basis for the new NGN test item types. These skills are sometimes referred to as Layer 3 of the NCJMM and are introduced in the next section of this chapter.

The NCJMM also identifies factors that influence the ability of nurses to make appropriate clinical judgments. Examples of these Environmental and Individual factors, sometimes referred to as Layer 4 of the NCJMM, are listed in Table 1.1. Individual factors are those related to the nursing graduate candidate taking the NGN.

What Are the Six NCSBN Clinical Judgment Measurement Model Cognitive Skills?

The NGN includes new test item types that measure the six cognitive skills of clinical judgment. Each of these thinking skills, sometimes referred to as cognitive processes,

TABLE 1.1	Example of Environmental and Individual Factors That Influence Clinical Judgment	
Examples of Environmental Factors	**Examples of Individual Factors**
Environment	Knowledge
Medical records	Skills
Time pressure	Specialty
Task complexity	Prior experience
Resources	Level of experience
Cultural considerations	Candidate characteristics
Client observation	
Consequences and risks	

BOX 1.3   Clinical Judgment Cognitive Skills With Key Questions
Recognize Cues: What matters most? **Analyze Cues:** What could it mean? **Prioritize Hypotheses:** Where do I start? **Generate Solutions:** What can I do? **Take Action:** What will I do? **Evaluate Outcomes:** Did it help?

is introduced in this chapter. Chapters 3 through 8 in this book describe these skills in more detail and present examples of NGN test items that are designed to measure each skill. The six cognitive skills essential for clinical judgment are listed in Box 1.3 with key questions that explain the focus of each skill.

Recognize Cues

For clients in any health care setting, the nurse collects client data from a number of sources. *Cues* are client findings or assessment data that provide information for nurses as a basis for decision making to make appropriate clinical judgments and can be divided into four major types as listed below. Chapter 3 describes these sources of cues in more detail.

- Environmental cues; e.g., presence of family member
- Client observation cues; e.g., signs and symptoms
- Medical record cues; e.g., lab values or vital signs
- Time pressure cues; e.g., rapid clinical decline

In actual clinical practice, the nurse reviews all client findings to determine which data are most important, relevant, and, in some cases, of immediate concern. To help you *Recognize Cues,* ask yourself which client data are most important in the presented clinical scenario. Carefully review the client's presenting data, such as vital signs and medical diagnosis, to determine their relevance. For example, a heart rate of 140 bpm would be of immediate concern for a middle-aged adult, but is within the typical range for a newborn.

In some clinical scenarios the client has a history of one or more acute and/or chronic health problems. For example, an older adult with a long history of COPD may have a Pao_2 of 65 mm Hg. This arterial oxygen level is abnormal because it is below the usual range of 80 to 100 mm Hg. However, for *this* client, the low arterial oxygen level is likely not important or of immediate concern because it is expected. Many clients with advanced COPD have chronically low arterial oxygen, but they compensate by using breathing techniques combined with low-flow supplemental oxygen.

Analyze Cues

After relevant cues have been identified in a clinical scenario, the nurse organizes and links them to the client's presenting clinical situation. Ask yourself: "What do the relevant client data mean or indicate at this time?" For example, consider a middle-aged

NGN TIP

Remember: To *Recognize Cues,* carefully review the client's assessment data like developmental age and history to help determine if findings are relevant or of immediate concern to the nurse.

BOX 1.4	Example of a Thinking Activity That Requires the Ability to *Analyze Cues*		
Client Finding	**Dehydration**	**Hypernatremia**	**Anemia**
Generalized weakness			
Acute confusion			
Dry mouth			
Increased heart rate			
Dyspnea on exertion			

BOX 1.5	Example of a Thinking Activity That Requires the Ability to *Analyze Cues*		
Client Assessment Finding	**Dehydration**	**Hypernatremia**	**Anemia**
Generalized weakness	X	X	X
Acute confusion	X	X	X
Dry mouth	X	X	
Increased heart rate	X	X	X
Dyspnea on exertion			X

client who had a small bowel resection 2 days ago and begins having increasing abdominal pain, distention, vomiting, and absent bowel sounds. These data, when grouped together, are consistent with a postoperative paralytic ileus. To link these assessment findings with an ileus, you need knowledge of pathophysiology, especially signs and symptoms.

In some clinical scenarios, the client may have *multiple* relevant cues that are associated with several different client conditions. The example in Box 1.4 illustrates this type of scenario for an older adult hospitalized for a urinary tract infection and sepsis. In this Thinking Activity, you would need to review each client finding to determine if it is consistent with one or more of the specified client conditions.

In this example, one finding may be linked with two or three client conditions, such as generalized weakness and acute confusion. However, dyspnea on exertion is associated with only one of the listed problems—anemia. The correct responses to the Thinking Activity are found in Box 1.5.

In other clinical scenarios, the client may not be experiencing an actual health problem, but is at risk for one or more potential complications. For example, the woman who recently had a spontaneous vaginal delivery is at risk for postpartum hemorrhage within the first 24 hours, particularly if the uterus becomes boggy (a client observation cue). In some clinical situations then, part of the thinking process to *Analyze Cues* is to identify if cues are linked to or associated with potential complications.

Prioritize Hypotheses

After organizing, grouping, and linking relevant client findings with actual or potential client conditions, the next cognitive skill requires you to narrow down what the data mean and prioritize the client's problems or needs. Although you may have learned about priority decision-making models such as the ABCs or Maslow's Hierarchy of Needs, these models are often not very useful in helping you make clinical judgments in more complex clinical situations.

To *Prioritize Hypotheses,* review and evaluate each of the client's needs or health problems in the clinical situation. Then rank them to decide what is *most likely* the priority

NGN TIP

Remember: To *Analyze Cues,* you are not required to make a medical diagnosis but rather will be expected to connect or link client findings with selected client conditions or health problems, either actual or potential.

health problem. Evaluate factors in the clinical situation such as urgency, risk, difficulty, and time sensitivity for the client. For example, consider this clinical situation:

A 42-year-old postpartum client who just gave birth to a third child in 4 years reports severe "afterbirth pains" of 9/10 on a 0 to 10 pain intensity scale. The client also reports having problems with getting the baby to latch for breast-feeding/chest-feeding. The nurse assesses that the client has a boggy uterus and is saturating a peri-pad every 20 to 30 minutes.

In this example, the client has three problems that you would evaluate and rank in this order:

1. Excessive postpartum bleeding due to boggy uterus
2. Severe abdominal pain due to uterine contractions
3. Difficulty with breast-feeding/chest-feeding due to inability of baby to latch

The priority for this client at this time is to manage excessive postpartum bleeding because the client could become hypovolemic and develop shock. In this situation, managing the client's bleeding is more *urgent* than managing severe pain or breast-feeding/chest-feeding difficulty to prevent the *risk* of a life-threatening complication.

Generate Solutions

After identifying the client's priority problem in a given clinical scenario, you want to think about all the possible actions that can be used to resolve or manage the problem. To assist in selecting the possible actions or approach to care you might include, first determine what outcomes are desired or expected for the client. For example, consider this scenario:

The birth parent of an 11-year-old brings the child to the ED for a right forearm injury experienced as a result of a scooter accident. The nurse observes that the child is crying and guarding the right arm, which is swollen, deformed, and bruised. The child is left-handed. During the head-to-toe assessment, the nurse notes old bruising on the left side of the child's chest and scarring on both upper thighs. Both knees have large abrasions with small stones and dirt embedded in them. The child denies having had any previous accidents or injuries. An x-ray confirms a right nondisplaced metaphyseal ulnar fracture.

In this example, the client has an acute injury and signs of previous injuries, possibly from abuse. The desired outcomes would include that the client:

■ States that pain is no more than a 2–3/10 on a 0 to 10 pain intensity scale
■ Does not experience compromised neurovascular compromise in the right arm
■ Has decreased swelling of the right arm
■ Will experience healing of bilateral knee abrasions without infection
■ Is safe at home (no neglect or abuse) with the birth parent or other family/significant other

The next step in this thinking process is to identify multiple potential actions or nursing interventions that could achieve the desired outcomes. Also identify which actions would be avoided or are contraindicated. To develop a list of actions or interventions for this pediatric client, you need knowledge of child development, fracture treatment, child abuse, and pain management.

Some nursing actions may focus on collecting additional information about the client. For instance, the nurse would likely want to interview the birth parent to obtain information about the old bruising and scarring observed on the child's chest and thighs. Other potential actions that could help achieve the desired outcomes in this clinical situation include:

■ States that pain is no more than a 2–3/10 on a 0 to 10 pain intensity scale
  ■ Administer nonopioid pain medication; avoid opioids if possible.
  ■ Provide distraction for the child, such as an iPad or gaming device.
  ■ Reassure the child that analgesics will be available as needed after discharge.

NGN TIP

Remember: The urgency of a clinical situation and risk to the client are important factors that will help you *Prioritize Hypotheses.*

NGN TIP

Remember: To *Generate Solutions* to meet a client's priority needs, determine the client's desired or expected outcomes first.

THINKING SPACE

- Does not experience compromised neurovascular compromise in the right arm
  - Assist in applying a right synthetic forearm cast.
  - Monitor the child's right arm neurovascular status after cast application.
- Has decreased swelling of the right arm
  - Apply ice pack to arm outside cast and teach child need to use ice for the next 24 hours.
  - Teach child to keep arm elevated as much as possible.
- Will experience healing of bilateral knee abrasions without infection
  - Clean both knees to remove debris and dirt.
  - Apply triple antibiotic cream on open areas and cover with clean gauze.
  - Apply topical lidocaine to knees to decrease pain.
- Is safe at home (no neglect or abuse) with the birth parent or other family/significant other
  - Communicate concern about child's safety to primary health care provider.
  - Consult with the social worker about the child's potential safety risk, family situation, and possible change in placement of the child.
  - Report potential child abuse to Child Protective Services (CPS).

After the list of potential actions has been identified for each desired outcome, determine which actions should be implemented to meet the priority needs of the client in the *Take Action* process.

Take Action

Deciding which action to implement is the focus of this clinical judgment thinking skill. After generating a list of possible interventions, determine the most appropriate intervention or combination of interventions that will resolve or manage the client's priority health problems or concerns. Also determine how each intervention will be implemented. Examples of methods to accomplish or implement interventions include what to communicate, document, perform, administer, teach, or request from a primary health care provider or other member of the health care team.

For example, in the pediatric clinical scenario described in the previous section on *Generate Solutions,* you might request a consultation with the social worker to interview the birth parent about the child's injuries and home situation. Social workers are experts in interviewing and addressing family situations, and can determine if the child's injuries are potentially consistent with abuse.

When deciding on how to implement interventions, avoid memorized textbook methods or procedures. Instead consider the elements of the clinical situation to determine which approach to use. For example, teaching the birth parent about the care of the child after discharge would be appropriate for most situations. However, in the pediatric clinical example, you might *not* want to teach the birth parent about home care after discharge from the ED until it is determined whether the child will go home with the birth parent. If abuse is suspected, the child would be removed from the current family situation.

NGN TIP

Remember: When deciding to *Take Action*, avoid memorized textbook methods and procedures; instead, customize your action to meet the needs of the client in the clinical scenario.

Evaluate Outcomes

The last clinical judgment thinking skill is to determine if the interventions implemented for the client resolved or effectively managed the health problem(s). The best way to make that determination is to compare what the desired or expected outcomes are with current client findings or observed outcomes. Ask yourself, "Which assessment findings/signs and symptoms indicate that the client's condition has improved?" "Which findings indicate that the client's condition has declined?"

For example, consider this clinical scenario:

A 78-year-old client has been hospitalized for 6 days for exacerbation of chronic heart failure. On admission the client was placed on supplemental oxygen and IV furosemide for peripheral edema and impending pulmonary edema. The primary health care provider adjusted the client's cardiac medications and restricted salt intake (no added table salt). The nurse preparing for the client's discharge performs a head-to-toe assessment to determine the effectiveness of heart failure management. The nurse documents the following client findings:

- *Lungs clear with no adventitious breath sounds*
- *No shortness of breath when walking short distances*
- *Lost 5 lb (2.3 kg) during hospital stay*
- *Bilateral ankle and foot edema decreased from 3+ to 1+*
- *States planning to continue using table salt at home*

In this example, all of the client assessment data at the time of discharge demonstrate that the interventions used to manage heart failure were effective because the client is improving. However, the client plans to continue using table salt at home, which could contribute to another exacerbation of heart failure. The nurse may need to reinforce teaching about the relationship of sodium to fluid retention or consult with the registered dietitian nutritionist to provide the teaching.

NGN TIP

Remember: To *Evaluate Outcomes*, compare desired or expected client outcomes with current observed outcomes.

How Will the Six Clinical Judgment Skills Be Measured on the NGN?

The new NGN exam is composed of current test item types and new test item types. The total number of test items should range between 85 and 150 total questions. The six NCJMM cognitive skills introduced in this chapter are measured on the NGN through use of a variety of new test item types that are embedded into two types of case studies—the Unfolding Case Study and the Stand-alone item. Both types of cases present a clinical scenario and include part of a medical record similar to the record shown in the figure.

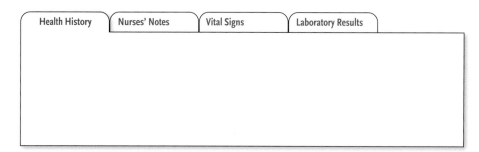

Additional medical record tabs may be included as the scenario requires.

The *Unfolding Case Study* presents the client over time through several phases of care in the clinical scenario. It is often referred to as the NGN Case Study. The time between phases can be minutes, hours, or even days. The client may initially be evaluated in an ED, acute care hospital, clinic, school, or urgent care center. As the scenario changes, or "unfolds," new NGN test items require that the candidate use the information in the current phase of the client's care to answer each question. Nursing candidates can expect to have three NGN Case Studies with six questions each. Each of the six questions represents one of the clinical judgment cognitive skills discussed earlier.

The *Stand-alone item* sometimes referred to as the Stand-alone clinical judgment item, presents a client at one point in time and includes one of the new NGN test item types. Each item measures one or more of the six clinical judgment cognitive skills. Nursing candidates are expected to have varying numbers of Stand-alone items on the NGN, depending on the candidate's ability in taking the exam. However, it is expected that most candidates will have about seven Stand-alone items.

How Can You Prepare for the NGN?

In addition to using this book, other resources such as the *Developing Clinical Judgment* workbooks written by one of this book's authors (D.D.I.) provide thinking exercises to help you master the six cognitive skills to make appropriate clinical judgments. If you need help with basic NCLEX® test-taking strategies and want beginning practice with NGN test items, two of this book's authors (L.A.S. and A.E.S.) created a book entitled *Clinical Judgment and Test-Taking Strategies.* All of these books are included in the NGN Resource list at the end of this book.

Another way to prepare for the NGN is to practice multiple test items in the Unfolding Case Study and Stand-alone item formats. NGN practice questions are located at the end of Chapters 3 through 8 of this book. Chapter 9 illustrates Stand-alone and Unfolding Case Studies with appropriate NGN test items. Chapter 10 is a comprehensive NGN Practice Test that includes questions in all specialty areas. Correct answers, rationales, test-taking strategies, specialty content area, selected concepts, and references are available for all NGN practice questions in the book.

In addition to the questions in this book, 50 Stand-alone items and Unfolding Case Studies with accompanying questions are available for your practice on the Elsevier Evolve site. Categories for selection of questions on Evolve include Content Area, Priority Concept, and Clinical Judgment Cognitive Skill.

Now that you have been introduced to the six cognitive skills needed to make appropriate clinical judgment, you are ready to learn about the new NGN test item types. The next chapter describes and illustrates examples of the new NGN test item types.

THINKING SPACE

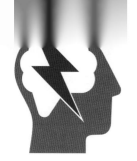

CHAPTER 2

Introduction to the NGN and the New NGN Item Types

NGN TIP

Remember: Data presented in the new NGN test item formats will usually be presented as part of a medical record as shown in the figure in Chapter 1. Many of the test items presented in this book are displayed in the medical record format.

NGN TIP

Remember: Expect each unfolding case on the NGN to present client data that change over time (minutes, hours, days) and six NGN test items, each measuring one of the six clinical judgment cognitive skills.

As described in Chapter 1, the NGN will be composed of current test item types and new test item types. The six NCJMM cognitive (thinking) skills introduced in Chapter 1 will be measured on the NGN through use of a variety of new test item types that are embedded into two types of cases—the Unfolding Case Study and the Stand-alone item. Both types of cases present a common, realistic clinical situation that new graduates will likely encounter.

This chapter describes the 15 new item types that will likely be part of the NGN. An example of each item type is presented and the correct responses are provided with brief rationales. Multiple examples of all item types, each with detailed Rationales, Content Area, Priority Concept, Cognitive Skill, and References, are presented throughout this book.

Unlike the current NCLEX® items, most new NGN items will be scored using partial credit rather than being completely correct or incorrect. This means that for most NGN items you will receive credit for any correct responses but will not receive credit for incorrect responses.

Test Item Types Used for Unfolding Case Studies

As described in Chapter 1, the *Unfolding Case Study,* also known as the NGN Case Study, presents a client and the initial data describing the clinical situation. These data will typically be part of a client medical record. The client either will be experiencing an urgent or emergent health problem or will be at risk for experiencing an urgent or emergent health problem. You'll need the information in the initial clinical scenario to answer the first NGN test item, which will measure the clinical judgment cognitive skill of *Recognize Cues.* The second NGN test item will likely measure your ability to *Analyze Cues.* As the clinical scenario continues, the client's condition will change over time through several phases of care in the clinical scenario. Four additional NGN test items will measure the other clinical judgment cognitive skills based on what client data are provided.

Twelve of the new item types on the NGN will be integrated into multiple unfolding case studies. The remaining two types will be used for the Stand-alone items discussed later in this chapter. Table 2.1 organizes these item types by major category and the cognitive skills that they best measure. Chapter 1 describes each of the six cognitive skills essential for making appropriate clinical judgment when caring for clients across the lifespan in a variety of health care settings.

Chapter 9 provides examples of complete unfolding cases with six accompanying test items and examples of the two types of Stand-alone items. The new item types that will be used as part of unfolding cases are described in the following sections.

Multiple Choice Test Items

Multiple choice test items have been a large part of the NCLEX® for many years. These items *currently* present a short clinical scenario and four choices with one correct response and three distractors (the wrong options) (see Box 1.2 in Chapter 1 for an example). For the NGN, there are two variations of the multiple choice item type: *Multiple Choice Single Response* and *Matrix Multiple Choice.*

TABLE 2.1   NGN Item Types for Unfolding Case Studies

NGN Item Types and Variations	Cognitive Skills That Can Be Optimally Measured
Multiple Choice	
Multiple Choice Single Response Matrix Multiple Choice	Recognize Cues Analyze Cues Prioritize Hypotheses (except Matrix Multiple Choice) Generate Solutions Take Action Evaluate Outcomes
Multiple Response	
Multiple Response Select All That Apply Multiple Response Select N Multiple Response Grouping Matrix Multiple Response	Recognize Cues Analyze Cues Prioritize Hypotheses (except Matrix Multiple Choice) Generate Solutions Take Action Evaluate Outcomes
Drop-Down	
Drop-Down Cloze Drop-Down Rationale Drop-Down in Table (may be replaced by a Drag-and-Drop in Table)	Recognize Cues Analyze Cues Prioritize Hypotheses Generate Solutions Take Action Evaluate Outcomes
Drag-and-Drop	
Drag-and-Drop Cloze Drag-and-Drop Rationale	Recognize Cues Analyze Cues Prioritize Hypotheses Generate Solutions Take Action Evaluate Outcomes
Highlight	
Highlight in Text Highlight in Table	Recognize Cues Evaluate Outcomes

Multiple Choice Single Response Item

On the NGN, the format for the Multiple Choice Single Response test item will be similar to the current NCLEX® format. However, the clinical scenario will be longer with more information about the client situation, usually within a portion of the medical record. In addition, the number of responses will *not* be restricted to four options, and as many as 10 options may be included. Sample Question 2.1 shows an example of this type of item to measure the clinical judgment cognitive skill of *Take Action* for an adult client with a mental health issue.

Sample Question 2.1   Multiple Choice Single Response

Health History	Nurses' Notes	Vital Signs	Laboratory Results

2245: A 28-year-old client is brought to the ED by friends, who state that the client became violent this evening in a local bar after a partner "break up." The client accused the partner of "cheating" and pulled out a knife. The client's friends were able to stop the client and take the knife before any harm occurred. They state that they have never seen the client act like this and are worried that something might be seriously wrong. Currently the client seems agitated and restless, and begins pacing in the ED demanding to "see my partner right now."

Based on the client information provided, what is the nurse's **first** *action?*

☐ Ask the client's friends to check the client for additional weapons.

☐ Reassure the client that the client is safe and secure in the ED.

☐ Call Security for assistance.

☒ Allow the client to vent own feelings.

☐ Administer an antianxiety medication.

☐ Distract the client and guide the client to practice coping skills.

NGN TIP

Remember: As with any client who is upset, paranoid, angry, or potentially violent, you would *first* allow the client to vent feelings, which may help diffuse the situation. Allowing a client to vent and keeping the client and staff safe are the initial focus of nursing care when encountering any client with an actual or potential mental health problem or crisis.

Rationale: The first nursing action is to allow the client to vent feelings. This action may help to de-escalate and decrease the client's agitation and restlessness. The nurse would not want to ask friends to check for weapons because they could possibly be harmed. Although calling Security may be needed later, the client may feel threatened by the presence of that authority figure and become more agitated or violent at this time. Reassuring the client that the client is safe does not address the concern. Although the client is agitated, distraction and practicing coping skills may be a better option at a later time after the current concern is addressed. Medication is usually the last resort unless needed to calm the client so that communication can occur. Although the client is restless and pacing in the ED, there is no evidence that the client would not vent feelings to the nurse.

Matrix Multiple Choice Item

The Matrix Multiple Choice test item is more complex than the Multiple Choice Single Response item. A Matrix Multiple Choice item provides a clinical scenario and selected data about the client. The test item is structured in a tabular format (matrix) with at least four rows and three columns. For this item, you would select only one response for each row. Sample Question 2.2 shows an example of this type of item to measure the clinical judgment cognitive skill of *Evaluate Outcomes* for an adult client who has had a surgical procedure.

Sample Question 2.2	Matrix Multiple Choice

The nurse provides health teaching for a 70-year-old client who had a TKA 3 days ago and is preparing to go home with a daughter.

*For each client statement, click or specify (with an **X**) whether the statement indicates **understanding or no understanding** of the teaching provided.*

Client Statement	Understanding	No Understanding
"I'll call my surgeon if my incision gets red or has drainage."	X	☐
"I can stop taking my blood thinner when I get home."	☐	X
"I'll have physical therapy for about a week."	☐	X
"I'm allowed to bear weight on my right leg."	X	☐
"I can probably drive in a few months."	X	☐

Rationale: As indicated in the test item, the client's statements that are not correct and show that the client does not understand the health teaching include: "I can stop taking my blood thinner when I get home," and "I'll have physical therapy for about a week." Clients who have total joint arthroplasty (especially knee and hip) are at a high risk for venous thromboembolism—DVT or PE. To help prevent these problems, the client is prescribed an oral anticoagulant, which is typically continued for 10 days to several weeks after surgery and should be taken after the client is home. The client would call the surgeon if the incision becomes red and/or has drainage because these symptoms indicate possible infection.

After surgery, most clients have 3 to 6 weeks of physical therapy depending on the type of prothesis and the client's overall health and tolerance. The surgical joint is often stiff, painful, and swollen, which limits the client's range of motion; however, weight bearing to tolerance helps promote ambulation and increase muscle strength. Physical therapy plus exercises that clients practice every day help to improve joint function and independence. The client will be allowed to drive when muscle strength and joint mobility improve. Driving is difficult until the surgical knee is able to flex more than 90 degrees. This goal may not be achieved for 6 to 8 weeks or more after surgery.

Multiple Response Test Items

Multiple Response test items have been a large part of the NCLEX® for many years. These items *currently* present a short clinical scenario with five or six options. The correct response(s) could be one, some, or all options (see Box 1.2 in Chapter 1 for an example). For the NGN, there are four variations of the Multiple Response test item:

- Multiple Response Select All That Apply Item
- Multiple Response Select N Item
- Multiple Response Grouping Item
- Matrix Multiple Response Item

Multiple Response Select All That Apply Item

On the NGN, the format for the Multiple Response Select All That Apply test item will be similar to the current NCLEX® format. However, the clinical scenario will be longer with more information about the client situation, usually within a portion of the medical record. The item will have at least five choices and no more than 10 choices. The correct response could be one, some, or all options. Sample Question 2.3 shows an example of this type of item to measure the clinical judgment cognitive skill of *Analyze Cues* for an older client who is residing in an assisted-living facility and who experiences acute confusion.

Sample Question 2.3	Multiple Response Select All That Apply

An 81-year-old client was admitted to an acute care unit from an assisted-living facility with a low-grade fever and acute confusion. The client's daughter tells the admitting nurse that the client's mother had a stroke 2 years ago that resulted in left hemiparesis and urinary incontinence, and the client has been in the assisted-living facility for the past 5 months. The client has a long history of DM type 2, which has been well controlled. Until this morning, the client's daughter had not been allowed to visit the facility due to the COVID-19 pandemic. During the visit today, the daughter noted that her mother was lethargic, confused, and unable to ambulate with a walker. POC testing in the ED indicated the presence of multiple bacteria in the client's urine and FSBG of 331 mg/dL (18.4 mmol/L). The client's BP is currently 96/48 mm Hg.

The nurse reviews the client assessment findings and determines that the client most likely has which of the following conditions? **Select all that apply.**

- ☒ Urosepsis
- ☒ Delirium
- ☒ Dehydration
- ☐ COVID-19
- ☐ DKA
- ☐ Transient ischemic attack
- ☒ Hyperglycemic hyperosmolar syndrome

Rationale: The client's assessment findings indicate that the client likely has a UTI (as evidenced by multiple bacteria in the urine). Fever, acute confusion, and a low BP suggest that the client is dehydrated and may have urosepsis. Acute confusion is also known as delirium, a common assessment finding in older clients who have a UTI. Because the client has type 2 diabetes, the client also is likely experiencing a diabetic complication called hyperglycemic hyperosmolar syndrome. The client's elevated blood glucose and dehydration are consistent with a hyperosmolar state. A low blood pressure is also consistent with dehydration.

Multiple Response Select N Item

The Multiple Response Select N test item is similar to the Multiple Response Select All That Apply item except that the number of required correct responses is specified in the question. This item will also have at least five options but no more than 10 options from which to choose. Sample Question 2.4 shows an example of this type of item to measure the clinical judgment cognitive skill of *Recognize Cues* for an adult client who has new onset of symptoms.

Sample Question 2.4	Multiple Response Select N

The nurse assesses a 53-year-old client whose partner brought the client to the ED with report of acute onset dyspnea and back pain that started about an hour ago. The client's medical history includes DM type 2, obesity, hypertension, hypercholesteremia, and asthma. The client's admission vital signs include:

- Temperature = 98.8°F (37.1°C)
- HR = 78 BPM and irregular
- RR = 26 bpm and slightly labored
- BP = 148/90 mm Hg
- SpO$_2$ = 95% (on RA)

The nurse reviews the client's assessment data. **Select 4 client findings that are relevant and of immediate concern to the nurse.**

- ☒ Dyspnea
- ☒ Back pain
- ☐ Temperature
- ☐ History of obesity
- ☐ History of diabetes
- ☒ Tachypnea
- ☐ History of asthma
- ☒ Elevated BP

Rationale: The client's new symptoms include dyspnea and back pain, which could indicate a possible MI and therefore are relevant in this clinical scenario. Women with an MI often present with symptoms that differ from those in men, including having back or jaw pain. The client's RR and BP are both elevated, but the temperature is normal. HR is within normal limits but is irregular. The medical history may help explain or predict the current client condition, but is not relevant at this time for planning nursing care.

Other examples of questions or statements that could be part of a Multiple Response Select N test item with their associated cognitive skills include:

- Select the three priority health problems that the client is experiencing. *Analyze Cues*
- What are the five assessment findings that indicate the client is improving? *Evaluate Outcomes*
- Select the four physician orders that the nurse would anticipate for this client. *Take Action*

NGN TIP

Remember: When reviewing client findings, first determine what is most relevant for that particular client in the clinical scenario. Organize these findings to determine which data are consistent with specific client conditions or health problems.

Multiple Response Grouping Item

The Multiple Response Grouping test item is similar to the Multiple Response Select All That Apply item except that the options are presented in categories or by group in a table with a minimum of two columns and five rows. Each category will have two to four options per row and require that at least one response option be selected. Sample Question 2.5 shows an example of this type of item to measure the clinical judgment cognitive skill of *Generate Solutions* for a pediatric client who has bacterial meningitis.

Sample Question 2.5	Multiple Response Grouping

The nurse admits an 11-month-old infant who has possible bacterial meningitis to the acute pediatric care unit.

*For each body system listed below, click or specify (with an **X**) the potential nursing interventions that are **appropriate** for the client's care. Each body system may support more than one potential intervention.*

Body System	Potential Nursing Interventions
Respiratory	☐ Incentive spirometer every 2 hours
	☒ Oxygen therapy via nasal cannula
	☐ Chest x-ray now and at bedtime
	☒ Continuous pulse oximetry monitoring
	☒ Droplet Precautions
Neurologic	☒ Seizure Precautions
	☐ Neurologic checks every day
Cardiovascular	☐ Type and crossmatch for 2 units of packed red blood cells (PRBCs)
	☒ Vital signs every hour
	☒ Contact physician if temperature above 102.4°F (39.1°C)
	☒ Begin IV cefotaxime infusion
	☒ Blood cultures

Rationale: Bacterial meningitis can be very contagious depending on the type, requiring Droplet Precautions to help prevent spread of the disease. The nurse would anticipate the immediate need for IV antibiotic therapy with either a cephalosporin or penicillin medication typically for 7 to 10 days, depending on the result of the blood cultures. The nurse would carefully monitor vital signs, especially temperature and BP. Complications of untreated or severe bacterial meningitis include sepsis, cardiovascular collapse, respiratory problems, and shock. Seizures and neurologic deterioration may also occur. Therefore the nurse would initiate Seizure Precautions and monitor the infant's neurologic status every hour (not daily) until the client is stabilized. Oxygen therapy via nasal cannula or with CPAP is frequently used unless the infant experiences more severe respiratory distress, which may necessitate intubation and mechanical ventilation. Monitoring the infant's pulse oximetry provides data on the oxygen saturation level.

NGN TIP

Remember: When selecting which nursing interventions are appropriate for a client in a clinical scenario on the NGN, consider the client's health problem and those actions that also require an order by a physician or other primary health care provider.

Matrix Multiple Response Item

The Matrix Multiple Response test item is similar to the Matrix Multiple Choice item in that they are both presented in a table format with multiple columns and rows. However, instead of selecting only one correct option per row as shown in Sample Question 2.6, you may select *more than one option* in each row. For this type item, each column must also have at least one option selected. Sample Question 2.6 shows an example of this type of item to measure the clinical judgment cognitive skill of *Analyze Cues* for an adult client who has abdominal pain.

Sample Question 2.6 | **Matrix Multiple Response**

The nurse is assessing a 63-year-old client who is admitted to the ED with report of acute severe abdominal pain and profuse vomiting. The client is jaundiced and has a gray-blue coloration of the periumbilical area. Current vital signs include:

- Temperature = 101.6°F (38.7°C)
- Apical pulse = 108 BPM
- RR = 26 bpm
- BP = 90/48 mm Hg
- SpO_2 = 96% (on RA)

For each client finding below, click or specify (with an X) if the finding is consistent with acute pancreatitis and/or dehydration. Each finding may support both client conditions.

Client Findings	Acute Pancreatitis	Dehydration
Fever	X	X
Tachycardia	X	X
Abdominal pain	X	☐
Hypotension	X	X
Vomiting	X	☐

Rationale: The client has classic signs and symptoms of acute pancreatitis, including an acute onset of severe abdominal pain, nausea and vomiting, and gray-blue coloration of the abdomen, especially around the umbilical area. Vomiting can cause dehydration but is not a symptom of dehydration. The client's vital signs reveal fever, tachycardia and hypotension, which are common in clients with pancreatitis. These vital sign changes are also common in clients who are dehydrated.

Drop-Down Test Items

For any Drop-Down test item, you will need to click on the word [Select] to determine what the options are for a fill-in-the-blank item to complete the information. For the NGN, there are three variations of the Drop-Down test item:

- Drop-Down Cloze item
- Drop-Down Rationale item
- Drop-Down in Table item (This variation may be changed to a Drag-and-Drop Table.)

Drop-Down Cloze Item

The Drop-Down Cloze and Drop-Down Rationale test items are very similar. Both variations present a sentence with blanks that you will need to fill in with options provided for each blank. The Drop-Down Cloze item has a minimum of one sentence and a maximum of five sentences with one or more drop-down menus per sentence. Sample Question 2.7 shows an example of this type of item to measure the clinical judgment cognitive skill of *Prioritize Hypotheses* for a pregnant woman.

Sample Question 2.7   **Drop-Down Cloze**

A woman who is 32 weeks pregnant visits her primary health care provider for the monthly OB visit. The nurse performs an initial assessment of the client prior to being examined by the provider and collects the following client data:

- States that she has had several mild to moderate headaches during the past week
- Gained 10 lb since last visit 4 weeks ago
- States that the baby is very active, especially at night
- FHR = 146 BPM
- Temperature = 98°F (36.7°C)
- HR = 82 BPM and regular
- RR = 18 bpm
- BP = 150/92 mm Hg
- Urine protein = 1+
- 1+ pitting edema on both feet and ankles

Based on the client findings, complete the following sentence by choosing from the lists of options provided.

The nurse reviews the client's assessment data and recognizes that she most likely has **preeclampsia**. The **priority** for this client's care is to **ensure maternal and fetal safety**.

Options for 1	Options for 2
CKD	Admit the client to the hospital
Gestational diabetes	Ensure maternal and fetal safety
Preeclampsia	Restrict her fluid intake
HELPP syndrome	Place her on a special diet

Rationale: As you probably determined, the client most likely has preeclampsia because she is in her third trimester of pregnancy, has an elevated BP, has dependent pitting edema, and is spilling protein in her urine. She has also had several headaches, which could be related to this complication of pregnancy. The most important desired outcome for the client is to ensure that she and her baby stay safe and healthy. Although urinary protein and edema may occur in clients who have CKD, additional signs and symptoms specific to CKD would be present. Likewise, there is no information presented in the clinical scenario that indicates the client has gestational diabetes. Hemolysis, elevated liver enzymes, and low platelets (HELPP) syndrome is a complication of hypertension during pregnancy. In this condition, HELPP develops before the 37th week of pregnancy but can occur shortly after the baby is delivered.

Drop-Down Rationale Item

The Drop-Down Rationale test item also uses a cloze (fill-in-the-blank) format in a cause-and-effect sentence. Using the clinical scenario and client data from the Drop-Down Cloze item in Sample Question 2.7, Sample Question 2.8 provides an example of this type of item to measure the clinical judgment cognitive skill of *Analyze Cues* for the client.

Sample Question 2.8   **Drop-Down Rationale**

The nurse reviews the client's assessment data and recognizes that she most likely has **preeclampsia** as evidenced by **hypertension** and **proteinuria**.

Options for 1	Options for 2
CKD	Pitting edema
Gestational diabetes	Hypertension
Preeclampsia	Weight gain
HELPP syndrome	Proteinuria

Rationale: The client most likely has preeclampsia because she is spilling protein in her urine and has an elevated BP. Having severe headaches would also be significant, but she describes her headaches as mild to moderate, which is not significant for a pregnant woman unless she develops additional visual changes. Having pitting edema does not necessarily indicate that the client is preeclamptic, but can occur in women with this complication.

Drop-Down in Table Item

The Drop-Down in Table test item provides categories of options from which you would need to choose. These options are often grouped by body system. Sample Question 2.9 shows an example of this type of item to measure the clinical judgment cognitive skill of *Take Action* for a pregnant woman.

Sample Question 2.9 — **Drop-Down in Table**

A woman who is 32 weeks pregnant visits her primary health care provider for the monthly OB visit. On assessment, the client is found to be hypertensive and has 1+ protein in her urine. The client has gained 10 lb over the past 4 weeks and has 1+ pitting edema in both feet and ankles. The physician recommends that the client be hospitalized for expectant management.

*For each body system listed below, select the potential nursing intervention(s) that would be **appropriate** for the care of the client. Each body system may support more than one potential nursing intervention, but at least one option in each category should be selected.*

Cardiovascular	<u>Antihypertensive drug therapy</u>
	<u>Vital signs every shift</u>
Neurologic	<u>Activity restriction</u>
Renal	<u>Weekly labs for creatinine</u>

Options for 1	Options for 2	Options for 3
Antihypertensive drug therapy	Seizure precautions	Weekly labs for creatinine
Vital signs every shift	Activity restriction	Urinary catheter
Daily labs for complete blood count	Ibuprofen for headaches	Diuretic therapy

---

Rationale: The client does not have severe preeclampsia at this time, so she can be monitored either at home or in the hospital. Her physician suggests hospitalization so that the client can be carefully monitored for more severe complications while she is receiving antihypertensive drug therapy and is on activity restriction. She would have admission lab work for a complete blood count (CBC), including platelets, creatinine to monitor kidney function, and liver function studies. After the admission labs, the client would then likely have weekly monitoring. Her BP and other vitals would be monitored frequently, at least once a shift. Unless her condition were to worsen or she were receiving intravenous magnesium sulfate, she would not need to be on seizure precautions or to have her reflexes monitored.

Drag-and-Drop Test Items

Drag-and-Drop test items are similar to current NCLEX® Drag-and-Drop/Order Response items in that you will need to click on several options and move them into part of one or more sentences to complete. At least two types of items will use this method: the Drag-and-Drop Cloze item and the Drag-and-Drop Rationale item.

Drag-and-Drop Cloze Item

The Drag-and-Drop Cloze test item is very similar to the Drop-Down Cloze. Instead of clicking on the blank to obtain a drop-down selection of options, you'll need to click on the correct responses to move them into the blanks to complete one or more sentences. Sample Question 2.10 displays an example of this type of item to measure the clinical judgment cognitive skill of *Analyze Cues* for a pregnant woman, using the clinical scenario in Sample Question 2.7.

Sample Question 2.10   Drag-and-Drop Cloze

A woman who is 32 weeks pregnant visits her primary health care provider for her monthly OB visit. The nurse performs an initial assessment of the client prior to her being examined by the provider and collects the following client data:

- States that she has had several mild to moderate head-aches during the past week
- Gained 10 lb since her last visit 4 weeks ago
- States that the baby is very active, especially at night
- FHR = 146 BPM
- Temperature = 98°F (36.7°C)
- HR = 82 BPM and regular
- RR = 18 bpm
- BP = 150/92 mm Hg
- Urine protein = 1+
- 1+ pitting edema on both feet and ankles

Drag (or select) words from the choices below to fill in the blank in the following sentences.

The nurse reviews the client's assessment data and determines that she has **gestational hypertension** and **preeclampsia**.

Options

HELPP syndrome	CKD
Gestational diabetes	Gestational hypertension
Preeclampsia	Heart failure

Rationale: The client has gestational hypertension as evidenced by her BP being elevated to above the normal range. In addition, she likely has preeclampsia because she is in her third trimester of pregnancy, when this complication most commonly occurs, and is spilling protein in her urine.

Drag-and-Drop Rationale Item

The Drag-and-Drop Rationale test item is very similar to the Drop-Down Rationale in that this item also uses a cloze format in a cause-and-effect sentence. Instead of clicking on the blank to obtain a drop-down selection of options, you'll need to click on the correct responses to move them into the blanks to complete the sentence. The sentence may have two blanks (dyad) or three blanks (triad) to complete. Using the clinical scenario and client data from the Drop-Down Rationale in Sample Question 2.8, Sample Question 2.11 provides an example of this type of item to measure the clinical judgment cognitive skill of *Analyze Cues* for the client.

Sample Question 2.11   Drag-and-Drop Rationale

Drag one condition and two client findings to fill in each blank in the following sentence.

The nurse reviews the client's assessment data and determines that she most likely has **preeclampsia** as evidenced by **elevated BP** and **proteinuria**.

Client Condition	Client Findings
HELPP syndrome	Increased FHR
Preeclampsia	Proteinuria
CKD	Weight gain
Heart failure	Elevated BP

NGN TIP

Remember: When answering either a Drop-Down Rationale or Drag-and-Drop Rationale test item that measures *Analyze Cues* or *Prioritize Hypotheses*, be sure that the client condition that you select is supported by the client findings presented in the clinical scenario in a cause-and-effect relationship.

Rationale: The client most likely has preeclampsia because she is spilling protein in her urine and has an elevated BP. The FHR is within normal limits, and she is expected to gain weight with pregnancy. However, part of her weight gain may be due to fluid retention as evidenced by pitting edema.

Highlight Test Items

Highlight test items require you to identify information in the clinical scenario to answer the question by highlighting with the computer mouse or, in a print product, with a marker. The two variations of this item are the Highlight in Text and Highlight in Table.

Highlight in Text Item

As discussed earlier for the new NGN, the clinical scenarios are presented as part of a client's medical record under tabs such as Nurses' Notes or Health History. This text is usually about a paragraph in length and presents client findings, including assessment data. To answer a Highlight in Text item, you would click on the computer mouse to answer the question, as shown in Sample Question 2.12. This example measures the clinical judgment cognitive skill of *Recognize Cues* for a young adult with type 1 DM.

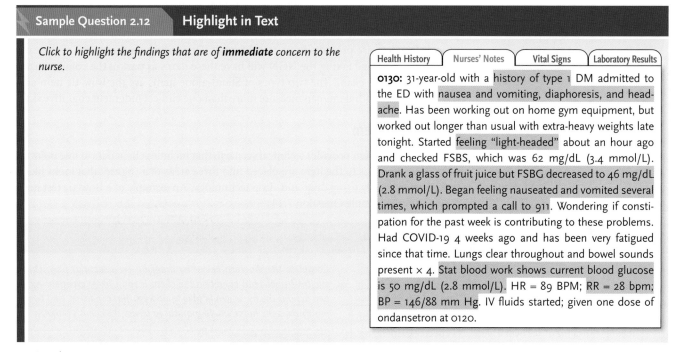

Sample Question 2.12	Highlight in Text

*Click to highlight the findings that are of **immediate** concern to the nurse.*

Health History	Nurses' Notes	Vital Signs	Laboratory Results

0130: 31-year-old with a history of type 1 DM admitted to the ED with nausea and vomiting, diaphoresis, and headache. Has been working out on home gym equipment, but worked out longer than usual with extra-heavy weights late tonight. Started feeling "light-headed" about an hour ago and checked FSBS, which was 62 mg/dL (3.4 mmol/L). Drank a glass of fruit juice but FSBG decreased to 46 mg/dL (2.8 mmol/L). Began feeling nauseated and vomited several times, which prompted a call to 911. Wondering if constipation for the past week is contributing to these problems. Had COVID-19 4 weeks ago and has been very fatigued since that time. Lungs clear throughout and bowel sounds present × 4. Stat blood work shows current blood glucose is 50 mg/dL (2.8 mmol/L). HR = 89 BPM; RR = 28 bpm; BP = 146/88 mm Hg. IV fluids started; given one dose of ondansetron at 0120.

Rationale: The client has DM type 1, indicating that the client is taking insulin for glucose control. The client began having symptoms that indicated the client's blood glucose was too low, including nausea and vomiting, diaphoresis, light-headedness, and headache. These findings prompted the ED nurse to perform a stat lab draw to confirm the blood glucose level, which was 50 mg/dL (2.8 mmol/L). Vital signs are within normal limits except for BP and respirations, which are elevated. Other client assessment data are not important at this time and could be addressed later.

Highlight in Table Item

The second variation of the Highlight test item is the Highlight in Table item. For this item type, the client findings are listed in a table format and often organized by body system, as shown in the example in Sample Question 2.13. This example uses the client findings in the clinical scenario described in Sample Question 2.12.

Sample Question 2.13	Highlight in Table

*Click to highlight the findings that require **immediate** follow-up by the nurse. Each body system will have at least one significant client finding.*

Body System	Client Findings
Gastrointestinal	Recent history of constipation, nausea and vomiting, abdominal bowel sounds present × 4
Neurologic	Reports headache and being light-headed, reports fatigue, blood glucose = 50 mg/dL (2.8 mmol/L)
Respiratory	Recent history of COVID; RR = 28 bpm
Cardiovascular	HR = 89 BPM, BP = 146/88 mm Hg

Rationale: The client has DM type 1, indicating the client is taking insulin for glucose control. The client began having symptoms that indicated the client's blood glucose was too low, including nausea and vomiting, diaphoresis, light-headedness, and headache.

NGN TIP

Remember: To answer a Bow-tie item, you'll first need to identify relevant data and organize those data to determine what the client's condition is in the clinical scenario. Then review the choices under Potential Conditions and select the one that best matches your analysis. After selecting or dragging the client condition into the middle section of the Bow-tie figure, decide on the Nursing Actions that would be appropriate to manage the client condition and the Parameters that a nurse would need to monitor to determine if those actions were effective.

These findings prompted the ED nurse to perform a stat lab draw to confirm the blood glucose level, which was 50 mg/dL. Vital signs are within normal limits except for BP and respirations, which are elevated. Other client assessment data are not important at this time and could be addressed later.

Test Item Types Used for Stand-alone Items

As described in Chapter 1, Stand-alone Clinical Scenarios, most often called Stand-alone items, present a client situation with assessment data, similar to that in the first phase of an Unfolding Case Study. However, the client's condition does not change over time unless data are presented in a trend format. Depending on the ability of the candidate, not everyone taking the NGN will have these items as part of the computerized adaptive licensure exam. The two types of Stand-alone items are the Bow-tie item and the Trend item. Both items can measure more than one clinical judgment cognitive skill.

Bow-tie Test Item

The Bow-tie test item provides a clinical scenario that includes client data at one point in time. The responses to the item are placed into three areas of a "figure" that looks like a bow-tie or butterfly using drag-and-drop technology. An example of a Bow-tie test item is presented in Sample Question 2.14.

Sample Question 2.14   Bow-tie

The nurse is assigned to a newly admitted 49-year-old client.

Health History	Nurses' Notes	Vital Signs	Laboratory Results

1530: Client admitted to the ED with partner with report of feeling "extra tired" for over a week. Has been experiencing intermittent chest pain and dyspnea today. Had a right ankle ORIF about 10 days ago. Other history includes several recent anginal episodes, DM type 1, and GERD. Admission blood glucose is 159 mg/dL (8.8 mmol/L).

The nurse is reviewing the client's admission note to prepare the client's plan of care.

Complete the diagram below by dragging (or selecting) from the choices below what condition the client is most likely experiencing, two actions the nurse would take to address that condition, and two parameters the nurse would monitor to assess the client's progress.

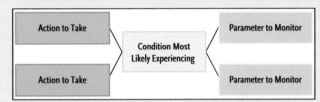

Nursing Actions	Condition Most Likely Experiencing	Parameters to Monitor
Start continuous IV heparin infusion	PE	POC glucose level
Give IV regular insulin	Upper GI bleeding	Oxygen saturation
Insert an NG tube to low continuous suction	Unstable angina	Pain level
Administer oxygen at 4 L/min via nasal cannula	DKA	Vital signs
Administer sublingual nitroglycerin		Serum creatinine

The correct responses for this Bow-tie test item are shown below.

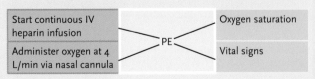

Rationale: The client had orthopedic surgery (ankle ORIF) within the last 2 weeks. Clients who have this type of surgery are at high risk for postoperative VTE, including PE, which typically manifests with sudden onset chest pain and dyspnea. Although the client has an elevated blood glucose level, there is no indication of DKA. Therefore IV insulin is not necessary at this time. The client's chest pain and dyspnea when resting might indicate unstable angina, but most clients with *stable angina* do not have dyspnea or shortness of breath. There is no evidence that the client has upper GI bleeding. The client does not have nausea or vomiting (hematemesis), which would be expected for clients who have active bleeding; therefore, there is no need for an NG tube. Once the diagnosis of a PE is confirmed by pulmonary angiography and V̇/Q̇ scan, the nurse would start a continuous IV heparin infusion to prevent the clot(s) from becoming larger and oxygen to manage the client's dyspnea. To ensure that the treatment is effective, the nurse would monitor the client's oxygen saturation levels via pulse oximetry and vital signs. Pain level would not be the most important parameter to monitor because it is more subjective than vital signs. There would be no need to monitor serum creatinine because there is no indication of possible kidney dysfunction.

THINKING SPACE

Trend Test Item

Similar to the Bow-tie item for the Stand-alone item, the Trend test item begins with a client situation that includes assessment data. These data, however, include multiple data points over time in the clinical scenario, such as vital signs, I&O, lab values, and Nurses' Notes entries. The test question for this type of item may be any of the 12 item types used for the Unfolding Case Studies. Sample Question 2.15 displays an example of a Trend item used for a Stand-alone item.

Sample Question 2.15 — Trend

The nurse is caring for a 15-year-old client who is admitted for observation due to moderate abdominal pain, loss of appetite, and nausea and vomiting, and is reviewing the medical record.

Health History	Flow Sheet	Nurses' Notes	Laboratory Results

Vital Signs	1900	0100	0700
Temperature	100°/37.8°	100.8°/38.2°	101.6°/38.7°
HR	82	90	80
RR	16	18	16
BP	112/74	96/58	102/64

Nurses' Notes

1900: Admitted with moderate abdominal pain (6/10) that started early this morning. Reports nausea with no appetite since yesterday, and vomited twice this morning. Bowel sounds present × 4; abdomen soft and slightly distended. Awaiting results of abdominal x-ray and ultrasound. IV of 5%D/0.45%NS infusing via left forearm catheter at 100 mL/h. Maintaining NPO. Given IV antiemetic.

0100: Imaging studies show excessive intestinal gas and enlarged appendix with inflammation. Resident on call notified. Increased IV rate to 125 mL/h. Lab called for stat results of CMP. Potassium and sodium slightly decreased; other labs WNL. Bowel sounds present × 4; abdomen more distended than at 1900. States pain is increasing. Placed in a high-Fowler position. No additional vomiting episodes.

0700: Surgical resident in to examine client. IV continuing to infuse at 125 mL/h. Remains NPO. Temperature increased. States nausea is improving.

The nurse consults with the surgical resident about the client's plan of care. Which of the following physician's orders would the nurse anticipate? *Select all that apply.*

- ☐ Obtain informed consent.
- ☒ Prepare client for surgery.
- ☐ Place a Salem sump tube and clamp.
- ☐ Type and crossmatch for 2 units packed RBCs.
- ☒ Administer IV antibiotic 1 hour prior to surgery.
- ☒ Change IV to Ringer's lactate at 125 mL/h.

NGN TIP

Remember: Before answering a Trend test item, review all information presented and determine the significance of changes in assessment data across time. The test question for this type of item may be any of the 12 types used for the unfolding case studies.

Rationale: The client has appendicitis and requires an appendectomy to remove the inflamed appendix before it could possibly rupture and cause peritonitis. The surgeon or surgical resident (not the nurse) is responsible for explaining the surgical procedure and potential complications, including death, and getting informed consent from the parents in this case. The nurse prepares the client for surgery by reinforcing health teaching and completing the preoperative checklist. The IV solution likely needs to be changed to Ringer's lactate because this isotonic solution is used to maintain or increase blood volume for clients who have or are at risk for low BP. An IV antibiotic may be given either an hour before surgery or at the surgical opening in the OR. The other orders are not required because this procedure will be performed laparoscopically and the client does not have peritonitis at this point. Because the client has not had additional vomiting, the Salem sump tube is not necessary. The client may be typed and crossmatched preoperatively in the event that blood is needed during surgery, but there is no information indicating that the client needs 2 units of packed RBCs.

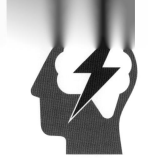

CHAPTER 3

Strategies for Answering NGN Questions: Recognize Cues

Recognize Cues is a CJ cognitive skill needed for nurses to make good clinical decisions. When clinical deterioration or a major change in a client's condition is not recognized, death or permanent disability from a complication of illness or care can result. This event is referred to as "failure to rescue." Preventing these negative client outcomes is crucial and requires that nurses have keen observation and thinking skills. Therefore being able to *Recognize Cues* is essential to ensure client safety and quality of care and will be measured both on the NGN and by your instructors on course exams.

 ## What Are Cues?

As we discussed in Chapter 1, *cues* are client findings or assessment data that provide information for nurses as a basis for decision making. Table 3.1 lists common sources and examples of client findings that may be presented as part of an NGN clinical scenario.

 ## How Are Client Findings (Cues) Presented in an NGN Clinical Scenario?

Unfolding Case Studies on the NGN will begin with a clinical scenario that could be presented in several ways. To make the scenario as realistic as possible, client findings are displayed as part of a medical record similar to the accompanying figure.

Health History	Nurses' Notes	Vital Signs	Lab Results

Admitting Problem: LUQ abdominal pain with rectal bleeding

History of Present Illness: Last week this 82-year-old widow residing in an independent living senior center began noticing bright red blood on tissue after having a BM. Since then the client has had bright red blood in the toilet every time the client defecates. Yesterday the client also started having LUQ abdominal pain, which worsens during the night. Admitted through the ED.

Current Medications:
- Acetaminophen 650 mg orally every 4–6 hours PRN for joint pain
- Metoprolol XL 100 mg orally every morning for hypertension
- Calcium carbonate 1000 mg chewable tabs twice each day for osteopenia
- Clopidogrel 75 mg orally every day for atrial fibrillation

NGN test items that measure the ability to Recognize Cues will require you to distinguish between which presented client findings are *relevant* (cues that are directly related to client outcomes or priority of care) and *not relevant* (cues that are *not* directly related to client outcomes or priority of care).

THINKING SPACE

 NGN TIP

Remember: Relevant client findings make a significant difference in achieving optimum outcomes for the client and help to determine the nurse's priority for client care.

TABLE 3.1	Common Sources and Examples of Client Assessment Findings	
Sources of Client Findings	**Examples of Client Findings**	
History data provided by client or family	History of past and present illness, family history, medications, allergies	
Physical assessment findings	VS, breath sounds, pain level	
Behavioral findings	Alcohol use, tobacco use, illicit drug use, mental health status	
Laboratory test results	Basic metabolic panel (BMP), complete blood count (CBC)	
Imaging test results	X-rays, CT scan impressions	

Which Client Findings Are Relevant?

When determining which client findings are relevant, you'll need to *first* consider if they are within the normal or usual parameters you learned from your nursing textbooks. For instance, consider the client findings in the following clinical situation:

A 91-year-old client has been brought by EMS to the ED after falling at home. The client's daughter explains to the nurse that the client has "always been stubborn by insisting on doing everything herself." While the daughter went out to buy groceries, the client climbed onto a stepstool to reach something in a cabinet over the refrigerator. The client apparently lost balance and was found on the kitchen floor. The nurse performs the initial assessment and documents these client findings:

- *Temperature: 96.8°F (36°C)*
- *HR: 90 BPM and regular*
- *RR: 22 bpm*
- *BP: 142/88 mm Hg*
- *SpO$_2$: 92% (on RA)*
- *Alert and oriented × 2 (person and place)*
- *States that pain is 10/10 (on a 0–10 pain intensity scale)*
- *Whimpering and holding right hip*
- *Right leg and foot externally rotated*
- *Right leg shorter than left leg*

In this situation, the findings that are *not* within the usual or normal range for an adult include:
- Temperature = 96.8°F (36°C)
- Respirations = 22 bpm
- BP = 142/88 mm Hg
- SpO$_2$ = 92% (on RA)
- Alert and oriented × 2 (person and place)
- States that pain is 10/10 (on a 0–10 pain intensity scale)
- Whimpering and holding right hip
- Right leg and foot externally rotated
- Right leg shorter than left leg

Although each of these findings is not within the usual or normal range for an adult and *could be* relevant, a body temperature of 96.8°F (36°C) is *expected* for older adults as a normal physiologic change associated with aging. So, for *this* client, a low body temperature is *not relevant* in this clinical situation. Another expected finding for any healthy adult is being alert and oriented × 3 (person, place, and time). However, this client is oriented to only person and place. After a fall with injury for an older adult, it would be *expected* that she might be disoriented, especially considering the amount of pain being experienced. Therefore the deficit in one aspect of orientation (time) is likely *not* relevant or of immediate concern to the nurse at this time.

Another example of an abnormal but expected finding for this client is the BP of 142/88 mm Hg, which is above the recommended normal range for adults. This elevation in BP could be relevant. However, this client is an older adult who is in severe pain owing to trauma from a fall, and the BP elevation is likely *not relevant*. As you may recall, when clients are in severe pain, they experience a sympathetic nervous system response. As a result, BP and HR increase. If this client's pain is effectively managed, the BP may return to a normal level or to the client's baseline.

The client's RR is slightly elevated (22 bpm) and the SpO_2 is slightly low at 92%. However, the client is in severe pain, so these data are probably not relevant in this clinical situation. An individual's oxygen saturation level tends to decrease with advanced age, so 92% may be expected and likely not relevant for this client.

The most relevant abnormal data are related to the client's trauma resulting from the fall. These data include:

- States that pain is 10/10 (on a 0–10 pain intensity scale)
- Whimpering and holding the right hip
- Right leg and foot externally rotated
- Right leg shorter than left leg

The CJ cognitive skill of *Recognize Cues* requires you to not only select relevant client findings, but also involves deciding which relevant findings are of *immediate* concern and *most* important to the nurse based on the clinical situation. This step determines how well you can identify client findings that must be followed up and managed immediately to prevent potential or actual harm.

NGN TIP

Remember: At this point, you should not interpret or analyze what is causing the client's findings or what nursing care may be required as a result.

Which Relevant Client Findings Are of Immediate Concern to the Nurse?

In some clinical scenarios, client findings may be relevant, but not of *immediate* concern or important at this time. For example, the nurse assessing a child who sustains multiple traumatic injuries after a motor vehicle accident would be immediately concerned about possible internal organ damage and hemorrhage. The child's history of well-controlled DM type 1 would be relevant for later in the client's plan of care, but is *not* an immediate concern to the nurse at this time.

NGN TIP

Use these strategies for NGN items that measure *Recognize Cues*:

1. Decide if each client finding is normal/usual or abnormal.
2. If the client finding is abnormal, determine if it is expected in the clinical scenario; if the client finding is *expected* in the clinical situation, it is likely *not relevant*. If the client finding is abnormal and *not expected*, it is likely *relevant* in the clinical scenario.
3. Decide which relevant client findings are most important, require follow-up, and/or are of immediate concern to the nurse for the client in the clinical scenario.

What Types of Clinical Scenarios May Be Included on the NGN?

As mentioned in Chapter 2, the test items on the *current* NCLEX-RN® and NCLEX-PN® are very concise and include only the relevant information needed for selecting a correct response. Similar to the items on the tests in your nursing program, most test questions are multiple choice. All current questions measure the ability of the test taker to ensure client safety. Box 3.1 presents an example of a *current* NCLEX®-style multiple choice item.

In this test question, the most relevant information that requires immediate attention of the nurse is provided in the brief clinical scenario. No additional client findings or other data are included. However, as described in Chapter 2, the new NGN items used to measure the cognitive skills of clinical judgment are lengthier than those on the current NCLEX® and usually require multiple answers rather than just one answer. Most importantly, NGN items present realistic and comprehensive clinical scenarios that nurses are likely to encounter as new graduates. Box 3.2 provides examples of common clinical problems requiring the ability to *Recognize Cues*.

What NGN Item Types Optimally Measure *Recognize Cues*?

Many NGN test item types may be used to measure the CJ cognitive skill of *Recognize Cues*. The best item types for measuring this skill are listed in Table 3.2.

Examples of these item types that best measure *Recognize Cues* are presented in this chapter.

THINKING SPACE

BOX 3.1   Example of Current NCLEX®-Style Multiple Choice Item

A client delivered a baby 4 hours ago and states she has saturated two peri-pads in the last hour. What is the nurse's **best** action at this time?
1. Document the client assessment in the medical record.
2. Massage the client's fundus until it is firm. ⟵
3. Administer supplemental oxygen at 2 L/min.
4. Increase the rate of the client's intravenous fluids.

Note: ⟵ indicates correct response.

BOX 3.2   Examples of Common Clinical Problems Requiring the Ability to Recognize Cues

- Dysrhythmias
- MI
- Heart failure
- Respiratory compromise
- Pneumonia
- Gastrointestinal bleeding
- Intestinal obstruction
- Bleeding, hypotension, hypovolemia, shock
- Stroke
- VTE (DVT and PE)
- Infection, sepsis, septic shock
- Arterial occlusion
- AKI
- Compartment syndrome
- Abdominal trauma
- Chest trauma
- Fluid and electrolyte imbalances
- Mental health crisis

TABLE 3.2   Test Items That Optimally Measure *Recognize Cues*

Type of Test Item	Item Variations
Highlight	Highlight in Text Highlight in Table
Drop Down	Drop-Down Cloze Drop-Down Rationale Drop-Down in Table (may be replaced by a Drag-and-Drop in Table)
Multiple Response	Multiple Response Select N Multiple Response Select All That Apply Multiple Response Grouping Matrix Multiple Response
Drag-and-Drop	Drag-and-Drop Cloze Drag-and-Drop Rationale

Highlight Items to Measure *Recognize Cues*

Highlight test items provide a clinical scenario with multiple client findings. When this item type is used to measure *Recognize Cues,* the test taker is required to highlight the relevant findings that require follow up or are of immediate concern to the nurse. The two variations of the Highlight test item are the Highlight in Text and Highlight in Table test items. Sample Question 3.1 illustrates a Highlight in Text item for an adolescent clinical scenario. The rationale and test-taking strategy to help you derive the correct responses in Sample Question 3.1 are also provided.

| Sample Question 3.1 | **Highlight in Text: Recognize Cues** |

A 16-year-old client is admitted to the acute behavioral health unit for observation and therapy. The nurse documents client findings in the medical record.

*Highlight the client findings below that require **immediate** follow-up by the nurse.*

| Health History | Nurses' Notes | Vital Signs | Lab Results |

1100: Alert and oriented × 3. Cut herself last night like before and doesn't understand why she was admitted. Client has been very depressed and was "planning to take parent's Xanax to help ease the emotional pain." Recognizes that her parents love her and are very supportive, but has no other support system. Thinks her boyfriend broke up with her because she is too fat. Has increased binge eating and purging. Height = 68 inches (173 cm); weight = 108 lb (49 kg). BMI = 16.4. Left upper thigh dressing from cutting intact with old bloody drainage. VS: T = 98°F (36.7°C); HR = 88 BPM; RR = 18 bpm; BP = 122/74 mm Hg.

Rationale: The client is a teenager who cuts herself and was planning to use her parent's antianxiety medication to manage emotional pain. The nurse would want to follow up on the client's self-mutilation behaviors and whether the client is suicidal or has suicidal tendencies now. The client thinks she is too fat, although her BMI is 16.4, below the desired level, and *expected* for a client with eating disorders. As a result, the client binge eats and then purges, which is a major concern for the nurse owing to potentially life-threatening risks for fluid and electrolyte imbalances. The nurse would want to collect more data about how long these eating behaviors have occurred and what previous body weights have been. The lack of support systems is a concern and needs to be addressed, but not immediately. The client's thigh dressing with old blood is expected because she has been cutting herself. This finding is also not concerning at this time because there is no active or new bleeding. VS are within normal range.

Test-Taking Strategy: Remember to first identify normal/usual or abnormal and expected (not relevant), and abnormal and not expected (relevant) client findings to determine which findings require immediate follow-up by the nurse. The client's findings can be categorized as shown in the table.

Test-Taking Strategy

Client Finding	Normal/Usual or Abnormal but Expected (Not Relevant) and Not Requiring Immediate Follow-up	Abnormal and Not Expected (Relevant) and Requiring Immediate Follow-up
Alert and oriented	☒	☐
Cuts herself	☐	☒
Depressed and planning to take medication	☐	☒
Parents loving and supportive	☒	☐
No other support system	☒	☐
Thinks her boyfriend broke up with her because she is too fat	☐	☒

Continued

Client Finding	Normal/Usual or Abnormal but Expected (Not Relevant) and Not Requiring Immediate Follow-up	Abnormal and Not Expected (Relevant) and Requiring Immediate Follow-up
Increased binging and purging	☐	☒
Underweight for height	☒	☐
Thigh dressing with old bloody drainage (from cutting)	☒	☐
VS: T = 98°F (36.7°C); HR = 88 BPM; respirations = 18 bpm; BP = 122/74 mm Hg	☒	☐

Next, recall that although teenage girls often have a poor self-image and self-esteem if they are rejected by their peers, it is *not* normal/usual or expected for them to self-mutilate, binge and purge, and take psychoactive drugs to manage their stress. For this clinical scenario, then, all of the relevant client findings require immediate follow-up by the nurse because they are of concern, with most being unhealthy coping behaviors that can cause self-harm.

Content Area: Mental Health Nursing
Priority Concept: Mood and Affect
Reference(s): Halter, 2022, pp. 247–254, 342–344, 483–484

Drop-Down Test Items to Measure *Recognize Cues*

Drop-down test items can be used to measure multiple cognitive skills needed to make clinical judgments, including *Recognize Cues*. Sample Question 3.2 presents a test item using the Drop-Down Cloze variation to assess whether you are able to identify the relevant client findings that are of immediate concern to the nurse. The rationale and test-taking strategy to help you derive the correct responses in Sample Question 3.2 are also provided.

Sample Question 3.2	Drop-Down Cloze: Recognize Cues

The nurse is reviewing the Nurses' Notes for an 84-year-old client admitted to a skilled nursing facility (SNF).

| Health History | Nurses' Notes | Vital Signs | Lab Results |

1100: Transfer from the community hospital following a right TKA for PT/OT. Daughter states that mother has been confused at times since surgery, but has no previous diagnosis of dementia. Needs supervision when transferring from bed to chair; incontinent of urine at times. Able to feed self and needs assistance with bathing. Fell yesterday while in bathroom while unattended with walker. VS: T = 98°F (36.7°C); HR = 88 BPM; RR = 18 bpm; BP = 102/64 mm Hg (sitting). Right knee incision dry and intact with Steri-Strips. Currently alert and oriented × 3. H/O hypertension, transient ischemic attack (TIA), stress incontinence, and osteoarthritis.

Based on the client findings, complete the following sentence by choosing from the lists of options provided.

The nurse recognizes that the relevant client findings that are of ***immediate*** concern to the nurse are <u>BP = 102/64 mm Hg (sitting)</u>, <u>confused at times since surgery</u>, and <u>fell yesterday</u>.

Options for 1	Options for 2	Options for 3
RR = 18 bpm	Confused at times since surgery	Fell yesterday
BP = 102/64 mm Hg (sitting)	H/O transient ischemic attack	Alert and oriented × 3
HR = 88 BPM	Admitted for PT/OT after a TKA	Incontinent of urine

THINKING SPACE

Rationale: The client is an older adult who had surgery several days ago before being admitted to the SNF. VS are within normal limits, but her sitting BP is a low normal reading of 102/64 mm Hg. When an individual changes from a sitting or lying position to standing, a slight decrease in systolic and/or diastolic BP is expected. An older adult, however, may have a major decrease in BP when changing positions, a condition known as orthostatic hypotension. Orthostatic hypotension is a decrease in systolic BP by at least 20 mm Hg or a decrease in diastolic BP by at least 10 mm Hg within 3 minutes of moving from a lying or sitting position to an upright position. This drop in BP is most common in older adults and can contribute to falls. The client's HR and RR are within normal limits.

According to the daughter, the client had no problems with cognitive state until surgery. Since that time, the client has apparently had episodes of confusion. Confusion is of immediate concern to the nurse because the client may try to get out of bed without supervision and experience a fall. The need for postoperative PT/OT is the purpose of admission; PT/OT should make the client stronger and able to ambulate and provide self-care, thus helping to prevent falls. The client's diagnosis of a previous TIA is not of immediate concern to the nurse, but the nursing staff would monitor for any new indications of a TIA or stroke while the client is in the SNF. The client experienced a fall the day before admission. A previous fall is a major risk factor for additional falls. Therefore the fall history is of immediate concern to the nurse. Urinary incontinence is also a risk factor for falls, but is not as important as the recent fall history. The client's current mental status of being alert and oriented × 3 is within normal limits and not a concern.

Test-Taking Strategy: Note that the word *immediate* requires you to review the client findings in the options and decide which findings need to be addressed now or at a later time. Some findings are normal and expected, and would not be a concern to the nurse in this clinical scenario. Use the table to help you answer this test item.

Test-Taking Strategy

Client Finding	Client Finding of Immediate Concern	Client Finding That Can Be Addressed at a Later Time or Is Not a Concern
RR = 18 bpm	☐	☒
BP = 102/64 mm Hg (sitting)	☒	☐
HR = 88 BPM	☐	☒
Confused at times since surgery	☒	☐
H/O transient ischemic attack	☐	☒
Admitted for PT/OT after a TKA	☐	☒
Fell yesterday	☒	☐
Alert and oriented × 3	☐	☒
Incontinent of urine	☐	☒

Content Area: Foundations of Nursing
Priority Concept: Mobility
Reference(s): Potter & Perry, 2021, pp. 404, 488, 824

Multiple Response Test Items to Measure *Recognize Cues*

Four variations of the Multiple Response test item can be used to measure any of the six CJ cognitive skills. When this type of item is used to measure *Recognize Cues,* a clinical scenario describing a client with multiple client findings is presented. Then these findings are listed in the test item, where you will be asked to select the relevant options that are of immediate concern to the nurse in the scenario. Sample Question 3.3 illustrates a Multiple Response Select N item for an older adult admitted to the ED. The rationale and test-taking strategy to help you derive the correct responses in Sample Question 3.3 are also provided.

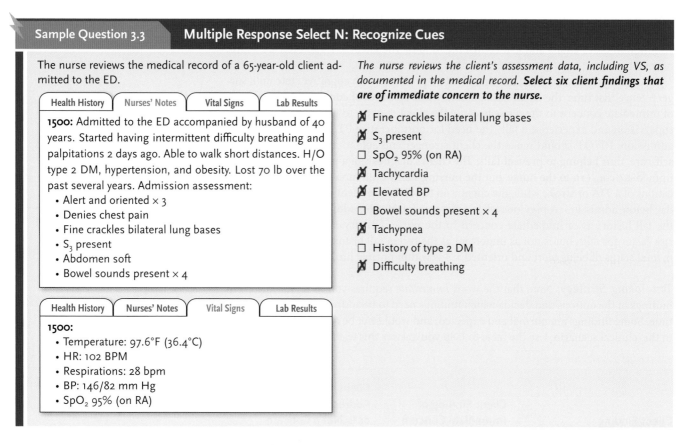

Sample Question 3.3 — Multiple Response Select N: Recognize Cues

The nurse reviews the medical record of a 65-year-old client admitted to the ED.

Health History	Nurses' Notes	Vital Signs	Lab Results

1500: Admitted to the ED accompanied by husband of 40 years. Started having intermittent difficulty breathing and palpitations 2 days ago. Able to walk short distances. H/O type 2 DM, hypertension, and obesity. Lost 70 lb over the past several years. Admission assessment:
- Alert and oriented × 3
- Denies chest pain
- Fine crackles bilateral lung bases
- S₃ present
- Abdomen soft
- Bowel sounds present × 4

Health History	Nurses' Notes	Vital Signs	Lab Results

1500:
- Temperature: 97.6°F (36.4°C)
- HR: 102 BPM
- Respirations: 28 bpm
- BP: 146/82 mm Hg
- SpO$_2$ 95% (on RA)

The nurse reviews the client's assessment data, including VS, as documented in the medical record. **Select six client findings that are of immediate concern to the nurse.**

- ☒ Fine crackles bilateral lung bases
- ☒ S$_3$ present
- ☐ SpO$_2$ 95% (on RA)
- ☒ Tachycardia
- ☒ Elevated BP
- ☐ Bowel sounds present × 4
- ☒ Tachypnea
- ☐ History of type 2 DM
- ☒ Difficulty breathing

Rationale: The client has adventitious breath sounds and an additional heart sound, which are not normal findings and are likely relevant. The BP of 146/82 mm Hg, HR of 102 BPM (tachycardia), and respirations of 28 bpm (tachypnea) are above normal or usual limits and are therefore relevant and of immediate concern to the nurse. The husband's report of the client's difficulty breathing is also concerning, given the presence of crackles. The nurse would recognize that all of these findings are indicative of impaired perfusion and gas exchange and could worsen. A history of DM may be a contributing factor to symptoms, but it is not of immediate concern to the nurse at this time. Many obese older adults have type 2 DM, which often contributes to cardiopulmonary health problems.

Test-Taking Strategy

Test-Taking Strategy: Remember to first identify normal/usual or abnormal and expected (not relevant), and abnormal and not expected (relevant) client findings. The client's findings can be categorized as shown in the table.

Client Finding	Normal/Usual or Abnormal but Expected (Not Relevant) and Not Requiring Immediate Follow-up	Abnormal and Not Expected (Relevant) and Requiring Immediate Follow-up
Fine crackles bilateral lung bases	☐	☒
S₃ present	☐	☒

Client Finding	Normal/Usual or Abnormal but Expected (Not Relevant) and Not Requiring Immediate Follow-up	Abnormal and Not Expected (Relevant) and Requiring Immediate Follow-up
SpO$_2$ 95% (on RA)	☒	☐
Tachycardia	☐	☒
Elevated BP	☐	☒
Bowel sounds present × 4	☒	☐
Tachypnea	☐	☒
History of DM	☒	☐
Difficulty breathing	☐	☒

Next review the findings that are abnormal and not expected for this particular client. These client findings are the significant cues in this clinical scenario and provide the correct responses to this test item measuring *Recognize Cues.*

Content Area: Medical-Surgical Nursing
Priority Concept: Perfusion
Reference(s): Ignatavicius et al., 2021, pp. 670–671

Drag-and-Drop Test Items to Measure *Recognize Cues*

As described in Chapter 2, Drag-and-Drop test items have at least two variations: Drag-and-Drop Cloze and Drag-and-Drop Rationale. A test item using the Drag-and-Drop Cloze item can assess whether you are able to identify the relevant client findings that require follow-up by the nurse (see Sample Question 3.4).

Sample Question 3.4	Drag-and-Drop Cloze: Recognize Cues

The nurse interviews the grandmother of a 10-month-old infant prior to being examined by the pediatrician.

| Health History | Nurses' Notes | Vital Signs | Lab Results |

1500: Grandmother states she brought the baby in to see the doctor because infant refused to eat or drink anything last night or this morning; vomited × 2. States that baby seems feverish with no interest in play; has had a cold with a "runny" nose and diarrhea for the last few days. Has a history of frequent upper respiratory infections. Grandmother is the baby's guardian because her daughter is a drug addict and lives with her boyfriend. States that she had to put the baby in day care last week because she went back to work to support her family. Blames herself that the baby may have gotten sick from day care. Baby's current axillary temperature = 103°F (39.4°C).

Drag and drop (or select) the correct responses from the list of client findings below to fill in the blanks in the following sentence.

The client findings that are of most concern to the nurse at this time are that the client **had vomiting × 2**, **has diarrhea**, **has an axillary temperature of 103°F (39.4°C)**, and **refuses to eat or drink**.

Client Findings

Had vomiting × 2
Attends day care
Has diarrhea
Has a "cold" with a runny nose
Has an axillary temperature = 103°F (39.4°C)
Refuses to eat or drink
Has history of frequent upper respiratory infections

Rationale: Infants and children have a greater need for water and are very vulnerable to altered fluid and electrolyte imbalances. When compared with adults, infants have a lower fluid volume, and therefore any loss of fluids can rapidly lead to dehydration. This infant presents with risk factors and assessment findings that place her at risk for

↘THINKING SPACE

dehydration. First, the infant lost fluid (and electrolytes) through vomiting and diarrhea. Second, the infant refuses to eat or drink, so she is not replacing fluids that were lost. The infant's temperature is elevated, which indicates that she is already likely dehydrated. Dehydration can lead to hypovolemic shock and if not treated could be life-threatening. These client findings indicate possible dehydration and would be of immediate concern to the nurse. Although attending day care places the infant at risk for infections, this finding is not of immediate concern. The infant's history of frequent respiratory infections, including a current cold with "runny" nose, is of interest but is not of immediate concern for the nurse.

Test-Taking Strategy

Test-Taking Strategy: The infant presents with multiple findings, including those that are consistent with a possible upper respiratory infection and those that are consistent with possible dehydration. Dehydration in an infant can be life-threatening. Therefore client findings that support or are risk factors for dehydration would be of immediate concern to the nurse. Use the table to determine which client findings are possibly associated with dehydration and would be of concern for the nurse at this time.

Client Finding	Possibly Associated With Dehydration: Yes or No?
Had vomiting × 2	Yes
Attends day care	No
Has diarrhea	Yes
Has a "cold" with a runny nose	No
Has an axillary temperature = 103° F (39.4°C)	Yes
Refuses to eat or drink	Yes
Has history of frequent upper respiratory infections	No

Once you have competed the table, select the options in the test item for the client findings for which you responded "Yes."

Content Area: Pediatric Nursing
Priority Concept: Fluid and Electrolyte Balance
Reference(s): Hockenberry et al., 2019, pp. 738–744

⚡ Practice Questions

Practice Question 3.1	Multiple Response Grouping

The nurse reviews the assessment findings for a newborn who was born 10 minutes ago via cesarean section at 35 weeks. The newborn's length is 19 in (48.3 cm) and weight is 4.4 lb (2000 g).

*For each body system listed below, click or specify (with an X) the newborn findings that are of **immediate** concern to the nurse. Each body system may support more than one relevant newborn finding.*

Body System	Newborn Finding
Respiratory	☐ Respirations: 40–60 bpm
	☐ Intermittent expiratory grunting
	☐ Fine crackles
	☐ Occasional apneic episodes
Neuromuscular	☐ Arms and legs relaxed
	☐ Crying
	☐ Relaxed body posture
	☐ Diminished reflexes
Cardiovascular	☐ Skin mottled
	☐ Axillary temperature: 96.7°F (35.9°C)
	☐ HR: 132 BPM and regular
	☐ Presence of murmur

Practice Question 3.2 — Highlight in Text

The nurse reviews selected data from the medical record of a 54-year-old client who was admitted to the ED with report of diarrhea and weakness.

*Highlight the client findings below in the Nurses' Notes and Laboratory Results that require **immediate** follow-up by the nurse.*

Health History	Nurses' Notes	Imaging Studies	Lab Results

1900: 54-year-old client admitted to the ED with report of severe, watery diarrhea, weakness, and occasional muscle twitching. Has no nausea and vomiting; alert and oriented × 3. Has stage 3 CKD, which has been well managed with diuretics, diet, and fluid restriction. Is not receiving kidney replacement therapy. HR 59 and irregular. Current ECG shows tall peaked T waves, flat P waves, and widened QRS complexes.

Health History	Nurses' Notes	Imaging Studies	Lab Results

1930: Stat lab results.

Laboratory Test Result	Normal Reference Range
Serum sodium 145 mEq/L (145 mmol/L)	136–145 mEq/L (136–145 mmol/L)
Serum potassium 5.9 mEq/L (5.9 mmol/L) **H**	3.5–5.0 mEq/L (3.5–5.0 mmol/L)
Hemoglobin 11.0 g/dL (6.83 mmol/L) **L**	14–18 g/dL (8.7–11.2 mmol/L)
Hematocrit 35% (0.35 volume fraction) **L**	42%–52% (0.42–0.52 volume fraction)
Blood urea nitrogen (BUN) 34 mg/dL (12.14 mmol/L) **H**	10–20 mg/dL (3.6–7.1 mmol/L)
Creatinine 2.8 mg/dL (247.58 mmol/L) **H**	0.6–1.3 mg/dL (53–106 mmol/L)

Practice Question 3.3 — Drag-and-Drop Cloze

A 78-year-old client has been hospitalized for the past week for evacuation of a subdural hematoma after a fall. Immediately after surgery, the client was alert and oriented with right-sided hemiparesis. The client's speech was slurred, but client could communicate needs without problem. The client was continent of bowel and bladder most of the time, and began rehabilitative therapies. On the third postoperative day, aspiration pneumonia was confirmed by x-ray and the client was placed on IV antibiotic therapy. Today the nurse reviews the last entry in the Nurses' Notes for an update of the client's condition.

Drag (or select) client findings from the choices below to fill in the blanks in the following sentence.

The nurse reviews the notes and recognizes that the client findings that are of **immediate** concern are _____[Select]_____, _____[Select]_____, _____[Select]_____, and _____[Select]_____.

Client Findings

Drowsiness
No adventitious or diminished breath sounds
Right arm weakness
Bowel sounds X 4
Incontinent diarrheal stools
Speech ability
Elevated temperature

Health History	Nurses' Notes	Imaging Studies	Lab Results

0730: Very drowsy this morning but can be aroused with gentle shaking. Remains oriented × 3. Does not readily respond when spoken to, but eventually answers in 1–2 words. No adventitious or diminished breath sounds. S_1, S_2 present; no additional heart sounds. BS present × 4 and abdomen soft. Had 2 incontinent diarrheal stools during the night. Able to move all extremities but right arm continues to be weak. Skin intact; no reddened areas noted. Plan to send to PT and OT this morning. Temperature this morning has increased from 98°F (36.7°C) last evening to 100.2°F (37.9°C).

Practice Question 3.4 — Multiple Response Select All That Apply

The nurse reviews part of a Nurses' Notes entry for a 48-year-old client admitted to the inpatient psychiatric unit after a suicide attempt.

| Health History | Nurses' Notes | Imaging Studies | Lab Results |

1100: Admitted to unit for observation and treatment related to a suicide attempt. Attempted to cut both wrists, which are currently bandaged. Client was in a severe motor vehicle accident 5 months ago, resulting in quadriplegia. Has been living in a group home with full-time caregiver for assistance with ADLs since discharge from rehabilitation. Has no family living in the area. Has stage 3 sacral pressure injury covered with gauze dressing. Recently completed a course of antibiotics for infected sacral wound. Wears an external condom catheter and follows bowel regimen but has frequent problems with urine leakage and bowel incontinence. Is able to transfer with supervision from bed to wheelchair using sliding board. Lost 20 lb (9.1 kg) since the accident and describes appetite as "fair." Does not want to be here because he is "sick of being in hospitals."

*Which client findings are of **immediate** concern to the nurse related to risk factors for additional or worsening pressure injuries? **Select all that apply.***

☐ Attempted suicide
☐ Quadriplegic
☐ Current stage 3 sacral wound
☐ ADL dependent
☐ Uses sliding board for transfers
☐ Urinary and bowel incontinence
☐ 48 years of age
☐ Weight loss of 20 lb (9.1 kg)
☐ Fair appetite

Practice Question 3.5 — Drop-Down in Table

The nurse reviews the Nurses' Notes documented by the nurse from the last shift who was assigned to care for a 70-year-old client. The client had a right THA 2 days ago and is planning to be discharged tomorrow.

| Health History | Nurses' Notes | Imaging Studies | Lab Results |

1805: Alert and oriented. Walked in hall tonight with walker independently. Reports increasing pain in right hip and "feeling funny" and anxious for the past hour. Is excited to go home tomorrow and follow up with PT. Husband states that the client has been coughing periodically since stopped walking and returned to the room. No adventitious or abnormal breath sounds. Current VS: T = 99.4°F (37.3°C); HR = 88 BPM; RR = 20 bpm; BP = 102/58 mm Hg; SpO$_2$ = 93% (on RA). Will recheck client and VS in 1 hour.
1922: Reports "a little" difficulty breathing but denies chest pain. VS: T = 99.4°F (37.3°C); HR = 94 BPM; RR = 26 bpm; BP 98/52 mm Hg; SpO$_2$ 88% (on RA). Oxygen initiated at 2/min via NC and HOB in Fowler position. MD notified and awaiting orders.

*For each body system listed below, select the client findings that would be of **immediate** concern to the nurse. Each body system may support more than one client finding, but at least one option should be selected for each system.*

Body System	Client Findings
Cardiovascular	_____ 1 [Select]_____
Neurologic	_____ 2 [Select]_____
Respiratory	_____ 3 [Select]_____

Options for 1	Options for 2	Options for 3
Tachycardia	Increased right hip pain	Difficulty breathing
Hypotension	Ambulating with walker	Tachypnea
Decreased oxygen saturation	Feeling anxious	Periodic coughing

Practice Question 3.6   Multiple Response Select N

The nurse reviews the admission note for a 13-year-old client in the Urgent Care Center.

Health History	Nurses' Notes	Imaging Studies	Lab Results

0850: Parent reports that son started having new GI symptoms 2 days ago, which were "due to something he may have eaten and didn't agree with him." Started with lack of appetite and nausea but has progressed to fever and vomiting with occasional diarrhea. Last night he went to bed earlier than usual and showed no interest in playing video games as he usually does before dinner every night. Parents are divorced; child is with one parent during the school week and the other parent every weekend. Parent is concerned that son does not eat a very healthy diet on the weekends. Both of them prefer "fast food," especially hamburgers. This morning parent noted dark urine in the toilet. Current temperature is 103.2°F (39.6°C). Child states he feels very tired and wants to go home to bed.

*Select four client findings that are of **immediate** concern to the nurse.*

☐ Anorexia

☐ Occasional diarrhea

☐ Nausea and vomiting

☐ Poor eating habits

☐ Elevated temperature

☐ Fatigue

☐ Wants to sleep

☐ Dark urine

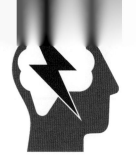

CHAPTER 4

Strategies for Answering NGN Questions: Analyze Cues

Analyze Cues is a cognitive skill nurses use to interpret the cues recognized in a clinical scenario and establish the significance of those cues. The nurse considers the context of the clinical scenario and thinks about what could be happening. The relevant cues are analyzed to determine supporting and opposing manifestations of an evolving client condition. Then, multiple factors are considered and potential complications that could be occurring are identified to guide subsequent planning and nursing actions. Applying the skill *Analyze Cues* is essential for making appropriate CJs and is a skill that will be measured both on the NGN and on your nursing course exams. When analyzing cues, you need to determine the meaning of the cues that are concerning. You need to connect or link these relevant cues to the client's scenario to determine their meaning.

 ## How Do You Analyze Cues?

The cognitive skill *Analyze Cues* requires a prompt and comprehensive examination of client data, fitting them into the bigger picture of the overall clinical scenario, and determining what the relevant cues mean. This requires considering multiple factors about what is occurring for the client and narrowing them down, serving as the basis for analysis and CJ. When analyzing cues, ask yourself two questions. First, ask yourself "What do these client findings mean?" Second, ask yourself "What is happening to the client?" Chapter 3 provides you with information about the cognitive skill *Recognize Cues*. Table 4.1 provides two examples of client findings that may be presented as part of an NGN clinical scenario. Relevant cues requiring application of the cognitive skill *Analyze Cues* are in boldface and italicized. All information in the client findings presented in these examples needs to be considered, but the relevant data are the focus to *Analyze Cues* and determine what these data mean for the client and how they fit into the bigger clinical picture.

 ## How Does Analyzing Cues Help You Guide Client Care?

The cognitive skill *Analyze Cues* requires you to examine the relevant data in a clinical scenario, link them to the client's clinical situation, and determine what these data mean. It is important to consider all factors presented in the clinical scenario to determine what is happening to the client. This is an important process because determining what relevant data mean tells you what is happening to the client. Once this is known, then you will be able to determine what you need to plan and do next to meet the client's needs.

NGN TIP

Remember: Analyzing cues and determining what relevant client data mean leads to formulating client needs, prioritizing client care, planning care, and clinical decision making with implementing care.

TABLE 4.1	Examples of Clinical Scenarios and How to Analyze Relevant Cues	
Clinical Scenario	**Analyze Cues**	
Scenario 1: A 5-week-old infant is brought by their parent to the clinic for a well-child check. The parent reports a **white coating on the tongue for the last 2 weeks.** The parent tried to clean the tongue with a washcloth but the **coating could not be removed.**	A white coating on the tongue of an infant could likely be milk residue or a sign of thrush. Factors to consider in analyzing these data are that the finding has lasted for 2 weeks and the coating could not be removed with a washcloth. *What do these data mean? What is happening to the infant?* Analysis of these data leads to a concern regarding the presence of thrush.	
Scenario 2: A client had a vaginal birth at home. The newborn's birth weight was 7 lb 11 oz (3.2 kg), and gestational age was 38 weeks 3 days. The newborn was transferred to the hospital immediately after birth. A **heart murmur was detected at the hospital, and the newborn was scheduled for a cardiology consultation.**	A heart murmur in a newborn may be an innocent murmur, meaning that it is not a cause for concern, or it could mean that there is a congenital cardiac condition, thus the need for cardiology consultation. *What do these data mean? What is happening to the newborn?* Analysis of these data leads to a concern regarding the possible presence of a congenital cardiac condition, and therefore further evaluation is required.	

How Do You Analyze Cues in an NGN Clinical Situation?

As noted in Chapter 3, NGN questions will begin with a clinical scenario presented as either a Stand-alone item or an Unfolding Case Study. Information about the client is presented, and you need to identify the relevant data. Once these relevant data are noted, you analyze the data and link these data to the client situation to determine what the data mean and what is happening to the client. Determining what these data mean and what is happening to the client is application of the cognitive skill *Analyze Cues*. The accompanying example provides you with a medical record and client data. After reviewing information in all tabs of the medical record provided, and once relevant cues are identified, you then analyze cues to determine what is happening to the client to guide client care. In this example, relevant data (cues) are in boldface and italicized. You need to analyze these data and make connections with the client situation to determine the meaning of the data. The cognitive skill *Analyze Cues* is required to ensure planning safe client care.

Example: Analyze Cues

Health History	Nurses' Notes	Vital Signs	Laboratory Results

A 65-year-old client presents to the ED at 1030 for *diarrhea 5 to 6 times daily × 1 week.* States that they get the urge to have a bowel movement suddenly and describes it as mixed, **both watery and formed at times.** Denies melena or blood in the stool. Doesn't recall eating anything that would cause the symptoms. Denies associated abdominal pain or colic and has no alleviating or aggravating factors. Has not taken any medication for the symptoms. Is still able to eat and drink, and appetite is unchanged. States they "just need to stay close to a bathroom." Denies recent travel and recent antibiotic use and states that they have no sick contacts. Current medications are reviewed, and none are associated with the complaints. The client is admitted to the observation unit for further testing.

Health History	Nurses' Notes	Vital Signs	Laboratory Results

1030: T = 98.2°F (36.8°C); *HR = 110 BPM; BP = 102/68 mm Hg;* RR = 16 bpm; SpO$_2$ = 98% on RA

THINKING SPACE

| Health History | Nurses' Notes | Vital Signs | Laboratory Results |

1100: Laboratory tests prescribed and stool culture for *Clostridium difficile*. Stool noted to be watery and tan in color. Specimen collected and sent to laboratory for testing.

| Health History | Nurses' Notes | Vital Signs | Laboratory Results |

Test	Result	Normal Reference Range
Red blood cells (RBCs)	4.8×10^{12} (4.8×10^{12})	4.2–6.2×10^{12}/L (4.2–6.2×10^{12}/L)
White blood cells (WBCs)	15,000/mm³ (15×10^9/L) H	5000–10,000/mm³ (5–10×10^9/L)
Segmented neutrophils	75% (8.3×10^9/L) H	62%–68% (2.5–7.5×10^9/L)
Band neutrophils	10% (1.1×10^9/L) H	0%–9% (0–1×10^9/L)
Lymphocytes	20% (0.1×10^9/L)	20%–40% (0.1–0.4×10^9/L)
Monocytes	2% (0.1×10^9/L)	2%–8% (0.1–0.7×10^9/L)
Eosinophils	1% (0.00×10^9/L)	1%–4% (0.00–0.5×10^9/L)
Basophils	1% (0.05×10^9/L)	0.5%–1% (0.02–0.05×10^9/L)
Platelets	200,000/mm³ (200×10^9/L)	150,000–400,000/mm³ (150–400×10^9/L)
Hemoglobin (Hgb)	17 g/dL (170 g/L)	12–18 g/dL (120–180 g/L)
Hematocrit (Hct)	46% (0.46)	37%–52% (0.37–0.52)
Albumin	4.2 g/dL (42 g/L)	3.5–5.0 g/dL (35–50 g/L)
Blood urea nitrogen (BUN)	24 mg/dL (8.64 mmol/L) H	10–20 mg/dL (3.6–7.1 mmol/L)
Calcium	10.2 mg/dL (2.7 mmol/L)	9–10.5 mg/dL (2.25–2.75 mmol/L)
Chloride	102 mEq/L (102 mmol/L)	98–106 mEq/L (98–106 mmol/L)
Creatinine	0.9 mg/dL (79.5 mcmol/L)	0.5–1.2 mg/dL (44–106 mcmol/L)
Glucose	87 mg/dL (4.8 mmol/L)	70–99 mg/dL (3.9–5.5 mmol/L)
Potassium	3.8 mEq/L (3.8 mmol/L)	3.5–5.0 mEq/L (3.5–5.0 mmol/L)
Sodium	142 mEq/L (142 mmol/L)	135–145 mEq/L (135–145 mmol/L)
Total bilirubin	0.3 mg/dL (5.1 mcmol/L)	0.3–1.0 mg/dL (5.1–17 mcmol/L)
Total protein	6.4 g/dL (64 g/L)	6.4–8.3 g/dL (64–83 g/L)
Alanine aminotransferase (ALT)	28 U/L (28 U/L)	4–36 U/L (4–36 U/L)
Aspartate aminotransferase (AST)	28 U/L (28 U/L)	0–35 U/L (0–35 U/L)
Stool culture C. difficile toxin	Detected	Negative

What Will You Think About to Analyze Cues in This Clinical Scenario?

To analyze cues, you will examine the relevant data and link these data to the clinical situation to interpret the data, determine what the data mean, and draw conclusions about what is happening to the client.

In this situation, the findings that are *not* within the usual or normal range include:

- Reports of frequent diarrhea; both watery and formed at times
- WBCs: 15,000/mm³ (15×10^9/L)

- Segmented neutrophils 75% (8.3×10^9/L)
- Band neutrophils 10% (1.1×10^9/L)
- BUN: 24 mg/dL (8.64 mmol/L)
- HR 110 BPM
- BP 102/68 mm Hg
- Stool culture *C. difficile* toxin: Detected

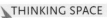
THINKING SPACE

To consider these findings in the bigger clinical picture, it is important to think about why these results may be out of range and how they are connected. Reports of frequent diarrhea as the primary client problem is a good starting point to frame the analysis. It helps to start thinking about possible causes of the diarrhea. Considering the information available in the medical record, a connection can be made that the ED physician is interested in exploring *C. difficile* infection as a cause.

From there, considering why the physician might be ordering a complete blood count or comprehensive metabolic panel will help progress the analysis. Specifically, a complete blood count will provide information about signs of infection. In this case, the WBC count is elevated and the differential, which breaks down the number of types of WBCs in the specimen, is also abnormal. With the segmented and band neutrophils being elevated, a bacterial infection would be suspected. This is often referred to as a "shift to the left."

A comprehensive metabolic panel will provide information on hydration status, electrolyte balance, and kidney and liver function. The BUN is elevated, and in the setting of a normal creatinine level, this indicates dehydration. This fits within the clinical context of multiple episodes of diarrhea as a result of suspected GI infection. The BP is lower than normal and the HR is elevated, also expected characteristics in dehydration. The potassium level and sodium level are in normal range but need to be monitored because these electrolytes are lost when a client has diarrhea. Last, the detection of the *C. difficile* toxin confirms the diagnosis of *C. difficile* infection.

Which Client Findings Are Most Important When Analyzing Cues?

The cognitive skill *Analyze Cues* requires you to interpret the meaning of client findings and create a bigger clinical picture to set the stage for making important decisions that inform and guide safe client care. All client findings are important, but those that are not normal or not expected are the most important when it comes to analyzing cues. You need to analyze these abnormal findings and ask "Is the abnormal finding acceptable or expected considering this client scenario, or is it not acceptable and an immediate concern for the nurse?" For example, the nurse assessing a client with an acute exacerbation of COPD would interpret acute shortness of breath as a manifestation of importance at this time and would determine that it requires *immediate* follow-up. However, noting a barrel chest when performing the physical assessment is relevant, but with further analysis the nurse knows that this is a long-term manifestation of the client's chronic disease.

When Might You Need to Analyze Cues in a Clinical Situation?

The ability to effectively apply the cognitive skill *Analyze Cues* is critical and is needed when answering both current NCLEX®-style questions and NGN questions. As a nurse, you need to always *Analyze Cues* in a clinical situation; this is an important part of your nursing practice. Knowledge about health problems and linking this knowledge to the interpretation of history and physical assessment findings, nursing assessment findings, and diagnostic test results are required to *Analyze Cues*. Table 4.2 provides examples of common health problems and diagnostic sources that would provide relevant data that link to the listed common health problem. These data are helpful when determining what is happening to the client with the listed health problem.

What NGN Item Types Optimally Measure *Analyze Cues*?

Four types of test items may be used to optimally measure the cognitive skill *Analyze Cues*. Variations of each type will be presented on the NGN. Table 4.3 presents these item types and their variations.

NGN TIP

Remember: Use these strategies for NGN items that measure *Analyze Cues*:

1. Examine the relevant cues or findings that are unexpected.
2. Determine client conditions that link or connect with the client findings or cues.
3. Ask yourself: What do these findings mean and what is happening to the client? Are there any findings or cues that support or oppose any client conditions?
4. Decide if any other information in the clinical situation would help establish the significance of the findings within the context of the bigger clinical picture.

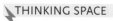
THINKING SPACE

TABLE 4.2   Examples of Common Health Problems and Diagnostic Sources for Analyzing Cues

Common Health Problems	Diagnostic Sources
Dysrhythmias	ECG results
MI	ECG results, laboratory results (e.g., cardiac markers, troponin levels)
Heart failure	ECG results, laboratory results (e.g., B-natriuretic peptide), imaging results (chest x-ray)
Respiratory compromise	Laboratory results (e.g., arterial blood gas levels)
Pneumonia	Laboratory results (e.g., white blood cell count, inflammatory markers), imaging results (e.g., chest x-ray)
GI bleeding	Laboratory results (e.g., hemoglobin level, hematocrit level, platelets, electrolytes), imaging results (e.g., abdominal CT scan, esophagogastroduodenoscopy [EGD])
Hypotension, hypovolemia, shock	Laboratory results (e.g., blood urea nitrogen [BUN] level, creatinine level, electrolytes)
Stroke	Imaging results (e.g., CT scan of the head)
VT (DVT and PE)	Laboratory results (e.g., prothrombin time [PT]/international normalized ratio [INR], partial thromboplastin time [PTT]), imaging results (e.g., Doppler ultrasound, CT scan of the lungs)
Sepsis	Laboratory results (e.g., white blood cell count, lactic acid level, glucose level)
Arterial occlusion	Imaging results (e.g., ultrasound)
Kidney dysfunction	Laboratory results (e.g., blood urea nitrogen [BUN] level, creatinine level), imaging results (e.g., renal ultrasound)
Compartment syndrome	Imaging results (e.g., x-ray, MRI, compartment pressure testing)
Abdominal trauma	Laboratory results (e.g., hemoglobin level, hematocrit level, platelets), imaging results (e.g., abdominal CT scan)
Chest trauma	Laboratory results (e.g., hemoglobin level, hematocrit level, platelets), imaging results (e.g., chest CT scan)

TABLE 4.3   Test Items and Variations That Optimally Measure _Analyze Cues_

Type of Test Item	Variations
Drop Down	Drop-Down Cloze Drop-Down Rationale Drop-Down in Table
Multiple Response	Multiple Response Select N Multiple Response Select All That Apply Multiple Response Grouping Matrix Multiple Response
Multiple Choice	Multiple Choice Single Response Matrix Multiple Choice
Drag-and-Drop	Drag-and-Drop Cloze Drag-and-Drop Rationale Drag-and-Drop in Table (may replace Drop-Down in Table)

All of these test item types are discussed in Chapter 2 with examples. The following sections explain the four major item types that best measure _Analyze Cues._

Drop-Down Test Items to Measure _Analyze Cues_

As mentioned in Chapter 2, Drop-Down items include Drop-Down Cloze, Drop-Down Rationale, and Drop-Down in Table. When the Drop-Down item type is used to measure _Analyze Cues,_ the test taker is required to complete a sentence or blank space by choosing from a list of options. Sample Question 4.1 illustrates a Drop-Down Rationale type of item. Rationale and test-taking strategy to help you derive the correct responses shown in Sample Question 4.1 are also provided.

NGN TIP

Remember: In a Drop-Down Rationale test item that requires completing a rationale, there is no partial credit. You must understand the full concept and the justification through the rationale to receive credit for your answer.

The nurse on a medical-surgical unit is caring for a postoperative 52-year-old client transferred from the PACU at 1100 following hiatal hernia repair using laparoscopic Nissen fundoplication (LNF). The client is on O_2 2 L per NC with orders to titrate based on SpO_2. The client has an NG tube attached to low intermittent suction (LIMS), and a PCA pump with hydromorphone for pain management.

Health History	Nurses' Notes	Vital Signs	Laboratory Results

1100: Arrived by bed from PACU and received bedside report from PACU nurse. Spouse is at bedside and engaged in teaching. VS stable on admission to postoperative unit. Surgical site dressings × 3: clean, dry, and, intact with topical adhesive in place, no drainage. NG tube in right naris to LIMS, 10 mL of gastric secretions in suction container. Pain reported as a 3/10 in surgical site. Oriented to room and to PCA use. Ice chips provided. Sequential compression devices in place as prescribed. Incentive spirometer teaching completed. Two side rails up, call light in reach. Demonstrates understanding of use of PCA pump and call light. VS: T = 98.2°F (36.8°C); HR = 90 BPM; BP = 128/74 mm Hg; RR = 16 bpm; SpO_2 = 99% 2 L per NC.

1115: Resting in bed comfortably with eyes closed. Pressed the PCA button one time with one dose delivered. Surgical site dressings × 3: clean, dry, and intact with no drainage, 10 mL of gastric secretions in suction container. VS: HR = 92 BPM; BP = 132/78 mm Hg; RR = 16 bpm; SpO_2 = 98% 2 L per NC. Reporting pain in abdomen 2/10.

1130: Resting in bed comfortably with eyes closed. Pressed the PCA button three times with two doses delivered. Surgical site dressing × 3: clean, dry, and intact with no drainage, 20 mL of gastric secretions in suction container. VS: HR = 92 BPM; BP = 130/78 mm Hg; RR = 16 bpm; SpO_2 = 98% 2 L per NC. Reporting pain in abdomen 2/10.

1145: Alert and oriented × 3, grimacing at times. Pressed the PCA button six times with three doses delivered. Surgical site dressings × 3: clean, dry, and intact with no drainage, 20 mL of gastric secretions in suction container. Reporting pain in abdomen 6/10. Reports no eructation or flatus. VS: HR = 90 BPM; BP = 148/80 mm Hg; RR = 20 bpm; SpO_2 = 97% 2 L per NC.

1200: Alert and oriented × 3. Grimacing frequently. Pressed the PCA button nine times with four doses delivered. Surgical site dressings × 3: clean, dry, and intact with no drainage, 30 mL of gastric secretions in suction container. Reporting pain in abdomen 8/10 with associated nausea; abdomen is distended. Reports no eructation or flatus. VS: T = 98.2°F (36.8°C); HR = 98 BPM; BP = 156/82 mm Hg; RR = 22 bpm; SpO_2 = 97% 2 L per NC.

Complete the following sentences by choosing from the list of options provided.

The nurse suspects **gas bloat syndrome** as a complication related to fundoplication. This suspicion is supported by **reports of no eructation or flatus** . The nurse would confirm the complication by **initiating early mobility** and reassessing the client.

Options for 1	Options for 2	Options for 3
Atelectasis	VS	Initiating early mobility
Gas bloat syndrome	Gastric output	Checking NG tube placement
Temporary dysphagia	Difficulty swallowing	Initiating NPO status
An obstructed NG tube	Reports of no eructation or flatus	Encouraging incentive spirometer use

Rationale: Complications of fundoplication procedures include temporary dysphagia, gas bloat syndrome, atelectasis, pneumonia, and obstructed NG tube. Based on the overall clinical scenario, including progressively increasing pain and overuse of the PCA; nausea; abdominal distention; lack of eructation or flatus; and increasing BP, RR, and pulse rate without abnormal changes in SpO_2 or temperature, the most likely complication is gas bloat syndrome. The defining manifestation for this complication is the report of no eructation or flatus, and the nurse would confirm this complication by initiating early mobility to promote peristalsis and monitor for improvement after mobility interventions. Atelectasis is often seen with dyspnea or chest pain, and pneumonia often presents with a fever. Use of incentive spirometry is encouraged to prevent and manage these complications. Temporary dysphagia is associated with difficulty swallowing, and NPO status may be needed until the dysphagia resolves. An obstructed NG tube may cause nausea, vomiting, abdominal distention, and a nondraining NG tube. If this is suspected, NG tube placement would be verified. In this case, the NG tube has been draining adequately.

Test-Taking Strategy

Test-Taking Strategy: First you need to identify the complications that can happen following this surgical procedure. Next, focus on the client information and think about what these data mean and what is happening to the client. Ask yourself if there are any findings or cues that support or oppose any complications. Decide which cues are of concern because they are relevant and not expected, and then establish the significance of the findings within the context of the bigger clinical picture. In a Drop-Down Rationale question, choosing correctly for the first option is the most important part, to guide you in selecting correct options for the remaining choices that follow.

To choose correctly in the first option for this situation, use the approach illustrated in the table, which categorizes the client's findings.

Client Finding	Supports Gas Bloat Syndrome	Opposes Gas Bloat Syndrome	Differentiates Gas Bloat Syndrome From Other Conditions
Excessive PCA use	☒	☐	Temporary dysphagia usually not associated with pain
Adequate gastric output	☒	☐	Obstructed NG tube would have inadequate gastric output
Location of pain (abdomen)	☒	☐	Pneumonia, atelectasis: pain usually located in the chest, not abdomen
Abdominal assessment (distention)	☒	☐	Pneumonia, atelectasis, temporary dysphagia: would not see abdominal distention
Lack of eructation or flatus with resulting abdominal distention	☒	☐	Pneumonia, atelectasis, temporary dysphagia: would not see abdominal distention
VS: no fever or abnormal oxygenation changes in this case	☒	☐	Pneumonia, atelectasis: likely would see fever or oxygenation changes

Categorizing the findings of each possible complication using this table will help you determine which client findings support or oppose the possible complications. The complication with the most findings in the "Supports Gas Bloat Syndrome" column is most likely the correct answer for the first option. You can decide which complications are differentiated based on the client findings, which will help to narrow down the answer.

The PCA use in this case supports gas bloat syndrome, and differentiates temporary dysphagia because temporary dysphagia does not usually cause pain. Gastric output, which is adequate in this case, supports gas bloat syndrome and differentiates obstructed NG tube, because with an obstructed NG tube there would be inadequate gastric output. The pain assessment supports gas bloat syndrome and differentiates pneumonia and atelectasis, because the pain reported with these complications is usually located in the chest and not the abdomen. The abdominal assessment supports gas bloat syndrome in that abdominal distention is noted, and differentiates pneumonia, atelectasis, and temporary dysphagia because this finding is not consistent with those complications. Lack of eructation and flatus also supports gas bloat syndrome because eructation and flatus relieve abdominal distention. This finding also differentiates pneumonia, atelectasis, and temporary dysphagia. Last, the VS support gas bloat syndrome and differentiate pneumonia and atelectasis because with these problems you would likely see a fever and changes with oxygenation.

Content Area: Medical-Surgical Nursing
Priority Concept: Fluid and Electrolyte Balance
Reference(s): Ignatavicius et al., 2021, pp. 1086–1087

NGN TIP

Remember: In a Drop-Down Rationale test item, it is critical to choose the first option correctly so that the remaining option choices are based on the correct foundation.

Multiple Response Test Items to Measure *Analyze Cues*

As mentioned in Chapter 2, Multiple Response test items include Multiple Response Select All That Apply, Multiple Response Select N, Multiple Response Grouping, and Matrix Multiple Response. When the Multiple Response item type is used to measure *Analyze Cues,* the test taker is required to follow the question directions regarding how to select options. Sample Question 4.2 illustrates a Matrix Multiple Response type of item. Rationale and test-taking strategy to help you derive the correct responses shown in Sample Question 4.2 are also provided.

Sample Question 4.2	Matrix Multiple Response: Analyze Cues

An 86-year-old client with COPD was admitted to the medical-surgical unit from the ED with complaints of increased shortness of breath, cough, heart palpitations, and more mucus production than normal.

| Health History | Nurses' Notes | Vital Signs | Laboratory Results |

H/O DM and COPD
Medications: Theophylline, short- and long-acting beta-adrenergic agonists, high-dose inhaled corticosteroid, prednisone, insulin glargine, and insulin aspart

| Health History | Nurses' Notes | Vital Signs | Laboratory Results |

1200: Color is pale, coughing and expectorating yellow-colored sputum, and complaining of chest tightness
Lung sounds reveal wheezing and diminished breath sounds bilaterally
POC blood glucose is 295 mg/dL (16.8 mmol/L)
VS: T = 101.8°F (38.8°C); apical HR = 120 BPM and regular; BP = 128/80 mm Hg; RR = 20 bpm; SpO$_2$ = 88% on RA

For each assessment finding below, click to specify if the finding is consistent with COPD exacerbation, pneumonia, or adverse effects of medications. Each assessment finding may support more than one condition.

Assessment Finding	COPD Exacerbation	Pneumonia	Adverse Effect of Medications
Increased shortness of breath	☒	☒	☐
Cough	☒	☒	☐
Increased mucus production	☒	☒	☐
Heart palpitations	☐	☐	☒
Blood glucose 295 mg/dL (16.8 mmol/L)	☒	☒	☒
Fever	☐	☒	☐
SpO$_2$ 88% on RA	☒	☒	☐

THINKING SPACE

Test-Taking
Strategy

Rationale: Manifestations of COPD exacerbation include increased coughing, wheezing, and more shortness of breath than usual. Other manifestations include changes in the color, thickness, or amount of mucus. In some COPD clients an SpO_2 of 88% could be normal, but it could also be an indication of exacerbation. In pneumonia the client presents with fever, a cough and mucus production, and shortness of breath. SpO_2 could be lower than normal because of the compromised respiratory status. Sharp or stabbing chest pain is also characteristic. The glucose level increases in the presence of infection such as pneumonia or in COPD exacerbation because the stress response in the body increases the amount of certain hormones such as cortisol and adrenaline. This leads to the body's increased production of glucose. Prednisone and other corticosteroids can cause a rise in blood glucose levels by making the liver resistant to insulin. Theophylline is a bronchodilator. Signs of toxicity are nausea, vomiting, abdominal pain, tachycardia, and muscle tremor. Heart palpitations are also a sign of toxicity.

Test-Taking Strategy: For each of the client conditions asked about in this question, you should ask yourself, based on the findings in the Health History and Nurses' Notes data, whether the assessment findings are specifically related or not specifically related to the suspected client condition and why you are interpreting the findings in this way. You can organize your thinking process as illustrated in the table.

Assessment Finding	COPD Exacerbation	Pneumonia	Adverse Effects of Medications
Increased shortness of breath	Related because of the added stress on the respiratory system	Related because of the added stress on the respiratory system	Not specifically related
Cough	Related as a chronic manifestation of COPD, worsened in exacerbation	Related as an acute manifestation of respiratory infection	Not specifically related
Increased mucus production	Related as a chronic manifestation of COPD, worsened in exacerbation	Related as an acute manifestation of respiratory infection	Not specifically related
Heart palpitations	Not specifically related	Not specifically related	Related to theophylline toxicity
Blood glucose 295 mg/dL (16.8 mmol/L)	High-dose inhaled and oral corticosteroid therapy can cause an increase in blood glucose; client has diabetes	Related as a manifestation of infection, especially in clients with DM	Related to prednisone
Fever	Not specifically related	Related as a manifestation of respiratory infection	Not specifically related
SpO_2 88% on RA	Related as a chronic manifestation of COPD, worsened in exacerbation	Related as an acute manifestation of respiratory infection	Not specifically related

NGN TIP

Remember: In a Matrix Multiple Response item there will be response columns, and each response column could have multiple correct responses.

Content Area: Medical-Surgical Nursing
Priority Concept: Gas Exchange
Reference(s): Burchum & Rosenthal, 2022, pp. 836, 928; Ignatavicius et al., 2021, pp. 573–577, 600

Drag-and-Drop Test Items to Measure *Analyze Cues*

Drag-and-Drop test items include Drag-and-Drop Cloze, Drag-and-Drop Rationale, and Drag-and-Drop in Table. When the Drag-and-Drop item type is used to measure *Analyze Cues,* the test taker is required to complete a sentence or fill in a blank space by choosing from a list of options and dragging that selected option to the answer space. Sample Question 4.3 illustrates a Drag-and-Drop Rationale type of item. Rationale and test-taking strategy to help you derive the correct responses in Sample Question 4.3 are also provided.

Sample Question 4.3 | **Drag-and-Drop Rationale Item: Analyze Cues**

The nurse conducts the admission assessment for a 72-year-old client admitted to the medical-surgical nursing unit with fever and shortness of breath. The medical record reveals the following findings.

| Health History | Nurses' Notes | Vital Signs | Diagnostic Results |

H/O present illness: 72-year-old client comes to the ED with complaints of fever and shortness of breath. Reports recent upper respiratory infection with fever and body aches diagnosed as influenza at the urgent care 3 days ago; oseltamivir was prescribed

Past medical history: Obesity, rheumatoid arthritis, stroke 4 years ago, type 2 DM, hyperlipidemia

Social history: Has smoked 1 pack of cigarettes per day for the past 42 years. Lives with child; does not drive owing to problems with eyesight and has limited mobility

Medications: Aspirin 81 mg daily, metformin 1000 mg twice daily, atorvastatin 10 mg daily, azathioprine 150 mg daily, oseltamivir (3 days remaining in course)

| Health History | Nurses' Notes | Vital Signs | Diagnostic Results |

T = 101.2°F (38.4°C); HR = 90 BPM; BP = 168/92 mm Hg; RR = 22 bpm; SpO$_2$ = 90% 2 L per NC
Weight: 220 lb (99.79 kg)
Height (reported): 5 feet 2 inches

| Health History | Nurses' Notes | Vital Signs | Diagnostic Results |

2-view chest x-ray: left lower lobe infiltrates

Drag one complication to option 1, one client finding to option 2, and one other client finding to option 3 to fill in each blank in the following sentence.

The client is at **highest** risk for developing <u>VTE</u> due to <u>acute infection</u> and <u>obesity</u>.

Options for 1	Options for 2 and 3
Aspiration	Body aches
Heart failure	Acute infection
Dysrhythmias	Inability to drive
VTE	Prescribed medications
Acute MI	Obesity

Rationale: Although the client has some risk factors for the other conditions (aspiration, heart failure, dysrhythmias, acute MI), the highest risk is for VTE. VTE history and risk are assessed at admission. Some risk factors include active cancer, previous VTE, reduced mobility, thrombophilic conditions, recent trauma or surgery, older age, cardiac and respiratory failure, acute MI, ischemic stroke, acute infection, rheumatologic disorders, obesity, and hormonal treatment. Client findings consistent with these risk factors include active infection, information noted in the past medical history (obesity, rheumatoid arthritis, cardiovascular disease, such as stroke), and social factors (smoking). The presence of body aches, although consistent with infection, is nonspecific and could be related to other problems. The inability to drive is not specifically related, and the medication regimen actually decreases the client's risk for this problem.

Test-Taking Strategy: First, focus on the client data, especially the relevant data and the abnormal and unexpected data, and determine what is happening to the client. Use thinking processes and determine what these data mean and how they affect the health of the client. Next, use knowledge and think about the complications that can occur with this client. Ask yourself if there are any findings or cues that support or oppose any

Test-Taking
Strategy

NGN TIP

Remember: For the Drag-and-Drop Rationale item, a full understanding of "paired" information is required in order to answer the question correctly. The concept needs to be justified by the rationale chosen. If a question is asking about a complication and associated client findings or associated risk factors, the complication needs to be correctly identified first. Then the client findings and risk factors associated with that complication need to be determined in order to receive credit for the answer.

complications. Decide which cues are of concern. In a Drop-Down Rationale question, choosing correctly for the first option is the most important part to guide you in selecting correct options for the remaining choices that follow. When answering a Drag-and-Drop Rationale item, it may be helpful to look at the options for the client findings first and then pair them with the possible complications. The complication with the most client findings is most likely the correct answer for the first option.

Client Finding	Complication
Body aches	Nonspecific to listed complications
Active infection	Risk factor for *VTE*
Inability to drive	Nonspecific to listed complications
Prescribed medications	Treatment for heart failure, dysrhythmias, acute MI, *VTE*
Obesity	Risk factor for heart failure, dysrhythmias, acute MI, *VTE*

As noted, the client presents with multiple risk factors for VTE compared with the other complications listed. The client's medication regimen is preventing or treating health problems. You may need to rely on your knowledge base related to risk factors for VTE and the other conditions to some extent to answer this question correctly.

Content Area: Medical-Surgical Nursing
Priority Concept: Clotting
Reference(s): Ignatavicius et al., 2021, p. 721

Multiple Choice Test Items to Measure *Analyze Cues*

Multiple Choice items include Multiple Choice Single Response and Matrix Multiple Choice. When these item types are used to measure *Analyze Cues,* the test taker is required to either select one option from a list of up to 10 options (Multiple Choice Single Response) or select one answer in each row of options (Matrix Multiple Choice). Sample Question 4.4 illustrates a Matrix Multiple Choice item. Rationale and test-taking strategy to help you derive the correct responses are also provided.

Sample Question 4.4	Matrix Multiple Choice: Analyze Cues

A 32-year-old client is admitted to the acute behavioral health unit for observation and therapy. The client is accompanied by their sibling, who tells the nurse that the client has had a noticeable, uncharacteristic change in behavior over the last 4 to 5 days. The nurse cares for the client during the daytime shift and provides the oncoming nurse with a report on the client.

Health History	Nurses' Notes	Vital Signs	Laboratory Results

Client talking and joking with everyone; demanding another client's attention
Making inappropriate sexual propositions to the other clients sitting in the day room
Telling everyone they are the child of the Vice President of the United States
Too distracted and disorganized to eat lunch
Writing numerous letters to famous people in Hollywood
Overactive and busily occupied with grandiose plans
Verbalizing crude and sexual remarks and profanities to the nursing staff

For each assessment finding, click to specify if the finding is consistent with hypomania or acute mania.

Assessment Finding	Hypomania	Acute Mania
Client talking and joking with everyone	☒	☐
Demanding another client's attention	☐	☒
Making inappropriate sexual propositions to the other clients sitting in the day room	☒	☐
Telling everyone they are the child of the Vice President of the United States	☐	☒
Too distracted and disorganized to eat lunch	☐	☒
Writing countless numbers of letters to famous people in Hollywood	☒	☐
Overactive and busily occupied with grandiose plans	☒	☐
Verbalizing crude and sexual remarks and profanities to the nursing staff	☐	☒

Rationale: Hypomania and acute mania are disorders related to bipolar spectrum disorders. Hypomania is a less severe and less intense form of mania and is characterized by a noticeable change in functioning that has lasted at least 4 days and that is uncharacteristic of the individual.

Acute mania is a more severe form of mania, and psychotic symptoms may be present. In hypomania the individual talks and jokes with everyone to be seen as the "life of the party," whereas in acute mania the individual becomes inappropriately demanding of people's attention, and their intrusive nature repels others. In hypomania the individual makes inappropriate sexual propositions to total strangers; talk is sexual and can be obscene. As the individual reaches acute mania, they verbalize crude and sexual remarks and profanities, especially to the nursing staff. In hypomania the individual has elaborate and grandiose schemes for becoming rich and famous and writes a large number of letters to rich and famous people about these schemes. These individuals are overactive and busily occupied with grandiose plans but are not delusional. In acute mania the individual has grandiose delusions and may come to believe that they are famous or especially gifted without any basis in fact. In hypomania the individual usually has a voracious appetite and eats on the run, gobbling food during brief periods. In acute mania the individual is too distracted and disorganized and has no time to eat.

Test-Taking Strategy: First note the difference in the terms *hypo*mania and *acute* mania. You can determine that hypomania assessment findings will be less severe than acute mania assessment findings. The easiest way to organize your thinking process for this question is to categorize the client findings as either "less severe" or "more severe" because these are the differentiating factors between hypomania and acute mania. Refer to the table as an example of applying these strategies. The client findings categorized as less severe would be answered as findings associated with hypomania, whereas those categorized as more severe would be answered as findings associated with acute mania.

Assessment Finding	Severity
Client talking and joking with everyone	Less severe
Demanding another client's attention	More severe
Making inappropriate sexual propositions to the other clients sitting in the day room	Less severe
Telling everyone they are the child of the Vice President of the United States	More severe
Too distracted and disorganized to eat lunch	More severe
Writing numerous letters to famous people in Hollywood	Less severe
Overactive and busily occupied with grandiose plans	Less severe
Verbalizing crude and sexual remarks and profanities to the nursing staff	More severe

Content Area: Mental Health Nursing
Priority Concept: Mood and Affect
Reference(s): Varcarolis & Fosbre, 2021, pp. 199–200, 227–229

THINKING SPACE

NGN TIP

Remember: In a Matrix Multiple Choice item, you need to select one option for each row.

Test-Taking Strategy

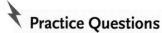

Practice Questions

A 45-year-old client diagnosed with CKD requires dialysis. As a candidate for both hemodialysis and peritoneal dialysis, the client decides that peritoneal dialysis is the better option for their lifestyle. The client is hospitalized and undergoes insertion of the peritoneal dialysis catheter, and the first dialysis procedure is ordered. The nurse documents predialysis assessment data and reviews laboratory results.

Health History	Nurses' Notes	Vital Signs	Laboratory Results

1100: T = 98.2°F (36.8°C); apical HR = 90 BPM and regular; BP = 146/98 mm Hg; RR = 16 bpm; breath sounds clear bilaterally. Weight = 160 lb (72.57 kg)

Health History	Nurses' Notes	Vital Signs	Laboratory Results

Test	Result	Normal Reference Range
Blood urea nitrogen (BUN)	30 mg/dL (10.8 mmol/L) H	10–20 mg/dL (3.6–7.1 mmol/L)
Creatinine	6.0 mg/dL (528 mcmol/L) H	0.5–1.2 mg/dL (44–106 mcmol/L)
Glucose	110 mg/dL (6.1 mmol/L) H	70–99 mg/dL (3.9–5.5 mmol/L)
Sodium	150 mEq/L (150 mmol/L) H	135–145 mEq/L (135–145 mmol/L)
Potassium	5.5 mEq/L (5.5 mmol/L) H	3.5–5.0 mEq/L (3.5–5.0 mmol/L)

During dialysis infusion, the nurse notes a slow inflow of the dialysate and the client complains of pain. On assessment of the catheter, the nurse notes some fibrin clot formation in the dialysis tubing. **Complete the following sentences by choosing from the list of options.**

The nurse recognizes that the slow inflow, presence of fibrin clots, and complaints of pain are **most likely** the result of _____1 [Select]_____ due to the _____2 [Select]_____.

Options for 1	Options for 2
Peritonitis	Catheter slippage
Initial dialysis treatment	Surgical procedure
Bowel perforation	Lack of aseptic technique
Abdominal pressure	Elevated BP and laboratory results

An 80-year-old client who had a cholecystectomy 2 weeks ago was admitted 2 hours ago to the medical-surgical unit from the ED with acute pain located in the left upper abdomen. The client had laboratory testing and contrast-enhanced CT scan of the abdomen. The nurse conducts an admission assessment and reviews the laboratory and diagnostic findings.

| Health History | Nurses' Notes | Vital Signs | **Diagnostic Results** |

Test	Result	Normal Reference Range
White blood cells (WBCs)	16,000/mm³ (16 × 10⁹/L) H	5000–10,000/mm³ (5–10 × 10⁹/L)
Hemoglobin (Hgb)	16 g/dL (160 g/L)	12–18 g/dL (120–180 g/L)
Hematocrit (Hct)	44% (0.44)	37%–52% (0.37–0.52)
Blood urea nitrogen (BUN)	18 mg/dL (6.48 mmol/L)	10–20 mg/dL (3.6–7.1 mmol/L)
Creatinine	0.8 mg/dL (70.6 mcmol/L)	0.5–1.2 mg/dL (44–106 mcmol/L)
Glucose	110 mg/dL (6.1 mmol/L) H	70–99 mg/dL (3.9–5.5 mmol/L)
Alanine aminotransferase (ALT)	80 U/L (80 U/L) H	4–36 U/L (4–36 U/L)
Aspartate aminotransferase (AST):	88 U/L (88 U/L) H	0–35 U/L (0–35 U/L)
Activated partial thromboplastin time (aPTT)	32 sec (32 sec)	30–40 sec (30–40 sec)
Prothrombin time (PT)	11.4 sec (11.4 sec)	11–12.5 sec (11–12.5 sec)
International normalized ratio (INR)	1.0 (1.0)	0.81–1.2 (0.81–1.2)
Amylase	800 U/L (800 U/L) H	60–120 U/L (60–120 U/L)
Lipase	320 U/L (320 U/L) H	0–160 U/L (0–160 U/L)

CT abdomen with contrast impression: Edema of the uncinate process of the pancreatic head, with peripancreatic fat, consistent with acute interstitial pancreatitis

| Health History | **Nurses' Notes** | Vital Signs | Diagnostic Results |

1100: T = 99.2°F (36.8°C); HR = 90 BPM; BP = 168/88 mm Hg; RR = 24 bpm; SpO₂ = 89% on RA; lung sounds clear but diminished to auscultation bilaterally and breathing is nonlabored. Bowel sounds are hypoactive in all quadrants. Abdominal pain is 4/10, client receiving prescribed morphine in the ED.

Based on the information in the Nurses' Notes and in the Diagnostic Results, complete the following sentence from the list of options provided.

As a complication of acute pancreatitis, the client is at **highest** risk for developing _____1 [Select] _____ as evidenced by _____2 [Select] _____.

Options for 1	Options for 2
Atelectasis	SpO₂ level
Bile duct calculi	PT/INR results
Pulmonary edema	CT abdomen results
Coagulation defects	BUN and creatinine levels

Practice Question 4.3 | Drag-and-Drop Cloze

The nurse working at the outpatient pediatric clinic is performing an admission assessment for a 7-year-old child who is accompanied by their parent. The child reports right ear pain for 3 days. The nurse documents the following assessment findings.

Health History	Nurses' Notes	Vital Signs	Diagnostic Results

Reports right ear pain × 3 days described as constant, aching, nonradiating; denies dry mucous membranes, eye drainage, nasal drainage, or throat pain; oropharynx pink, moist, with no redness, swelling, exudate

Reports no sick contacts and has been attending full days of school; reports swimming daily for the past week

Denies neck stiffness; no swelling of the neck, or swollen lymph nodes

Denies cough, wheezing, difficulty breathing; lung sounds clear

Tenderness noted on palpation and manipulation of right auricle with ear canal erythema; no discharge; left auricle nontender

Immunizations up-to-date

Allergies: No known allergies

Health History	Nurses' Notes	Vital Signs	Diagnostic Results

Weight: 55 lb (59th percentile)
Height: 49.25 inches (55th percentile)
BMI: 15.94 (58th percentile)
T: 97.9°F (36.6°C) temporal
HR: 98 BPM
RR: 18 bpm
BP: 108/70 mm Hg

Complete the following sentence. Drag the words from the options below to fill in each blank.

The nurse determines that the child is experiencing otitis externa based on assessment findings that include _____1 [Select] _____, _____2 [Select] _____, and _____3 [Select] _____.

Options for 1	Options for 2	Options for 3
No sick contacts	Denies neck stiffness	Denies cough
Ear pain without fever	Immunizations up-to-date	No lymphadenopathy
Attends full school days	Swimming daily for the past week	Tenderness on manipulation of right auricle
Left auricle is nontender to manipulation	Lack of nasal drainage or throat pain	Lung sounds clear to auscultation bilaterally

Practice Question 4.4 — Multiple Response Select All That Apply

Every 30 minutes the nurse is monitoring a 28-year-old client who was admitted 3 hours ago to the labor and delivery unit in the first stage of labor. The nurse suddenly notes late decelerations and frequent episodes of fetal tachycardia in response to FHR decelerations on the monitor.

The nurse determines that these findings indicate which of the following conditions? **Select all that apply.**

☐ Breech baby

☐ Fetal hypoxemia

☐ Metabolic fetal acidemia

☐ Strong uterine contractions

☐ Uteroplacental insufficiency

Practice Question 4.5 — Multiple Choice Select All That Apply

A 45-year-old client is admitted to the ED because of frequent episodes of chest pain unrelieved by sublingual nitroglycerin. The ECG shows ST segment elevation. Troponin levels are elevated. While awaiting results of diagnostic studies and transfer to the cardiac unit, the nurse monitors the client.

Vital signs reveal the following:

Health History	Nurses' Notes	Vital Signs	Laboratory Results

1200: HR = 88 BPM; RR = 22 bpm; BP = 142/86 mm Hg
1215: HR = 92 BPM; RR = 24 bpm; BP = 120/82 mm Hg
1230: HR = 106 BPM and weak; RR = 28 bpm; BP = 100/62 mm Hg
1245: HR = 120 BPM and weak; RR = 32 bpm; BP = 90/58 mm Hg

The nurse determines that these vital sign findings **most likely** *indicate which complication(s)?* **Select all that apply.**

☐ Dysrhythmias

☐ Pulmonary edema

☐ Cardiogenic shock

☐ Cardiac tamponade

☐ Pulmonary embolism

☐ Dissecting aortic aneurysm

Practice Question 4.6 — Matrix Multiple Response

At 1300 hours an 86-year-old client with altered mental status who is accompanied by their child is admitted to the medical-surgical unit, and the nurse is performing an assessment. The client has an IV solution of a 1000-mL bag of 0.9% sodium chloride hung at 1200 in the ED that is infusing at 100 mL/hr. One hour after admission the client's child calls the nurse and reports that the client has a pounding headache, is having trouble breathing, and seems scared.

Health History	Nurses' Notes	Vital Signs	Laboratory Results

1300: Client is weak and reports has not been able to eat or drink in the past 3 days because of anorexia.
Skin is very dry, dry mucous membranes, sleepy.
The child reports that the client has a H/O heart failure, hypertension, and hyperlipidemia.
Breath sounds clear bilaterally.
Medications include lisinopril, carvedilol, and digoxin.
1400: Client is dyspneic and complaining of chest tightness, coughing and is pale, neck vein distention is seen. Breath sounds wheezing and congestion bilaterally. 500 mL remaining in the IV bag.

Health History	Nurses' Notes	Vital Signs	Laboratory Results

Test	Result	Normal Reference Range
Blood urea nitrogen (BUN)	24 mg/dL (8.64 mmol/L) H	10–20 mg/dL (3.6–7.1 mmol/L)
Creatinine	1.8 mg/dL (159.4 mcmol/L) H	0.5–1.2 mg/dL (44–106 mcmol/L)
Digoxin level	2.2 ng/mL (2.8 nmol/L) H	0.5–2.0 ng/mL (0.64–2.56 nmol/L)
Sodium	148 mEq/L (148 mmol/L) H	135–145 mEq/L (135–145 mmol/L)
Potassium	5.2 mEq/L (5.2 mmol/L) H	3.5–5.0 mEq/L (3.5–5.0 mmol/L)

Health History	Nurses' Notes	Vital Signs	Laboratory Results

1300: T = 100.2°F (36.8°C); apical HR = 72 BPM and regular; BP = 100/68 mm Hg; RR = 24 bpm; SpO$_2$ = 90% on RA
1400: T = 100.2°F (36.8°C); apical HR = 110 BPM and regular; BP = 152/98 mm Hg; RR = 28 bpm; SpO$_2$ = 89% on RA

*For each assessment finding below, click to specify if the finding is **most likely** consistent with dehydration, circulatory overload, or digoxin toxicity.*

Assessment Finding	Dehydration	Circulatory Overload	Digoxin Toxicity
Anorexia	☐	☐	☐
Dry mucous membranes	☐	☐	☐
BUN and creatinine levels	☐	☐	☐
Sodium and potassium levels	☐	☐	☐
Digoxin level	☐	☐	☐
Elevation in BP and RR	☐	☐	☐
Wheezing and congestion bilaterally in lungs	☐	☐	☐
Neck vein distention	☐	☐	☐

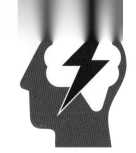

CHAPTER 5

Strategies for Answering NGN Questions: Prioritize Hypotheses

Prioritize Hypotheses is a cognitive skill nurses use to establish and rank client needs or hypotheses in order of priority. When prioritizing hypotheses, the nurse considers potential occurrences such as the likelihood of what could happen in a specific scenario, the urgency of it, and associated risks. In addition, environmental factors and individual factors need to be considered when you are prioritizing hypotheses. These factors are described in this chapter.

THINKING SPACE

What Do Hypotheses Mean?

You may ask, "What are *hypotheses*?" A *hypothesis* (singular) or *hypotheses* (plural) are in part a prediction that you make about a clinical scenario to determine the client's priority needs. Once you interpret the relevant data in a clinical scenario and consider all possibilities or predictions about what is occurring, you then rank these predictions according to their urgency and risks for the client, in order to decide on the priority needs. You need to determine which needs are *most immediate* and *most serious,* and why. You need to ask yourself, "What could explain what I am seeing with my client? Which explanations are most likely? Which explanations are least likely? Which of these explanations are the most immediate and serious?" and "Where do I start with planning care?"

What Does Prioritizing Mean?

Prioritizing means that you need to rank the client's needs in order of importance. It is important to focus on all the information in the clinical scenario because the order of importance may vary depending on the health problems, the environmental setting, and the client's condition. When a clinical situation is presented, you may also need to consider what the client deems a priority, which may be quite different from what you think is most important.

NGN TIP

Remember: When you prioritize, you are deciding which client needs or problems are primary and require immediate attention and which ones could be delayed until a later time because they are not urgent.

What to Consider When Prioritizing Hypotheses

Applying the skill *Prioritize Hypotheses* is essential for making appropriate clinical judgments, and is a skill that will be measured both on the NGN and on your nursing course exams. When prioritizing hypotheses, in addition to the information in the clinical scenario, you need to consider external factors and connect or link these factors to the clinical scenario in order to determine priority client needs. Considering external factors is important when applying every cognitive skill. The cognitive skill *Prioritize Hypotheses* is the skill that involves considering all possibilities or predictions about what is occurring, ranking these predictions by their urgency and risks for the client, and deciding where to start with planning care. A description of how each external factor affects your thinking process in determining priority client needs is discussed in this chapter. See Box 5.1 for the possible external factors you may be asked about or need to consider in a clinical scenario.

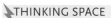THINKING SPACE

BOX 5.1 External Factors to Consider When Prioritizing Hypotheses	
Environmental Factors	**Individual Factors**
Environment	Knowledge
Client observation	Skills
Resources	Specialty
Medical records	Candidate (test-taker) characteristics
Consequences and risks	Prior experience
Time pressure	Level of experience
Task complexity	
Cultural considerations	

From National Council of State Boards of Nursing (NCSBN). (2019). *Next Generation NCLEX® News, Winter 2019.* <https://www.ncsbn.org/NGN_Winter19.pdf>

External Factors and Prioritizing Hypotheses

The cognitive skill *Prioritize Hypotheses* asks you to determine priority client needs in a specific clinical scenario. In doing so, you need to consider the context of any external factors presented. The NCSBN notes that there are environmental factors and individual factors that need to be considered (see Box 5.1). Following is a description of how each external factor affects your thinking process in determining priority client needs.

Environmental Factors

Environment

The environment refers to the setting in which client care is taking place. The environment is important to think about because you may need to establish priority client needs and approach answering a question in the ED differently than in a community-based clinic. For example, a client experiencing an emergent problem, such as symptoms of acute coronary syndrome, or a heart attack, would need to have care prioritized differently based on the resources available in the environment in which the care is taking place. In a clinic setting the nurse would be calling EMS to transport the client to the hospital as a priority, whereas in the ED setting the nurse would be facilitating management of the problem, such as obtaining diagnostic testing and analyzing the results, and initiating the treatment plan.

Client Observation

The nurse's observations of the client need to be considered in order to establish hypotheses and then rank them in order of priority, which will be necessary to guide further client care. Your thinking process should be focused on "Where do I start?" For example, when caring for a client who is in pain, the nurse would prioritize by first conducting a thorough and comprehensive pain assessment. This would help the nurse to determine the most appropriate solutions and interventions and allow for a connected follow-up assessment after pain medication or other pain-relieving measures are instituted.

Resources

Availability of resources will affect the way you answer a question about a clinical scenario. For example, if you were a first responder to a mass casualty site, you would triage victims differently than you would if the victims were brought to the ED because the available resources would be quite different and much more limited at the mass casualty site. Also, think about this situation: If a cardiac arrest was discovered, you would answer a question differently if you had additional personnel to assist than if you (the nurse) were the only personnel available.

Medical Records

NGN test items will present a medical record as part of the question, and this is another external factor you need to consider before answering the question about the clinical scenario. All information provided in the medical record needs to be reviewed and critically analyzed before you determine the urgency of findings, think about explanations of those findings, and establish priority client needs. Refer to Chapter 3, which discusses the cognitive skill *Recognize Cues,* and Chapter 4, which discusses the cognitive skill *Analyze Cues*—both of which need to be applied when considering information in a medical record before applying the skill *Prioritize Hypotheses.*

Consequences and Risks

While thinking about explanations for client findings and establishing and ranking hypotheses based on the explanations, you need to think about the consequences and risks associated with the findings. This will guide you in prioritizing. For example, the nurse caring for a client with dehydration will think about the risks and consequences associated with the fluid volume deficit being left untreated or unmanaged while considering the urgency or priority of subsequent nursing actions. Another example may be a client with a UTI, who would be monitored for signs and symptoms of sepsis and shock.

Time Pressure

Time pressure is another external factor to consider when applying the skill *Prioritize Hypotheses.* If time is part of the data presented in the question, it may be a factor to consider as you are deciding on the answer or answers to the question. As an example, a nurse taking care of a postoperative client will consider client data findings differently and consider different explanations of the findings based on whether the client just came out of surgery, has been out of surgery for 8 hours, or had the surgery several days before. Another example may be related to how long it may take to meet a client need. If you had a client experiencing dyspnea, you would consider elevating the head of the client's bed right away to alleviate the respiratory distress, which takes seconds to do, before listening to lung sounds, which will take more time.

Task Complexity

Task complexity is a measure of the difficulty of a task that the nurse considers and takes into account in order to complete the task. For example, with regard to prioritizing hypotheses, one factor a home care nurse would think about is how much time would be needed and how involved the client's needs are for each assigned client for the day, and would organize the schedule according to the clients' needs and the complexity of the care to be provided. The nurse may have a client who needs an admission assessment completed, a client who needs a wound irrigation, and a client requiring teaching about a simple dressing change. The nurse would take into consideration the complexity of the tasks involved with the care being provided as one factor to decide how to prioritize.

Cultural Considerations

The last environmental factor to think about is cultural considerations. If information related to the client's culture is included in the clinical scenario, it will be important to consider these factors as you are answering test questions. As an example, the nurse may need to consider dietary preferences as they relate to culture in order to provide nutrition that is aligned with these important values and meet the client's needs while the client is in the nurse's care. Or you may need to consider higher-risk health problems that are specific to a cultural group when you are prioritizing hypotheses.

Individual Factors

Knowledge and Skills

Nursing knowledge and skills are individual factors considered when nursing exam questions are developed for your nursing courses and for the NGN. Intuitively, exam questions will be written to test specific nursing knowledge and skills, based on expected

THINKING SPACE

activities performed by new graduate nurses. When caring for a client, you need to use nursing knowledge when applying all cognitive skills including prioritizing hypotheses. In your nursing program it is critical that you *not* learn just by memorizing concepts. Learning by memorization is short-lived and is a superficial type of learning that does not require any thinking. You need to approach the learning process so that you will be able to make connections from what you learned to a new situation you may encounter and be able to know what is most urgent when prioritizing hypotheses. This type of learning is called deep learning, and requires thinking. For example, you are presented with a situation in which a client has an MI. You will need to recall many previously learned concepts and skills in order to prioritize hypotheses and safely care for that client. Some concepts you need to recall are the anatomic structure of the heart and coronary arteries, their function, cardiac rhythms, emergency treatments, and complications associated with an MI.

Specialty

Another individual factor is the nursing specialty. With regard to nursing exams and NGN test items, you will be presented with questions about foundations of care, pharmacology, medical-surgical nursing, or mental health nursing. Exam questions may also be written based on the population being cared for, such as children (pediatrics) or pregnant individuals (obstetric or maternity nursing). As noted earlier, deep learning is important because you may, for example, need to apply physical assessment concepts or foundational concepts previously learned to a new situation. Consider this scenario when prioritizing hypotheses: An 85-year-old client is admitted to the nursing unit with weakness, confusion, an elevated temperature, tachycardia, and hypotension. You need to consider all possibilities or predictions about what is occurring in this client, such as possible dehydration or even infection; you then rank these predictions according to their urgency and risk(s) for the client in order to decide on the priority need(s). You need to determine which needs are *most immediate* and *most serious,* and why. You would need to recall previously learned knowledge to then prioritize hypotheses.

Candidate Characteristics, Prior Experience, and Level of Experience

Candidate characteristics, such as prior experience and level of experience, are additional individual factors considered with the application of cognitive skills and clinical judgment. As an example, a new nursing graduate may not be as skilled as an experienced nurse about actions to take when the nurse notices a change in a client's clinical condition. This could depend on their prior experience and current level of experience. However, it is important to remember that regardless of prior or level of experience, client safety is the priority, and the nurse needs to be able to rank priority needs swiftly if a client's condition deteriorates. Nurses with less experience can always use the guidance of more experienced nurses as an invaluable resource.

 ## How Do You Know That You Need to Prioritize?

As a nurse, you will be prioritizing all the time; this skill is a critical one to ensure safety for each client. For example, when you receive an assignment for the nursing shift you will need to prioritize client needs for a group of clients and determine which assigned client you will need to assess first, second, third, and so on. Look at the following scenario about prioritizing for a group of clients.

Scenario 1: The nurse is assigned the following three clients on the 0600–1400 shift. Who would the nurse assess first, second, and third?

Client 1: Client who was admitted to the nursing unit during the night because of difficulty breathing

Client 2: Client on IV antibiotics and due to receive a dose at 0900

Client 3: Client being discharged to home today who needs further teaching about insulin administration and diet

In addition, as a nurse, you will also need to prioritize client needs for one client. On NCLEX®, prioritizing client needs for one client will most likely be presented. Look at the following example of prioritizing for a single client.

THINKING SPACE

*Scenario 2: The client is experiencing a sickle cell crisis. What are the **immediate** priority client needs? **Select all that apply.***

Client Need 1: Pain
Client Need 2: Fluids
Client Need 3: Oxygen
Client Need 4: Nutrition
Client Need 5: Electrolyte balance

Questions that require prioritization will include strategic words or strategic phrases in the question that indicate the need to prioritize. Be sure to look for these specific words or phrases. What are these words or phrases? Box 5.2 lists some of the common strategic words or phrases.

What Three Strategies Can You Use to Prioritize Hypotheses?

First and foremost, it is important to think and use your nursing knowledge. Nursing knowledge provides information that you need to process and think about critically in order to answer the question. If you can use your nursing knowledge to answer the question, then by all means do so!

Next, three strategies that you can use to assist in prioritizing client needs are the *Priority Classification System; Airway, Breathing, and Circulation;* and *Physiological and Safety Needs.* These strategies are described in the following sections.

Priority Classification System

There are some strategies that you can use to prioritize hypotheses. To start, try to use the Priority Classification System and rank hypotheses as a high (top), intermediate (middle), or low (last) priority. Your high-priority hypotheses then become your primary and urgent client needs. Your intermediate hypotheses are the client's needs that are less urgent but still important, and can wait to be addressed. Your low-priority hypotheses are those client needs that are either unrelated to the client's health problem or can wait to be addressed until after attending to the high- and intermediate-priority hypotheses. Box 5.3 provides a description of the three types of classifications.

BOX 5.2 Common Strategic Words or Phrases		
Best	Initial	Essential
First	Immediate	Most likely
Primary	Next	Most important

BOX 5.3 Priority Classification System
High (Top) Priority: A client need that is life-threatening, or if untreated could result in harm to the client
Intermediate (Middle) Priority: A nonemergency and non–life-threatening client need that does not require immediate attention and can wait to be addressed
Low (Last) Priority: A client need that is not directly related to the client's illness or prognosis, is not urgent, and can wait until high and intermediate client needs are addressed

Airway, Breathing, and Circulation

Airway, breathing, and circulation is abbreviated as the ABCs. You can use the ABCs to help you determine the priority client needs. Airway is always a priority in caring for any client. Think about it: If a client does not have a patent airway and breathing is ineffective to oxygenate body tissues, will any other client need matter? Breathing is the next priority because breathing is needed to oxygenate tissue; again, if the airway is not patent, then the client will not be able to breathe. Finally, circulation: Circulation is critical but requires oxygenated blood to effectively oxygenate tissue. Note that there is one exception, and that is if you are prioritizing client needs in a cardiopulmonary resuscitation scenario. For these scenarios, remember to follow CAB—circulation (compressions), airway, and breathing—to prioritize. Consider the clinical scenario in which a client with COPD is experiencing difficulty breathing and the SpO_2 level is lower than the baseline level. This scenario would take high priority because the airway (and breathing and circulation as well) is involved. When ranking in the context of other client's needs, consider this clinical scenario for the client with COPD and at the same time a postoperative client complaining of pain of 5/10 at the operative site who is asking for pain medication. Because the second clinical scenario does not involve the ABCs, the nurse would appropriately rank the client with difficulty breathing ahead of the client having pain.

Physiological and Safety Needs

A physiological client need and safety are always priorities. It is important to consider all client needs in any clinical scenario, but most likely you will need to address physiological needs. Remember that physiological integrity is necessary for survival. Along with this priority need is the need for safety. In fact, client safety must be at the top of your list when caring for each and every client.

For example, you have a client who is being discharged from the hospital and needs teaching about administering insulin, so you identify teaching as a priority client need. Safety must be considered along with the teaching. Your client suddenly develops weakness, shakiness, and hunger, and you determine that the client is experiencing hypoglycemia. At that time your priority client need switches from teaching to one that is addressing the physiological need of hypoglycemia, but, in addition, safety is a priority. It is important to remember that in a clinical scenario the priority order of client needs is not static. In other words, as a client's condition changes, whether that be improvement or deterioration, the priority of needs can change.

How Do You Prioritize Hypotheses in an NGN Clinical Situation?

As noted in Chapter 3, NGN questions will begin with a clinical scenario presented as either a Stand-alone item or an Unfolding Case Study. Information about the client is presented, and you need to identify the relevant data. As noted in Chapter 4, once these relevant data are noted, you analyze the data and link these data to the client situation to determine what the data mean and what is happening to the client. Then, based on your judgment of what you think is happening to the client, you assign priority or urgency to those client needs, which exemplifies application of the skill *Prioritize Hypotheses*. The following example provides you with client data. After reviewing information in all tabs of the medical record, and once relevant cues have been identified and analyzed, you then prioritize hypotheses. You need to determine the urgency of the identified client needs to guide the next steps in client care. The cognitive skill *Prioritize Hypotheses* is required to ensure planning safe client care. Remember to consider the external factors previously discussed when considering the priorities of care.

Example—Prioritize Hypotheses: A 45-year-old client is preparing for discharge following a 2-month hospitalization and will need long-term IV antibiotics. The client has a central line in place. The client has a past medical history of DM, and takes insulin with meals and at bedtime.

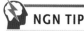

NGN TIP

Remember: *Prioritize Hypotheses* is the cognitive skill in which you rank the urgency of client needs. This leads to formulating the plan of care based on those needs (*Generate Solutions*), and clinical decision making with implementing care (*Take Action*).

THINKING SPACE

During this hospitalization the client has become very weak and needs PT and OT to help improve functional ability. The client will be moving in with family, who will be the primary caregivers. The client will have home health support services to help manage medications. The client is anxious about going home and having to rely on others to help with care.

What Will You Think About to Prioritize Hypotheses in This Clinical Scenario?

To *Prioritize Hypotheses,* you would need to think about the client's needs based on the information provided in the scenario. As the nurse preparing the client for discharge, you would consider what the client will need in the first few days at home, until the client's new routine is established and home health care services and other supports are in place.

Begin by considering the external factors that may be important in the scenario. Thinking about these factors before looking at the question you are being asked will help your thinking process as you answer. Consider the environment—a hospital setting. This helps to frame your thinking in terms of what the role of the nurse is in providing teaching and support to the client during this time. Think about any client observation data—the client will need long-term IV antibiotics, is weak after a prolonged hospitalization, has a past medical history of DM and takes insulin, and is anxious about going home. These client needs will be important to address as priorities in the discharge teaching. This scenario mentions the resources of home health care and family support. As you think about answering questions about this, consider these resources and how they may factor into the way the questions are answered. Other considerations as you prioritize hypotheses for this scenario may be task complexity and consequences and risks. The client will need IV antibiotics and insulin. These are important interventions where very clear and understandable teaching will need to be provided in order to promote safety and mitigate risk and any unintended consequences. In this scenario, thinking also about the external factors, you would consider the following as priority hypotheses:

- Safety in the home environment
- Discharge needs
- Establishing care with home health support
- Maintaining a central line
- Administering antibiotics
- Complications of a central line
- Side effects of medications
- Client and caregiver teaching

What NGN Item Types Optimally Measure *Prioritize Hypotheses?*

Three types of test items may be used to measure the cognitive skill *Prioritize Hypotheses.* Variations of each type will be presented on the NGN. Table 5.1 presents these item types and their variations.

All of these test item types are discussed in Chapter 2, and some examples are provided. The following section explains the three major item types that best measure *Prioritize Hypotheses.*

NGN TIP

Remember: Use these strategies for NGN items that measure *Prioritize Hypotheses:*

1. Examine the clinical scenario and any relevant external factors.
2. Determine urgency of client findings as you assign priority in planning subsequent client care.
3. Ask yourself: Which needs are most immediate and most serious, and why?
4. Think about: What could explain what I am seeing with the client, and what explanations are most likely or least likely?
5. Ask yourself: Where do I start with planning care?

TABLE 5.1 Test Items and Variations That Optimally Measure *Prioritize Hypotheses*	
Type of Test Item	**Variations**
Drop Down	Drop-Down Cloze
	Drop-Down Rationale
	Drop-Down in Table
Multiple Response	Multiple Response Select N
	Multiple Response Select All That Apply
	Multiple Response Grouping
Drag-and-Drop	Drag-and-Drop Cloze
	Drag-and-Drop Rationale
	Drag-and-Drop in Table (may replace Drop-Down in Table)

Drop-Down Test Items to Measure *Prioritize Hypotheses*

NGN TIP

Remember: In a Drop-Down Cloze test item the maximum score is equivalent to the number of drop downs, and partial credit for correct responses is given.

As discussed in Chapter 2, Drop-Down items include Drop-Down Cloze, Drop-Down Rationale, and Drop-Down in Table. When the Drop-Down item type is used to measure *Prioritize Hypotheses,* the test taker is required to complete a sentence or blank space by choosing from a list of options. Sample Question 5.1 illustrates a Drop-Down Cloze type of item to measure the cognitive skill *Prioritize Hypotheses.* The rationale and test-taking strategy to help you derive the correct responses in Sample Question 5.1 are also provided.

Sample Question 5.1	Drop-Down Cloze Item: Prioritize Hypotheses

A 32-year-old client visits the physician because of vomiting and severe watery diarrhea for the previous 3 days. Following an initial assessment, the physician prescribes hospital admission for further evaluation and treatment. The nurse conducts an initial assessment and reviews the physician's orders and results of preadmission laboratory tests.

Physician's Orders	Nurses' Notes	Vital Signs	Lab Results

Contact Precautions
Stool culture: Call with results as soon as known
Call with result of laboratory studies
Blood culture × 3 for temperature >100.2°F (37.9°C)
Clear liquid diet
IV 1000 mL D$_5$W in 0.9% NS at 100 mL/hr
Ondansetron 4 mg IV stat then 8 mg sublingual every 6 hr
Loperamide 4 mg oral stat then 2 mg oral after each
    unformed stool; daily dose not to exceed 16 mg
VS every 4 hours
Strict intake and output measurements

Physician's Orders	Nurses' Notes	Vital Signs	Lab Results

1400: T = 101.2°F (38.4°C); HR = 102 BPM; BP 100/66 mm Hg; RR = 20 bpm; SpO$_2$ = 96% on RA; abdominal pain = 4/10

Physician's Orders	Nurses' Notes	Vital Signs	Lab Results

1400: States vomiting and diarrhea began 3 days ago shortly after eating cheese manicotti and tossed salad at a local restaurant. Vomit is described as mostly bile and is unable to hold down any liquids or food. Stool is watery and now tan to yellow in color. Has experienced frequent chills and fever. Reports no blood in vomit or stool. Has diffuse abdominal pain rated currently as 4/10 and states it is continuous.
Appears pale, skin and mucous membranes dry, feeling tired and light-headed.
Urine output 45 mL since 0900, dark yellow, strong smelling; states urinating in small amounts about 3 times daily.
Current medications: No regular medication regimen and states tried some loperamide with no effect.
Denies recent travel and states has not been in contact with any sick persons. Is an insurance agent and has been working from home for the past 10 months because of the pandemic.
Stool sent for culture.
Laboratory called for blood culture draws.

Health History	Nurses' Notes	Vital Signs	Lab Results

Test	Result	Normal Reference Range
White blood cells (WBCs)	15,000/mm³ (15 × 10⁹/L) **H**	5000–10,000/mm3 (5-10 × 10⁹/L)
Hemoglobin (Hgb)	17 g/dL (170 g/L)	12–18 g/dL (120–180 g/L)
Hematocrit (Hct)	46% (0.46)	37%–52% (0.37–0.52)
Blood urea nitrogen (BUN)	24 mg/dL (8.64 mmol/L) **H**	10–20 mg/dL (3.6–7.1 mmol/L)
Creatinine	0.9 mg/dL (79.5 mcmol/L)	0.5–1.2 mg/dL (44–106 mcmol/L)
Potassium	3.1 mEq/L (3.1 mmol/L) **L**	3.5–5.0 mEq/L (3.5–5.0 mmol/L)
Sodium	147 mEq/L (147 mmol/L) **H**	135–145 mEq/L (135–145 mmol/L)
Stool culture	Pending	Negative
Blood culture	Pending	No growth

Complete the following sentences by choosing from the list of options.

The *immediate* client needs to address on admission are

<u>hypokalemia</u> as evidenced by **potassium level** and

<u>dehydration</u> as evidenced by **urine output** .

Options for 1	Options for 2	Options for 3	Options for 4
Renal injury	Sodium level	Anemia	Urine output
Hypokalemia	Potassium level	Infection	Temperature
Hypernatremia	Blood urea nitrogen level	Dehydration	WBC count

Rationale: When a client experiences vomiting and severe watery diarrhea over a period of time, one primary client need and concern is that the client is dehydrated. In addition, electrolytes, specifically potassium, are lost whenever a client experiences diarrhea. The client exhibits signs of dehydration, such as paleness, dry skin and mucous membranes, tiredness and light-headedness, small amounts of urine output, dark color and strong odor of urine, and infrequent voiding. The BUN is slightly elevated, and in the setting of a normal creatinine level this indicates dehydration. The potassium level is low, indicating hypokalemia, and needs to be immediately addressed because of the risk of dysrhythmias. There is no evidence of kidney injury; the slightly elevated BUN and low urine output are associated with dehydration. Therefore dehydration and hypokalemia are the immediate client needs to be addressed on admission. Although an elevated temperature may occur in dehydration, here it is more likely an indication of infection because the WBC count is also elevated; infection is a concern but cannot be treated until blood culture and stool culture results are known. The Hgb and Hct are normal and this is expected because the client reports no evidence of blood in the vomit or stool; therefore anemia is not a concern. The sodium level is elevated and this is another sign of dehydration. The pulse rate is elevated and the BP is lower than normal; these findings are associated with the dehydration. The nurse would immediately report the laboratory results to the physician and point out that the potassium level is low. The physician may prescribe potassium to be added to the IV solution. Once the dehydration is treated, other abnormal findings will resolve and return to normal range. The potassium level will also return to normal once potassium is administered.

Test-Taking Strategy: Focus on the information in the scenario. Remember that with questions that require prioritizing, there will be options that are pertinent, but you need to decide which options take priority. As illustrated in the table, consider each client condition, whether it is present or not present, the evidence supporting each condition, and assign priority to those conditions based on safety.

Test-Taking Strategy

Client Condition	Present/ Not Present	High Priority/ Low Priority	More Information Needed
Renal injury	Not present	N/A	N/A
Hypokalemia	Present	High priority	No
Hypernatremia	Present	Low priority	No
Anemia	Not present	N/A	N/A
Infection	Present	High priority	Yes
Dehydration	Present	High priority	No

N/A, Not applicable.

This thinking process will help you answer the first part of each question. Renal injury and anemia are not present and can be eliminated first. Hypokalemia is present and is a high priority because it can lead to life-threatening dysrhythmias if not treated. Hypernatremia is present but is of low priority because it is expected with the client's condition. Infection is present and is a high priority because of complications that can occur, such as sepsis and shock, but additional information is needed, such as the blood culture and stool culture results, before treatment can begin. Dehydration is present and is a high priority because it can lead to other life-threatening complications as well. To decide between dehydration and infection, ask yourself if you have all the information you need in the clinical scenario, and then rank accordingly. You do not have all the needed information to address the infection, so the higher priority should be assigned to dehydration at this time. Next, using concepts of pathophysiology, connect each prioritized client condition with the evidence in the scenario that supports that condition.

Content Area: Medical-Surgical Nursing
Priority Concept: Fluid and Electrolyte Balance
Reference(s): Ignatavicius et al., 2021, pp. 247–248, 253, 925, 1135–1137

NGN TIP

Remember: In a Multiple Response Select All That Apply test item, there may be only one correct response or multiple correct responses. In addition, all responses presented could be correct.

Multiple Response Test Items to Measure *Prioritize Hypotheses*

As discussed in Chapter 2, Multiple Response test items include Multiple Response Select All That Apply, Multiple Response Select N, and Multiple Response Grouping. When the Multiple Response item type is used to measure *Prioritize Hypotheses* or other cognitive skills, the test taker is required to follow the question directions regarding how to select options. Sample Question 5.2 illustrates a Multiple Response Select All That Apply type of item. Rationale and test-taking strategy to help you derive the correct responses in Sample Question 5.2 are also provided.

Sample Question 5.2	Multiple Response Select All That Apply: Prioritize Hypotheses

A 34-year-old client is brought to the ED by EMS. The client fell while downhill skiing and hit a tree. EMS reports that the client was unconsciousness when they arrived at the scene. VS were as follows: BP 100/70 mm Hg, HR 98 BPM, and RR 30 bpm. Pupils were reactive bilaterally. GCS score was reported as 3, in which there was no response to eye opening, and no verbal or motor response. The client was placed on a spinal backboard and the neck was immobilized at the site of the injury. EMS applied oxygen at 2 L/min per NC and inserted an IV line. No open wounds or obvious injuries or fractures noted by EMS. The initial assessment on arrival at the ED reveals the following findings. Physician's orders are initiated.

Physician's Orders	Nurses' Notes	Vital Signs	Test Results

T = 98.2°F (36.7°C); HR = 100 BPM; BP 90/40 = mm Hg; RR = 32 bpm and labored; SpO$_2$ = 91% on 2 L/min per NC

Physician's Orders	Nurses' Notes	Vital Signs	Test Results

Combative and unresponsive to commands.
GCS = 8: no appropriate motor response, opens eyes spontaneously, verbal responses are inappropriate.
Patent IV line.
Lying on spinal backboard; neck immobilized.
No open wounds seen and no obvious deformities noted.
Purple bruising noted on right hip area and right lower abdomen.

Physician's Orders	Nurses' Notes	Vital Signs	Test Results

CT scan of the head
Chest, pelvic, and spinal x-rays
Arterial blood gas (ABG) analysis
Maintain a patent IV line
Insert Foley catheter; obtain urinalysis
White blood cell (WBC) count, hemoglobin (Hgb) and hematocrit (Hct), electrolytes, blood urea nitrogen (BUN) and creatinine

Physician's Orders	Nurses' Notes	Vital Signs	Test Results

Test	Result	Normal Reference Range
White blood cells (WBCs)	9,000/mm³ (9 × 10⁹/L)	5000–10,000/mm3 (5–10 × 10⁹/L)
Hemoglobin (Hgb)	10 g/dL (100 g/L) **L**	12–18 g/dL (120–180 g/L)
Hematocrit (Hct)	33% (0.33) **L**	37%–52% (0.37–0.52)
Blood urea nitrogen (BUN)	10 mg/dL (3.6 mmol/L)	10–20 mg/dL (3.6–7.1 mmol/L)
Creatinine	0.5 mg/dL (44 mcmol/L)	0.5–1.2 mg/dL (44–106 mcmol/L)
Potassium	4.0 mEq/L (4.0 mmol/L)	3.5–5.0 mEq/L (3.5–5.0 mmol/L)
Sodium	142 mEq/L (142 mmol/L)	135–145 mEq/L (135–145 mmol/L)
ABG	pH 7.40 PaCO$_2$ 40 mmHg PaO$_2$ 90 mmHg HCO$_3$ 23 mEq/L	7.35–7.45 PaCO$_2$ 35–45 mmHg PaO$_2$ 80–100 mmHg HCO$_3$ 22–27 mEq/L
Urinalysis	Bilirubin: Negative Glucose: Negative Blood: Negative pH: 5.0 Protein: **Trace** Specific gravity: 1.010	Bilirubin: Negative Glucose: Negative Blood: Negative pH: 4.6-8.0 Protein: Negative Specific gravity: 1.005–1.030

CT scan of the head: Left temporal cerebral contusion with a midline shift of brain structures. Left temporal parietal subdural hematoma.
Chest, pelvic, and spinal x-rays: No fractures or abnormalities seen. Negative x-rays.

*What are the **immediate** concerns for the client?* ***Select all that apply.***

- ☒ Bleeding
- ☐ Infection
- ☐ Kidney injury
- ☒ Cerebral edema
- ☐ Perforated bladder
- ☐ Electrolyte imbalance
- ☒ Respiratory compromise
- ☐ Spontaneous pneumothorax
- ☒ Increased ICP

►THINKING SPACE

Rationale: The client sustained a severe head injury. The immediate concerns for this client are bleeding, cerebral edema, increased ICP, and respiratory compromise. The GCS is a useful and quick tool to use to determine a client's neurologic condition. The scale assesses eye opening, verbal response, and motor response. Scores range from 3 to 15; the lower the score, the more critical the condition. A score between 3 and 8 indicates a severe head injury. The client currently has a GCS score of 8. The CT scan shows a temporal cerebral contusion with a midline shift of brain structures and a left temporal parietal subdural hematoma. Brain shifts can lead to edema, shearing of brain structures and bleeding, and brain ischemia. Therefore the nurse would be most concerned about bleeding in the brain, swelling and cerebral edema, and a resultant increase in ICP. The client's pulse is at 100 BPM, very slightly elevated from that measured at the scene of the accident. The BP is lower at 90/40 mm Hg, and respirations are increased at 32 bpm and labored. The client's Hgb and Hct are lower than normal. Normal Hgb is 12–18 g/dL (120–180 g/L). Normal Hct is 37%–52% (0.37–0.52). Therefore the nurse would be concerned about bleeding. The respiratory center is located in the brain, so the nurse would be very concerned about respiratory compromise. Cerebral edema can cause pressure on the respiratory center, resulting in a life-threatening condition. It is critical for the nurse to continuously monitor the VS and neurologic status so that any subtle changes that indicate deterioration in the client's condition can be detected early. Infection is not a concern at this time; the client's temperature is normal, there are no open wounds, and the WBC count is normal. Because the pelvic and spinal x-rays are normal, kidney injury and bladder perforation are not an immediate concern, although follow-up monitoring would be important. In addition, the urinalysis is normal without blood present. Laboratory studies reveal normal electrolytes, so electrolyte imbalance is not a concern. The chest x-ray is normal, so spontaneous pneumothorax is not an immediate concern.

Test-Taking Strategy: Note the strategic word *immediate.* Think about the scenario and the effects of the injury. Look at each option provided and make an association with the information presented in the medical record, as illustrated in the table.

Test-Taking Strategy

Option	Evidence From Medical Record
Bleeding	BP: 90/40 mm Hg RR: 32 bpm and labored SpO$_2$: 91% on 2 L/min per NC Hgb: 10 g/dL (100 g/L) Hct: 33% (0.33) CT scan results
Infection	None—WBC count and temperature are normal
Kidney injury	None—BUN, creatinine, urinalysis normal
Cerebral edema	Neurologic changes GCS scores
Perforated bladder	None—urinalysis normal
Electrolyte imbalance	None—potassium, sodium normal
Respiratory compromise	RR: 32 bpm and labored SpO$_2$: 91% on 2 L/min per NC CT: scan results
Spontaneous pneumothorax	Negative chest x-ray
Increased ICP	CT scan results

Note that for infection, kidney injury, perforated bladder, and electrolyte imbalance, there is no evidence that these problems exist. The respirations are elevated and labored and the SpO$_2$ is low; because the chest x-ray is negative, this rules out a spontaneous pneumothorax as a concern. The correct options are supported by clear evidence or data, and therefore would be considered the immediate concerns.

Content Area: Medical-Surgical Nursing
Priority Concept: Safety
Reference(s): Ignatavicius et al., 2021, pp. 912–922

Drag-and-Drop Test Items to Measure *Prioritize Hypotheses*

NGN TIP

Remember: In a Drag-and-Drop Cloze test item you will be asked to drag an option from a list of choices to fill in the blank in a sentence.

As discussed in Chapter 2, Drag-and-Drop test items include Drag-and-Drop Cloze, Drag-and-Drop Rationale items, and Drag-and-Drop in Table. When the Drag-and-Drop item type is used to measure *Prioritize Hypotheses,* the test taker is required to follow the question directions regarding how to select options. Sample Question 5.3 illustrates a Drag-and-Drop Rationale type of item, and Sample Question 5.4 illustrates a Drag-and-Drop Cloze type of item. The rationale and test-taking strategy to help you derive the correct responses in Sample Question 5.3 and Sample Question 5.4 are also provided.

| **Sample Question 5.3** | **Drag and Drop Rationale: *Prioritize Hypotheses*** |

The nurse working in the outpatient dialysis center is assisting in performing hemodialysis. The client's BP during dialysis decreased to 82/54 mm Hg. The nurse intervened by reducing the temperature of the dialysate, adjusting the rate of the dialyzer blood flow, placing the client in Trendelenburg position, and administering albumin as prescribed. The BP after these interventions was 80/52 mm Hg, and the client started complaining of light-headedness.

Based on this clinical scenario, drag one condition and one underlying cause to fill in each blank in the following sentence.

The client is **most** at risk for developing **myocardial injury** due to **pericardial disease**.

Condition	Potential Underlying Cause
Hypoglycemia	Fluid shifts
Myocardial injury	DM
Infectious disease	Pericardial disease
Fluid volume imbalances	Frequent blood transfusions
Disequilibrium syndrome	Rapid reduction of electrolytes

Rationale: Certain adverse effects can occur during hemodialysis, including hypotension, disequilibrium syndrome, cardiac events, and reactions to dialyzers. Hypotension is a common complication caused by heat transfer resulting in vasodilation. Initially the nurse would reduce the temperature of the dialysate; adjust the rate of the dialyzer blood flow; place the client in Trendelenburg position; and administer a fluid bolus, albumin, or mannitol as prescribed. If these interventions do not resolve the problem and if hypotension persists, the nurse would consider myocardial injury and possible underlying pericardial disease as a cause. The other conditions noted can occur with hemodialysis; however, the client findings in this clinical scenario and the fact that the interventions were ineffective indicate a cardiac event.

Test-Taking Strategy: Note the strategic word *most,* and remember that this word indicates the need to prioritize. This likely means that some or all of the options are correct or make sense in the clinical scenario, but you need to decide which condition the client is most at risk for. Note that the interventions were ineffective, and even though a cardiac history is not noted, this points to pericardial disease as the underlying cause. In the table, begin by matching the condition on the left with the potential underlying cause on the right.

Condition	Matched Potential Underlying Cause
Hypoglycemia	DM
Myocardial injury	Pericardial disease
Infectious disease	Frequent blood transfusions
Fluid volume imbalances	Fluid shifts
Disequilibrium syndrome	Rapid reduction of electrolytes

From here, based on the data in the clinical scenario, you need to decide which condition the client is most at risk for developing, knowing that these are all possible with hemodialysis. Note that the nurse already reduced the temperature of the dialysate, adjusted the rate of the dialyzer blood flow, placed the client in Trendelenburg position, and administered albumin as prescribed, and the BP was still low. This will direct you to consider myocardial injury caused by pericardial disease as the priority client need.

Content Area: Medical-Surgical Nursing
Priority Concept: Perfusion
Reference(s): Ignatavicius et al., 2021, p. 1416

NGN TIP

Remember: A Drag-and-Drop Rationale test item requires full understanding of paired information and justification through a rationale. Both the concept and the rationale must be correct to earn credit.

A 38-year-old client presents to the ED complaining of severe back pain in the right flank area rated 9/10 on a 0 to 10 pain intensity scale. The client has a history of hypertension, DM, hyperlipidemia, hypothyroidism, arthritis, and renal calculi. The CT scan of the abdomen shows a 10-mm renal calculus in the right kidney with hydronephrosis. The client is requesting ketorolac for the pain, stating that this has worked well in the past. Home medications include lisinopril, metformin, atorvastatin, levothyroxine, and ibuprofen. The ED physician resumes all home medications except for the ibuprofen, adds tamsulosin daily and ketorolac as needed for pain, orders laboratory testing, and arranges for urology consultation. The urologist assesses the client and adds morphine as needed for pain to the medication regimen, and orders extracorporeal shockwave lithotripsy (ESWL) for the following day. Laboratory results return, and the nurse reviews the results and physician's orders.

Health History	Nurses' Notes	Vital Signs	Lab Results

Test	Result	Normal Reference Range
Red blood cells (RBCs)	5.8×10^{12} (5.8×10^{12})	$4.2–6.2 \times 10^{12}$/L ($4.2–6.2 \times 10^{12}$/L)
White blood cells (WBCs)	9,000/mm³ (9×10^9/L)	5000–10,000/mm3 ($5–10 \times 10^9$/L)
Platelets	200,000/mm³ (200×10^9/L)	150,000–400,000/mm3 ($150–400 \times 10^9$/L)
Hemoglobin (Hgb)	17 g/dL (170 g/L)	12–18 g/dL (120–180 g/L)
Hematocrit (Hct)	50% (0.50)	37%–52% (0.37–0.52)
Albumin	3.6 g/dL (36 g/L)	3.5–5.0 g/dL (35–50 g/L)
Blood urea nitrogen (BUN)	32 mg/dL (11.52 mmol/L) **H**	10–20 mg/dL (3.6–7.1 mmol/L)
Calcium	10.2 mg/dL (2.7 mmol/L)	9–10.5 mg/dL (2.25–2.75 mmol/L)
Carbon dioxide (bicarbonate)	27 mmol/L (27 mmol/L)	22–27 mmol/L (22–27 mmol/L)
Chloride	102 mEq/L (102 mmol/L)	98–106 mEq/L (98–106 mmol/L)
Creatinine	2.2 mg/dL (194.3 mcmol/L) **H**	0.5–1.2 mg/dL (44–106 mcmol/L)
Glucose	80 mg/dL (4.45 mmol/L)	70–99 mg/dL (3.9–5.5 mmol/L)
Potassium	4.4 mEq/L (4.4 mmol/L)	3.5–5.0 mEq/L (3.5–5.0 mmol/L)
Sodium	140 mEq/L (140 mmol/L)	135–145 mEq/L (135–145 mmol/L)
Total bilirubin	0.3 mg/dL (5.1 mmol/L)	0.3–1.0 mg/dL (5.1–17 mcmol/L)
Total protein	6.5 g/dL (65 g/L)	6.4–8.3 g/dL (64–83 g/L)
Urinalysis	Bilirubin: Negative Glucose: Negative Blood: **Positive** pH: 5.0 Protein: **Trace** Specific gravity: 1.012	Bilirubin: Negative Glucose: Negative Blood: Negative pH: 4.6-8.0 Protein: Negative Specific gravity: 1.005-1.030

Based on this clinical scenario, drag one client need to fill in each blank in the following sentence.

The **priority** client need would be **pain management** followed by **preparation for ESWL**.

Options for 1	Options for 2
Pain management	Pain management
Stone analysis	Stone analysis
Preparation for ESWL	Preparation for ESWL

THINKING SPACE

Rationale: Calculi (also known as stones) are deposits of minerals that form into stones inside the urinary tract, and can be found in the kidneys, ureters, or bladder. When the calculus moves, it can cause pain that is often described as unbearable. Medications are integral to the treatment of someone with this problem, particularly for the management of pain. Because the client is experiencing such severe pain, the priority need is pain management, and the nurse would administer prescribed pain medication as a priority. Ketorolac can be very effective for pain associated with renal calculi. It is classified as an NSAID. This medication can be problematic in the setting of impaired renal function. Because the client's BUN and creatinine levels are elevated and there is blood noted on the urinalysis, NSAIDs should be avoided, and the nurse would opt for another pain management choice, such as the prescribed morphine. Opioid analgesics are often needed for the client experiencing renal colic from calculi. The nurse would need to contact the physician to inform them of the abnormal renal function and to clarify whether the ketorolac should be discontinued as an option for pain management. ESWL uses shock waves to break a kidney stone into small pieces that can more easily travel through the urinary tract and pass from the body. The nurse would prepare the client for this procedure next. Tamsulosin is classified as an alpha-adrenergic antagonist; it works by relaxing the smooth muscle in the bladder neck and thereby assists with passing the stone. This medication would be administered, but not as the priority need in this scenario. A 10-mm stone may be difficult to pass, but after ESWL the stone fragments will pass and may pass more easily if tamsulosin is part of the treatment plan. The stone then can be analyzed for composition and type, and this information will assist with determining the best treatment.

Test-Taking Strategy: Note the strategic word *priority* in this question. The ability to use judgment and prioritize client needs is needed to answer this question correctly. Considering the client's needs in the context of the health problem the client is experiencing can help you decide on priorities of care. Using a thinking process as illustrated in the table may be helpful.

Test-Taking
Strategy

Plan/Intervention	Assists With Immediate Client Need	Does Not Assist With Immediate Client Need
Pain management	☒	☐
Stone analysis	☐	☒
Preparation for ESWL	☒	☐

Once you determine that pain management and preparation for ESWL are the priorities because they assist with immediate client needs, you need to rank order these and decide which one should come first and which should follow. Focusing on the client and the client's experience will help you decide on pain management as the first priority, followed by preparation for ESWL.

Content Area: Medical-Surgical Nursing
Priority Concept: Elimination
Reference(s): Burchum & Rosenthal, 2022, p. 162; Ignatavicius et al., 2021, p. 1362

Practice Questions

Practice Question 5.1   **Multiple Response Grouping**

A 12-year-old client visits the health care clinic for a follow-up visit after laboratory and other testing. The client is accompanied by a parent. The client tells the nurse about an increase in appetite lately and about urinating more frequently than usual. The nurse reviews the client's test results and collects data from the client prior to the client being seen by the physician. The following is documented in the medical record.

Health History	Nurses' Notes	Diagnostic Tests	Lab Results

VS: T = 98.2°F (36.6°C); HR = 78 BPM; BP = 118/70 mm Hg; RR = 16 bpm; SpO$_2$ = 96% on RA; denies pain.
Skin: Warm, dry, intact.
Respiratory: Dry cough. Reports sputum expectoration of white thick mucus following respiratory treatments. Lung sounds clear to auscultation in all lung fields.
GI: Increased appetite. Reports taking pancreatic enzymes with all meals and snacks. Bowel sounds active × 4 quadrants. Regular bowel movements that are brown and fatty.
Weight: 91.5 lb (41.5 kg)
Height: 59.0 inches (149.8 cm)
Parent states that client was diagnosed at 3 years of age with cystic fibrosis (CF).

Health History	Nurses' Notes	Diagnostic Tests	Lab Results

Chest x-ray: Mild lung hyperinflation; no chest infiltrates, atelectasis, or bronchiectasis
Oral glucose tolerance test (OGTT): glucose 240 mg/dL (13.37 mmol/L) 2 hours after administration of the glucose liquid

---

*For each body system, click to select the **priority** client need to prevent a complication of the client's health problem. **Each body system supports one priority client need.***

Body System	Priority Client Need
Respiratory	☐ Oscillatory positive expiratory therapy (PEP)
	☐ Oxygen administration
GI	☐ Pancreatic enzyme therapy
	☐ Low-fat diet
Immune	☐ Prophylactic antibiotic therapy
	☐ Contact precautions with separation from others with CF by at least 6 feet
Endocrine	☐ Insulin administration
	☐ Recombinant human growth hormone administration
Integumentary	☐ High-sodium foods
	☐ Oatmeal baths

Multiple Response Select N

A 68-year-old client complaining of chest pain is admitted to the medical-surgical nursing unit for acute coronary syndrome. The cardiologist prescribes a continuous IV heparin infusion per protocol. The client weighs 165 lb (74.8 kg), and baseline partial thromboplastin time (PTT) is 32 seconds. A bolus is administered as prescribed and a continuous infusion is initiated based on the protocol noted in the Medication Administration Record.

Health History	Nurses' Notes	Vital Signs	Med Admn Record

Baseline PTT and every 6 or 12 hours after start of continuous infusion based on protocol

Heparin 80 units/kg IV bolus prior to start of continuous infusion

Start heparin 25,000 units in 250 mL D_5W (concentration 100 units/mL) continuous infusion 18 units/kg/hr

Adjust continuous infusion based on the following:
- PTT less than 35 seconds: IV bolus 80 units/kg, increase rate by 4 units/kg/hr, PTT in 6 hours
- PTT 35–45 seconds: IV bolus 40 units/kg, increase rate by 2 units/kg/hr, PTT in 6 hours
- PTT 46–70 seconds (goal): No bolus, no rate change, PTT in 12 hours
- PTT 71–90 seconds: No bolus, decrease rate by 2 units/kg/hr, PTT in 12 hours
- PTT above 90 seconds: No bolus, stop infusion

The next day, the oncoming nurse assigned to monitor the client assesses the client and checks laboratory results. The client states, "I feel OK, I just have a hard time sleeping since I've been in the hospital. My chest pain is better. I had a nosebleed this morning but it stopped. I'm ready for breakfast; it should be here soon." The most recent PTT from 1 hour ago was 92 seconds. The heparin infusion is running at 13.5 mL/hr.

*Select the three priority needs that are of **immediate** concern.*

☐ Appetite
☐ Chest pain
☐ Nosebleed
☐ PTT results
☐ Heparin infusion
☐ Difficulty sleeping

Practice Question 5.3   Drag-and-Drop Rationale

A 70-year-old client had an exploratory laparotomy with colectomy due to small bowel obstruction. The surgery was completed, and the client has been transferred to the postoperative medical-surgical nursing unit. The client received general anesthesia and has a PCA pump with hydromorphone for pain control. The client has been using the PCA pump every 10 minutes for the last 8 hours. The oncoming nurse receives report and is assessing the client.

Physical Assessment	Nurses' Notes	Vital Signs	Lab Results

T = 98.2°F (36.7°C); HR = 80 BPM; BP = 138/78 mm Hg; RR = 18 bpm; SpO$_2$ = 96% on 2 L/min per NC; pain rated as a 2/10 on a 0 to 10 rating scale

Physical Assessment	Nurses' Notes	Vital Signs	Lab Results

Skin: Warm, dry, intact.
Respiratory: RR 18 bpm, unlabored. SpO$_2$ 96% on 2 L/min per NC. Dry cough, no sputum. Lung sounds clear to auscultation in all lung fields.
Cardiovascular: Apical pulse rate 80 BPM. Heart sounds, regular rate and rhythm.
GI: Bowel sounds active × 4 quadrants. Abdomen rigid to palpation. Dressing over midline abdominal incision intact with scant amount of serosanguineous drainage noted. Dressing changed per surgeon's order, wound cleansed with normal saline, and dressing reapplied. Incision is well approximated; no redness, swelling, tenderness at incision site. Pain 2/10 at the incision site.
Genitourinary: Unable to urinate since arrival to unit 8 hours ago.
Neurologic: Alert and oriented × 3.

Based on the client findings, complete the following sentence by choosing from the lists of options provided.

The client is at **highest** risk for developing _____1 [Select]_____ as evidenced by _____2 [Select]_____.

Options for 1	Options for 2
Infection	Urine output
Atelectasis	Temperature
Hemorrhage	BP
Urinary retention	RR
Wound dehiscence	Drainage on dressing

Practice Question 5.4 | Multiple Response Select All That Apply

A 22-year-old client is brought to the ED by EMS. The client's parent found the client slumped over and unconscious. The client was sitting in the wheelchair eating breakfast when the parent last saw the client, 15 minutes prior. The client was bleeding profusely from both wrists, and the parent reports immediately placing pressure on both wrists and screaming to the spouse for help and to call EMS. At the scene, EMS reports that the client was unconscious but that the bleeding was controlled and pressure dressings and continuous pressure to both wrists were maintained. EMS reports that the client's BP was 98/60 mm Hg, apical HR was 120 BPM, RR was 16 bpm. Oxygen at 3 L per NC was administered, an IV line was inserted, an infusion of lactated Ringer's was initiated, and the client was transferred to the ED.

On arrival at the ED, the client is arousable but sleepy. Assessment and treatment are immediately initiated, and the client is stabilized and admitted to the hospital. The admission nurse reviews the medical record, performs an assessment, and documents in the Nurses' Notes.

Health History	Nurses' Notes	Vital Signs	Lab Results

This 22-year-old client sustained a spinal cord injury in the lower thoracic region 1 year ago from a motor vehicle crash. Client has paraplegia.
No other medical problems.

Health History	Nurses' Notes	Vital Signs	Lab Results

T = 101°F (38.3°C); HR = 96 BPM; BP = 116/78 mm Hg; RR = 20 bpm; SpO$_2$ = 94% on RA; wrist pain = 4/10

Health History	Nurses' Notes	Vital Signs	Lab Results

Client is alert and oriented. Is sleepy but easily arousable. States is "sick and tired of living this way and is too young to have to be in a wheelchair for the rest of my life." States, "It is my own fault that I am this way, and I am so sorry that they found me this morning. I slashed my wrists using my breakfast knife. I am so useless and do nothing right, even with trying to kill myself."

Has no appetite and is refusing to eat. States wants to sleep and not be bothered by anyone.

Dressings on both wrists are dry and intact. No redness or break in skin integrity noted in other skin areas.

No sensation felt in lower extremities. Unable to move lower extremities.

Last bowel movement 1 day ago. Bowel sounds present in all 4 quadrants.

Abdomen firm. Urinary output 200 mL in the ED via catheterization. States needs to self-catheterize every 6 hours depending on intake.

No respiratory distress. RR = 20 bpm; SpO$_2$ = 94% on RA; wrist pain = 4/10. Pain medication administered in the ED 2 hours ago.

No chest pain; pulse 96 BPM.

Health History	Nurses' Notes	Vital Signs	Lab Results

Test	Result	Normal Reference Range
Red blood cells (RBCs)	4.7 × 10^{12} (4.7 × 10^{12})	4.2–6.2 × 10^{12}/L (4.2–6.2 × 10^{12}/L)
White blood cells (WBCs)	12,000/mm^3 (12 × 10^9/L) **H**	5000–10,000/mm^3 (5–10 × 10^9/L)
Platelets	160,000/mm^3 (160 × 10^9/L)	150,000–400,000/mm^3 (150–400 × 10^9/L)
Hemoglobin (Hgb)	14 g/dL (140 g/L)	12–18 g/dL (120–180 g/L)
Hematocrit (Hct)	42% (0.42)	37%–52% (0.37–0.52)

*Which of the following are the priority client needs of **immediate** concern?* ***Select all that apply.***

☐ Pain

☐ Appetite

☐ Infection

☐ Bleeding

☐ Paraplegia

☐ Suicide risk

☐ Urinary output

Practice Question 5.5 — Drop-Down in Table

A 59-year-old postmenopausal client with stage IV bilateral breast cancer had a double mastectomy. The biopsy showed a hormone receptor–positive tumor, and the client was prescribed tamoxifen therapy. One month later the client visits the clinic for a follow-up and tells the nurse completing the intake about experiencing the following over the past month since the last visit:

- Pelvic pain, vaginal discharge, burning on urination
- Hot flashes, dizziness, tenderness and warmth to the left leg
- Weakness, bone pain, joint stiffness
- Constipation, stomach cramps, nausea and vomiting

*For each body system below, click to specify one **priority** concern specific to a complication of tamoxifen therapy.*

Body System	Priority Concern
Genitourinary	☐ Pelvic pain
	☐ Vaginal discharge
	☐ Burning on urination
Cardiovascular	☐ Hot flashes
	☐ Dizziness
	☐ Tenderness and warmth to left leg
Musculoskeletal	☐ Weakness
	☐ Bone pain
	☐ Joint stiffness
GI	☐ Constipation
	☐ Stomach cramps
	☐ Nausea and vomiting

Practice Question 5.6 — Multiple Response Select N

A 30-year-old pregnant client (G2P1) who is at 35 weeks of gestation presents to the labor and delivery triage unit stating that a sudden gush of fluid occurred 1 hour ago. The nurse collects data and documents the following in the Nurses' Notes.

Health History	Nurses' Notes	Vital Signs	Lab Results

1400:
Client states that they noticed a sudden gush of fluid 1 hour ago at 1300
Has continued to notice fluid leakage sporadically since that time
States that prior to becoming pregnant, smoked cigarettes, 1 pack per day for 13 years; has not smoked during pregnancy
States was diagnosed with chlamydia early in the pregnancy, which was treated with doxycycline

*Based on this clinical scenario, select four potential complications that are of **highest priority** to the nurse.*

☐ Preeclampsia
☐ Client sepsis
☐ Chorioamnionitis
☐ Client hypertension
☐ Umbilical cord prolapse
☐ Fetal pulmonary hypoplasia
☐ Umbilical cord compression

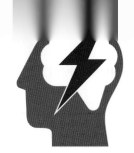

CHAPTER 6

Strategies for Answering NGN Questions: Generate Solutions

Generate Solutions is a cognitive skill nurses use to create the plan of care. When generating solutions, the nurse uses knowledge of treatments and interventions that would address identified client needs and modifies them to meet priorities of care. The nurse needs to be able to generate the best possible evidence-based solutions to provide safe care.

 ## What to Consider When Generating Solutions

Applying the skill *Generate Solutions* is essential for planning and making appropriate clinical judgments and is a skill that will be measured both on the NGN and on your nursing course exams. When generating solutions, you need to consider the information in the clinical scenario, and connect appropriate actions to your ranked hypotheses. You will use the hypotheses to identify interventions that would achieve an expected client outcome. Because the cognitive skill *Generate Solutions* is the skill that involves thinking through several care options to create the plan of care, you will need to decide which actual or potential interventions are acceptable in that scenario and which are potentially harmful and therefore need to be avoided. See Box 6.1 for examples of acceptable and contraindicated interventions in a plan of care for a client with heart failure exacerbation with fluid volume overload.

 ## The Plan of Care and Generating Solutions

The cognitive skill *Generate Solutions* asks you to determine outcome criteria based on priority client needs while planning care. In doing so, you need to think about appropriate interventions, the evidence that will help to determine whether the client has met outcomes and to what extent, followed by communicating and documenting the plan of care.

 ## How Do You Know That You Need to Generate Solutions?

As a nurse, you will be problem solving and using your nursing knowledge to create evidence-based plans of care based on previous client data and presenting hypotheses. For example, when you assume care for your assigned clients, you will look at the previously established plan of care, and consider current hypotheses to determine the appropriateness of the interventions in the plan of care. You may need to revise a plan of care based on evolving client needs. As the nurse, you need to think about what you would plan to do, as well as what you would plan not to do, in order to meet the client's needs. Ask yourself: *What are the desirable outcomes for this client? What interventions will achieve those outcomes? What interventions need to be avoided?* Box 6.2 lists some important considerations related to *Generate Solutions* that will help you to effectively apply this cognitive skill.

 NGN TIP

Remember: When you *Generate Solutions*, you are using your nursing knowledge of evidence-based practice to decide which interventions or actions need to be taken in a clinical scenario.

 NGN TIP

Remember: Generating solutions requires the nurse to identify expected outcomes by using established priorities to define a set of interventions that will achieve outcomes.

BOX 6.1 Heart Failure Exacerbation With Fluid Overload: Examples of Acceptable and Contraindicated Interventions

Acceptable Interventions	Contraindicated Interventions
Monitor for edema	Provide sodium in the diet
Monitor daily weight	Encourage fluid intake
Monitor I&O	Administer IV fluids
Monitor labs (B-natriuretic peptide [BNP], electrolytes)	Maintain the same position in bed
Assess lung and heart sounds	Promote high activity level
Administer diuretics	
Encourage activity as tolerated	
Position upright	
Assess VS	

Data from Ignatavicius, D.D., Workman, M.L., Rebar, C.R., et al. (2021). *Medical-surgical nursing: Concepts for interprofessional collaborative care* (10th ed.). St. Louis: Elsevier, p. 691.

BOX 6.2 Considerations Related to Generate Solutions

- Use known client data and prioritized hypotheses.
- Decide on expected outcomes of safe client care.
- Create a list of multiple actual and potential interventions—not just the best intervention.
- Remember that actual and potential interventions could be actions or collecting more information.
- Communicate and document expected outcomes clearly.
- Revise interventions as client needs evolve.

How Do You Generate Solutions in an NGN Clinical Situation?

As noted in Chapter 2, NGN questions will begin with a clinical scenario presented as either a Stand-alone item or an Unfolding Case Study. Chapter 3 discusses the cognitive skill, *Recognize Cues*; information about the client is presented and you need to identify the relevant data. As discussed in Chapter 4, once these relevant data are noted, you analyze the data and link these data to the client situation to determine what the data mean and what is happening to the client. Then, as stated in Chapter 5, based on your judgment of what you think is happening to the client, you identify client needs and assign priority or urgency to those needs. At this point, you are ready to begin thinking about outcome criteria and developing a plan of care consisting of evidence-based nursing interventions, applying the skill *Generate Solutions*. The following example provides you with a clinical scenario in which you use client data to *Generate Solutions*. Remember to consider both acceptable and contraindicated interventions as you apply this cognitive skill.

Example: *Generate Solutions*

An 88-year-old client is on the medical-surgical nursing unit with acute confusion. The client's children brought the client to the ED when the client wasn't making sense on the phone one evening. The children report that when arriving at the client's home, the client was in disarray, was very weak, and was speaking incoherently. The children tell the nurse that the client has a history of stroke 2 years ago and has type 1 DM. The client's spouse died from breast cancer in the last year. The client's appetite is very poor. The client is diagnosed with acute delirium related to hypoglycemia. The physician has prescribed continuous IV fluids with dextrose 10% in water.

What Will You Think About to Generate Solutions in This Clinical Scenario?

To generate solutions, you need to think about the client's problem based on the information provided in the scenario. As the nurse caring for the client, you would consider what client outcome data would demonstrate improvement in the acute confusion, and what interventions you would need to perform to promote attainment of this goal.

Begin by considering the outcome data. What would tell you that the acute confusion is improving? It would be important to know this client's cognitive baseline. You could ask the children if the client has any confusion at baseline or if the client is alert and oriented. Next, you could consider outcome criteria based on level of consciousness and cognition. Perhaps a return to the client's baseline cognition would be an appropriate outcome to consider in the plan. Another appropriate outcome would be for the client to remain safe and free from injury. With these outcomes in mind, you would think about the nursing interventions or actions that will assist in achieving these goals. Remember that some interventions may be focused on assessment and others on actions. Nursing interventions to consider in this clinical scenario might be:

- Perform a mental status assessment every shift.
- Assess for hypoglycemia and hyperglycemia and treat accordingly with available prescribed interventions.
- Identify contributing factors, such as medications, hypoglycemia, infection, or other problems that may result in acute confusion.
- Promote adequate hydration, nutritional intake, and sleep.
- Facilitate sensory awareness and use sensory aids as appropriate, such as glasses and hearing aids.
- Provide orientation to surroundings as often as needed.
- Encourage visitation from family and support persons.
- Assist with toileting needs frequently.
- Communicate and document changes with cognition.

 NGN TIP

Remember: With NGN item types that measure *Generate Solutions,* you could be asked about planning assessment-related interventions and action-related interventions.

What NGN Item Types Optimally Measure *Generate Solutions?*

Four types of test items optimally measure the cognitive skill *Generate Solutions.* Variations of each of these types will most likely be presented on the NGN. Table 6.1 presents these item types and their variations. Each of these test item types is discussed in Chapter 2, and some examples are provided. The following section explains the four major item types that best measure *Generate Solutions.*

Drag-and-Drop and Drop-Down Test Items to Measure *Generate Solutions*

As discussed in Chapter 2, Drag-and-Drop and Drop-Down items include Cloze, Rationale, and Table. When the Drag-and-Drop item type is used to measure *Generate Solutions,* the test

 NGN TIP

Remember: In a Drag-and-Drop Cloze item, the maximum score is equivalent to the number of targets for answer boxes, and partial credit is given for correct responses.

TABLE 6.1   Test Items and Variations That Optimally Measure *Generate Solutions*

Type of Test Item	Variations
Drag-and-Drop	Drag-and-Drop Cloze Drag-and-Drop Rationale Drag-and-Drop in Table (may replace Drop-Down in Table)
Drop Down	Drop-Down Cloze Drop-Down Rationale Drop-Down in Table
Multiple Response	Multiple Response Select N Multiple Response Select All That Apply Multiple Response Grouping Matrix Multiple Response
Multiple Choice	Multiple Choice Single Response Matrix Multiple Choice

taker is required to drag words from a list of choices to fill in the blank of a sentence or sentences. When a Drop-Down item type is presented, the test taker is required to select words from a drop-down menu to fill in the blank of a sentence or sentences. Sample Question 6.1 illustrates a Drag-and-Drop Cloze type of item to measure the cognitive skill *Generate Solutions.* Rationale and test-taking strategy to help you derive the correct responses are also provided.

Sample Question 6.1	Drag-and-Drop Cloze Item: Generate Solutions

0900: A 32-year-old client G2P1 is admitted to the labor and delivery unit, and the nurse assigned to care for the client reviews the health history.

Health History	Nurses' Notes	Vital Signs	Lab Results

32-year-old G2P1. First delivery was vaginal and uncomplicated. Has a history of uncomplicated mitral valve stenosis that is currently being monitored. No other medical history. No prescribed medication taken except for prenatal vitamins. Uterine ultrasound done 1 week ago showed normal progression of pregnancy, and examination revealed effacement 100% with 4 cm dilation.

Health History	Nurses' Notes	Vital Signs	Lab Results

1400: The client delivers a 7 lb 4 oz (3.35 kg) baby via an uncomplicated vaginal delivery. Postdelivery VS: T = 98.6°F (36.0°C); HR = 92 BPM; BP = 132/78 mm Hg; RR = 20 bpm; SpO_2 = 95% on RA. The client is breast-feeding/chest-feeding the baby.

1500: The client's spouse calls the nurse because the client is complaining of abdominal cramping and complains that the peripad feels wet. The nurse checks the pad and finds that it is saturated with blood. The nurse assesses the fundus while another nurse checks VS. VS: HR = 120 BPM; BP = 98/62 mm Hg; RR = 24 bpm; SpO_2 = 92% on RA. The fundus is soft and 4 fingerbreadths above the umbilicus and deviated to the right.

Complete the sentence. Drag one intervention listed in Options for 1 and one intervention listed in Options for 2 if the intervention is required to meet the client's immediate needs.

To meet the client's needs the nurse would **immediately** plan for <u>uterine massage</u> and <u>IV infusion of oxytocin</u>.

Options for 1	Options for 2
Uterine massage	Hysterectomy
Rapid administration of blood	Uterine tamponade
Administration of methylergonovine	Oxygen administration
Manual exploration of the uterine cavity	IV infusion of oxytocin

Rationale: The initial intervention in management of excessive postpartum bleeding focuses on interventions to contract the uterus and stop the bleeding. Immediate interventions if the bleeding is due to uterine atony is firm massage of the uterine fundus, expression of any clots in the uterus, elimination of bladder distention, and continuous IV infusion of oxytocin. It may be necessary to insert an indwelling urinary catheter to prevent bladder distention and to monitor urine output as a measure of renal perfusion to vital organs. Laboratory studies will be monitored and usually include a complete blood cell count with platelet count, fibrinogen, fibrin split products, prothrombin time, and partial thromboplastin time. Blood type and antibody screen are done if not previously performed. Rapid administration of crystalloid solutions or blood products or both may be necessary to restore intravascular volume, but this is not the immediate intervention. Methylergonovine is a medication that is administered intramuscularly to produce sustained uterine contractions; however, this medication is contraindicated in the presence of hypertension or cardiovascular disease because it can induce vasoconstriction, so this is not a safe option for this client because of the history of mitral valve stenosis. Oxygen may be administered by nonrebreather facemask to enhance oxygen delivery to the cells, but this is not the immediate intervention. In addition, the SpO_2, although lower than the previous reading, is still a normal value. If the uterus does not become firm and bleeding persists, the PHCP may perform manual exploration of the uterine cavity for retained clots or placental fragments. If treatment measures are ineffective, uterine tamponade or surgical management may be necessary and a hysterectomy may be needed.

Test-Taking Strategy: First it is important to note the word *immediately* in the question. This tells you that some or all of the options may be correct, and you need to select the option for each blank area that would be a first action. Retrieving your knowledge on the causes of postpartum bleeding, think about what would be immediate or primary actions as part of the plan of care in this particular clinical scenario, as illustrated in the table. Note that in the first column, you are presented with a set of actions. You need to decide if each listed action is primary for the client in this question, or if there are any data in the client's history that would make any of the actions unsafe actions and contraindicated.

Nursing Action	Primary	Contraindicated
Uterine massage	Yes	No
Rapid administration of blood	No	No
Administration of methylergonovine	Yes	Yes
Manual exploration of the uterine cavity	No	No
Hysterectomy	No	No
Uterine tamponade	No	No
Oxygen administration	No	No
IV infusion of oxytocin	Yes	No

For those options that are primary and not contraindicated, these are the actions you would consider as being the correct answers to this question. If an action is not a primary action, but rather a later action if other interventions were unsuccessful, or if the action is contraindicated, then these are probably not the correct answers to this question.

Content Area: Maternal-Newborn Nursing
Priority Concept: Perfusion
Reference(s): Lowdermilk et al., 2020, pp. 724–725

Multiple Response Test Items to Measure *Generate Solutions*

As discussed in Chapter 2, Multiple Response test items include Multiple Response Select All That Apply, Multiple Response Select N, Multiple Response Grouping, and Matrix Multiple Response. When the Multiple Response item type is used to measure *Generate Solutions* or other cognitive skills, the test taker is required to follow the question directions regarding how to select options. Sample Question 6.2 illustrates a Multiple Response Select All That Apply type of item. The rationale and test-taking strategy to help you derive the correct responses are also provided.

NGN TIP

Remember: In a Multiple Response Select All That Apply item, credit is given for correct responses, and credit is deducted for incorrect responses.

Sample Question 6.2	**Multiple Response Select All That Apply: Generate Solutions**

A 68-year-old client presents to the ED complaining of numbness and tingling of the left side of the face and the left arm that started 2 hours ago. The ED nurse performs a focused assessment and notes focal neurologic deficits on the left side of the body. The ED physician orders a stat CT scan of the brain, which confirms ischemic stroke affecting the middle cerebral artery. The ED nurse assesses VS. The client has no known past medical history and does not take any medications on a routine basis.

Health History	Nurses' Notes	Vital Signs	Lab Results

BP = 152/84 mm Hg; HR = 98 BPM; RR = 20 bpm; T = 97.5°F (36.4°C); SpO$_2$ = 96% on RA

*Which of the following actions would the ED nurse plan for the client? **Select all that apply.***

☒ Complete a swallow screen.
☐ Allow thickened liquids only.
☒ Administer fibrinolytic therapy.
☒ Obtain an electronic infusion pump.
☒ Perform a cardiovascular assessment.
☐ Insert an indwelling urinary catheter.
☐ Administer IV antihypertensive medication.
☒ Perform frequent neurologic assessments.

▶THINKING SPACE

Rationale: An ischemic stroke is caused by a blockage of a cerebral or carotid artery. Multiple interventions are needed for the client experiencing a stroke, in order to ensure safety. The client with an ischemic stroke may experience impaired swallowing as a complication of the stroke. The nurse needs to complete a swallow screen per facility protocol, to determine any impairments with swallowing. This action will prevent complications such as pneumonia from aspiration. The nurse needs to keep the client NPO until the appropriate diagnostic testing is completed, such as a video fluoroscopic swallow study usually performed by a speech-language pathologist; therefore, thickened liquids would not be given at this time until this workup has been done. The nurse would anticipate a prescription to administer fibrinolytic therapy. This is the standard of practice for clients experiencing ischemic strokes who meet specified criteria. Exclusionary criteria include more than 4.5 hours from onset of symptoms, older than 80 years, anticoagulant use, ischemic injury to greater than one-third of the brain, significant neurologic impairment, and history of both stroke and DM. This client does not meet any of these exclusionary criteria and therefore would be considered a candidate for fibrinolytic therapy. To safely administer this therapy, the nurse needs to use an electronic infusion pump and double-check the dose with another licensed nurse. A cardiovascular assessment is important to assess for heart murmurs, dysrhythmias such as atrial fibrillation, and hypertension. With an ischemic stroke, a BP of approximately 150/100 mm Hg is needed to maintain cerebral perfusion. With a BP of 152/84 mm Hg, an IV antihypertensive medication would not be indicated. For a client receiving fibrinolytic therapy, invasive tubes such as indwelling urinary catheters should not be placed for at least 24 hours or until the client is stable, in order to prevent bleeding. Frequent neurologic assessments per facility protocol are important for a client with ischemic stroke and for clients receiving fibrinolytic therapy, to detect further clinical deterioration early.

Test-Taking Strategy

Test-Taking Strategy: Note that the question is asking about nursing actions to plan care for the client experiencing an ischemic stroke. Think about the scenario and the potential effects of these interventions on the health problem presented. Look at each option provided, and make an association with the information presented in the medical record, as illustrated in the table.

Intervention	Potential Effects on Ischemic Stroke
Complete a swallow screen.	Ensure safety in the event of dysphagia as a complication of the stroke.
Allow thickened liquids only.	Is unsafe and could result in aspiration; need to wait until further work-up and consultation are done.
Administer fibrinolytic therapy.	Would promote a better outcome for a client with ischemic stroke meeting criteria.
Obtain an electronic infusion pump.	Needed to safely administer fibrinolytic therapy.
Perform a cardiovascular assessment.	Important information such as heart sounds and BP are needed to monitor for complications in a client with ischemic stroke.
Insert an indwelling urinary catheter.	No indication that this is necessary, and it could pose a risk for UTI and bleeding.
Administer IV antihypertensive medication.	A BP of 150/100 mm Hg is needed to maintain cerebral perfusion; BP is not high enough for an IV antihypertensive medication.
Perform frequent neurologic assessments.	Assists in detecting clinical deterioration early.

The correct options are those that ensure safety, monitor for complications or clinical deterioration, or promote a better outcome of care. The options that are unsafe and could result in additional complications or that do not have the data to support the interventions are the incorrect options.

Content Area: Medical-Surgical Nursing
Priority Concept: Clotting
Reference(s): Ignatavicius et al., 2021, pp. 928–934

Multiple Choice Test Items to Measure *Generate Solutions*

As discussed in Chapter 2, Multiple Choice test items include Multiple Choice Single Response and Matrix Multiple Choice test items. When the Multiple Choice item type is used to measure *Generate Solutions,* the test taker is required to select a single option from a list of several options or from a table with rows. Sample Question 6.3 illustrates a Matrix Multiple Choice type of item. The rationale and test-taking strategy to help you derive the correct responses are also provided.

NGN TIP

Remember: In a Matrix Multiple Choice item type, each row must have an option selected in order for the test taker to move on, and each row should be treated as its own multiple choice question.

Sample Question 6.3	Matrix Multiple Choice: Generate Solutions

A client who is 5 days postoperative following a right colectomy to remove a bowel tumor calls the nurse and states that they felt a popping sensation in the incision after an episode of forceful coughing. The nurse removes the abdominal dressing and notes that the incision has opened, wound layers are separated, and a portion of the bowel is protruding from the wound.

Place an X to indicate whether each potential intervention listed below is either Indicated (appropriate or necessary), or Contraindicated (could be harmful) for the plan of care for the client at this time.

Potential Intervention	Indicated	Contraindicated
Place the client with the head and body flat and with the hips and knees bent.	☐	☒
Place a sterile warm saline–soaked dressing over the open wound.	☒	☐
Don sterile gloves and gently reinsert the protruding bowel into the wound.	☐	☒
Provide the client with small amounts of water or juice to stay hydrated.	☐	☒
Notify the surgeon.	☒	☐
Prepare the client for surgery.	☒	☐
Assess VS every 10 minutes.	☒	☐

Rationale: Evisceration is the total separation of wound layers and the protrusion of internal organs through the wound. It usually occurs between the fifth and tenth days after surgery. The separation of wound layers occurs most often in clients who have diabetes, are obese, are malnourished, have an immune deficiency, or use steroid medication. Evisceration is a surgical emergency, and the nurse would stay with the client and have another nurse notify the surgeon and/or Rapid Response Team immediately and bring any needed supplies. The nurse would provide reassurance to the client and position the client in a supine position with the hips and knees bent and with the head of the bed at 15 to 20 degrees. This position prevents stretching of the abdominal tissues and prevents pressure on the incision line, which would worsen the condition. Using sterile technique, the nurse would apply one to two large abdominal dressings saturated with warm normal saline to the wound. This will prevent hypothermia and provide moisture to the tissues and protruding organ. The nurse would not attempt to reinsert the protruding organ because this could cause trauma. The nurse would monitor the client's VS every 5 to 10 minutes until the surgeon arrives and would monitor for signs of shock. The client is not allowed to have anything by mouth, to decrease the risk of aspiration if surgery is necessary.

NGN TIP

Remember: In a Matrix Multiple Choice item, you will be asked to select one option per row, and there can be up to 10 rows in an item.

Test-Taking Strategy

THINKING SPACE

Test-Taking Strategy: Note that this question is asking about interventions that are either indicated or contraindicated, based on the clinical scenario involving evisceration. Using a thinking process as illustrated in the table, you can decide whether each of the options would be a part of a safe and effective plan of care for a client in this situation, and then think about what the outcome of that action might be.

Potential Intervention	Safe and Effective	Potential Outcome
Place the client with the head and body flat and with the hips and knees bent.	No	Lying flat could cause further tissue disruption from pressure on the incision line.
Place a sterile warm saline–soaked dressing over the open wound.	Yes	Will prevent hypothermia and will provide moisture to the affected organs and tissues.
Don sterile gloves and gently reinsert the protruding bowel into the wound.	No	Could cause trauma.
Provide the client with small amounts of water or juice to stay hydrated.	No	Aspiration could occur in the event surgery is needed.
Notify the surgeon.	Yes	Obtain additional orders; determine details for likely surgery.
Prepare the client for surgery.	Yes	Repair the surgical site.
Assess VS every 10 minutes.	Yes	Monitor for clinical deterioration, early detection of shock.

Organizing the information in this way will allow you to then decide whether these potential interventions are indicated or contraindicated in this clinical scenario. You will need to rely on your nursing knowledge of the care involved with this postoperative complication in order to answer this question correctly.

Content Area: Medical-Surgical Nursing
Priority Concept: Tissue Integrity
Reference(s): Ignatavicius et al., 2021, pp. 177, 181

Sample Question 6.4 illustrates a Multiple Choice Single Response item type, in which the test taker is presented with a clinical scenario and asked to select the correct option from a list of several options.

Sample Question 6.4   Multiple Choice Single Response: Generate Solutions

A 3-month-old infant diagnosed with heart failure due to ventricular septal defect (VSD) at birth is being seen by the cardiologist in the pediatric intensive care unit (PICU). The nurse performs an assessment and documents the findings in the Nurses' Notes. The pediatric cardiologist prescribes digoxin, enalapril, carvedilol, and furosemide.

Health History	Nurses' Notes	Vital Signs	Diagnostic Results

Tachycardic, tachypneic, cool extremities, hypotensive, weak peripheral pulses, prolonged capillary refill time, irritability, feeding difficulties

Health History	Nurses' Notes	Vital Signs	Diagnostic Results

RR = 64 bpm; HR = 164 BPM; T = 97.8°F (36.5°C); BP = 78/48 mm Hg; SpO$_2$ = 91% on RA

Health History	Nurses' Notes	Vital Signs	Diagnostic Results

Chest radiograph impression: Cardiomegaly, marked left atrial enlargement

Based on this clinical scenario, select one intervention that the nurse would plan for the infant.

☐ Maintain a fluid restriction

☐ Administer sodium bicarbonate.

☐ Administer potassium supplements.

☒ Plan feedings around the infant's sleep schedule.

☐ Allow the infant to cry for 5 minutes before feeding.

☐ Monitor for bradycardia, bradypnea, and hypertension.

Rationale: Heart failure is the inability of the heart to pump an adequate amount of blood to the rest of the body to meet metabolic demands. Heart failure can occur as a consequence of congenital heart disease, such as VSD. Clinical manifestations of heart failure may include tachycardia, tachypnea, cool extremities, hypotension, weak peripheral pulses, prolonged capillary filling time, irritability, and feeding difficulties, among other findings. Even though fluid volume overload is a problem with heart failure, fluid restriction is often not needed in infants because of their feeding difficulties. Medication therapy is a mainstay of heart failure management for an infant with congenital heart disease. Medications that improve cardiac function include digoxin, angiotensin-converting enzyme inhibitors such as enalapril, and beta blockers such as carvedilol. In management of heart failure exacerbation, diuretics such as furosemide may be prescribed. Monitoring the potassium level is very important for anyone taking furosemide, because it is a potassium-wasting diuretic. Often, potassium supplementation is needed; however, for the infant being given enalapril, potassium supplementation is usually not needed even when the infant is taking furosemide, because the enalapril also blocks the action of aldosterone, which can lead to hyperkalemia, especially if potassium supplementation is given. Sodium bicarbonate is a medication used in chronic kidney disease; although renal impairment can occur with heart failure, sodium bicarbonate is not part of the treatment regimen for heart failure. An important part of care for the infant with heart failure is maintaining nutritional status. The metabolic rate for these infants is greater because of poor cardiac function; therefore their caloric needs are higher. Feeding difficulties occur because of lack of energy related to the cardiac problem. Feedings need to be planned around the infant's sleep schedule so that energy can be conserved for feedings and feedings can be most effective. The infant needs to be fed soon after awakening so that energy is not depleted from crying.

Test-Taking Strategy: Note that this question asks you to select one correct option. The ability to use clinical judgment and determine whether listed interventions would be safe and effective is needed to answer this question correctly. Using a thinking process as illustrated in the table may be helpful.

Test-Taking Strategy

Intervention	Assists With Health Problem	Indicated	Not Indicated or Contraindicated
Maintain a fluid restriction.	No	☐	☒
Administer sodium bicarbonate.	No	☐	☒
Administer potassium supplements.	No	☐	☒
Plan feedings around the infant's sleep schedule.	Yes	☒	☐
Allow the infant to cry for 5 minutes before feeding.	No	☐	☒
Monitor for bradycardia, bradypnea, and hypertension.	No	☐	☒

For each intervention, decide whether it would be indicated or not indicated or contraindicated in this scenario. To decide that, think about whether that intervention assists with the health problem. If so, then it would be indicated. If not, it would be not indicated or contraindicated.

Content Area: Pediatric Nursing
Priority Concept: Gas Exchange
Reference(s): Hockenberry et al., 2019, pp. 741–752

Practice Questions

Multiple Response Grouping

A 58-year-old client is recovering from an L4–L5 spinal fusion completed 3 hours ago. The client is on the medical-surgical nursing unit, and is prescribed hydromorphone via PCA, 0.2 mg every 10 minutes, with a 4-mg lock-out dose in 4 hours. The nurse is preparing a plan of care for this client.

For each body system below, click to specify the potential intervention that would be appropriate for the initial plan of care to monitor for or prevent adverse effects of hydromorphone. **Each body system may support more than one potential nursing intervention.**

Body System	Potential Nursing Intervention
Renal	☐ Assess renal function.
	☐ Monitor I&O.
	☐ Maintain fluid restriction.
Respiratory	☐ Assess RR frequently.
	☐ Ensure naloxone is available.
	☐ Place the PCA on hold if RR is less than 18 bpm.
Cardiovascular	☐ Encourage brisk walking.
	☐ Instruct the client to change positions slowly.
	☐ Assess BP and HR frequently.
Gastrointestinal	☐ Administer methylnaltrexone.
	☐ Administer ondansetron as indicated.
	☐ Ensure adequate intake of fluids and fiber.
Urinary	☐ Assess the bladder frequently.
	☐ Prompt the client to void every 4 hours.
	☐ Perform straight catheterization every 4 hours.

Multiple Response Select N

A 72-year-old client with a history of peripheral vascular disease has an arterial leg ulcer that is open and draining copious amounts of drainage. The client is admitted to the medical-surgical nursing unit for wound care management. The initial plan is to pack the wound with sterile saline–moistened gauze and then cover with a dry sterile dressing, with daily dressing changes and as needed. The nurse noted that the client was requiring multiple dressing changes each day owing to the excessive drainage, and initiates a wound care team consultation. The client is seen by the wound care team, and the physician prescribes negative-pressure wound therapy (NPWT).

Which five interventions would the nurse include in the plan of care for the client to maintain and ensure a good seal during NPWT?

☐ Identify air leaks using a stethoscope.

☐ Shave the hair on the skin around the wound.

☐ Make sure the periwound skin surface area is dry.

☐ Avoid wrinkles when applying the transparent film.

☐ Fill uneven skin surfaces with a skin barrier product.

☐ Frame the periwound area with a hydrocolloid dressing.

☐ Cut the transparent film to extend ½ inch beyond the wound perimeter.

☐ Use as many additional dressing layers as needed for identified air leaks.

| Practice Question 6.3 | **Drag-and-Drop Rationale** |

A 44-year-old postoperative client returned to the nursing unit from the PACU following bilateral mastectomy. The client has four Jackson-Pratt drains from the incisional areas on the chest. The nurse assesses VS and performs the physical assessment.

Based on the client findings, complete the following sentence by choosing from the lists of options provided.

To ensure client safety, the nurse plans to *first* _____1 [Select] _____ to address _____2 [Select] _____.

Options for 1	Options for 2
Administer enoxaparin	Pain
Administer pain medication	Infection
Increase supplemental oxygen	Hypoxemia
Empty and compress surgical drains	Thrombus risk

Health History / Physical Assessment / Vital Signs / Orders

Alert and oriented. Incisional pain rated 2/10.
Bilateral incisions on the chest covered with a dry sterile dressing, clean, dry, and intact.
Lung sounds clear to auscultation bilaterally. S1S2, no S3S4. +2 peripheral pulses, no edema.
4 Jackson Pratt drains from the incisional areas: #1 with 5 mL of sanguineous drainage, #2 with 10 mL of sanguineous drainage, #3 with 5 mL of sanguineous drainage, #4 with 10 mL of sanguineous drainage, compressed for suction.

Health History / Physical Assessment / Vital Signs / Orders

BP = 146/72 mm Hg; HR = 70 BPM; RR = 20 bpm; T = 98.2°F (36.8°C); SpO_2 = 97% at 3 L per NC

Health History / Physical Assessment / Vital Signs / Orders

Monitor VS per unit protocol
Titrate oxygen to maintain SpO_2 greater than 92%
Monitor incision site for signs of bleeding
Monitor and maintain surgical drains
Enoxaparin 40 mg subcutaneously daily
Apply sequential compression devices (SCDs) below the knee bilaterally for venous thrombosis prevention
Pan management via PCA pump
Clear liquids advance to regular as tolerated
Incentive spirometry per unit protocol
Ondansetron 4 mg IV every 4 hours as needed for nausea

| Practice Question 6.4 | **Multiple Response Select All That Apply** |

A 22-year-old client presents to the outpatient clinic reporting feeling "down" and stating having difficulty maintaining responsibilities with school. States experiencing a hard time finding friends, that peers in class don't think the client is smart, and that they make fun of the client behind the client's back. When asked about family dynamics, the client states is not speaking to parents and that the only support system is the client's partner. States "putting myself through school." Describes not being able to meet assignment deadlines and thinks about considering quitting school. The client is referred to the counseling and psychological center and is beginning group therapy.

Based on this scenario, which of the following interventions would the psychiatric nurse plan for the client? **Select all that apply.**

☐ Set realistic goals for behavior modification.
☐ Reward the client for practicing new behaviors.
☐ Provide positive regard for adaptive behaviors only.
☐ Encourage the client to practice behavior modifications.
☐ Help the client identify negative qualities and experiences.
☐ Help the client identify their own behaviors needing change.
☐ Reinforce self-worth with time and attention by giving one-to-one time.

Practice Question 6.5   Matrix Multiple Choice

A 32-year-old client is in the neurologic unit after sustaining a head injury after falling from a ladder while working in the garage. The client is unable to eat or drink because of unconsciousness. The intensivist prescribes central line insertion and total parenteral nutrition (TPN) to be administered for nutritional support.

*Place an X to indicate whether each potential intervention listed below is either **Anticipated** (appropriate or necessary) or **Contraindicated** (is unnecessary or is harmful) for the client's plan of care at this time.*

Potential Intervention	Anticipated	Contraindicated
Administer insulin.	☐	☐
Assess for diaphoresis.	☐	☐
Monitor IV site.	☐	☐
Follow Droplet Precautions.	☐	☐
Monitor blood glucose level every 6 hours.	☐	☐
Shut the infusion off if the bag is empty while waiting for the next TPN bag to become available.	☐	☐

Practice Question 6.6   Multiple Response Select N

A 46-year-old client was admitted to the hospital after reporting increased thirst, increased hunger, and increased urination for the last 7 days. On admission, the client's blood glucose level was significantly elevated, and the client was treated for DKA. After being stabilized, the client was discharged to home with a diagnosis of new-onset DM. The home care nurse is visiting the client and is providing teaching on self-management and measures to prevent hospitalization. The client tells the home care nurse about often feeling hungry, irritable, shaky, and weak and having a headache.

Based on the client's reported symptoms, which five measures would the home care nurse plan to teach this client to implement when these symptoms occur?

☐ Eat 6 saltine crackers.

☐ Eat 3 graham crackers.

☐ Drink 120 mL of fruit juice.

☐ Drink 240 mL of skim milk.

☐ Consume 6 to 10 hard candies.

☐ Consume 4 tablespoons of honey.

☐ Drink 120 mL of a diet soft drink.

☐ Decrease intake of carbohydrates.

☐ Administer insulin based on sliding scale.

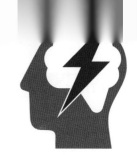

CHAPTER 7

Strategies for Answering NGN Questions: Take Action

Take Action is a cognitive skill that is activity oriented and involves the nurse performing appropriate and necessary interventions based on the client's situation and generated solutions. Thus this cognitive skill involves the nurse undertaking an action or multiple actions. Necessary nursing actions can be those interventions that prevent health problems, maintain client stability, improve the client's condition, prevent complications of a health problem, or manage an emergency situation such as a deterioration in a client's condition. The ability to make decisions using clinical judgment about essential actions to take in a clinical situation is a crucial nursing responsibility to promote safe client care.

The cognitive skill *Take Action* requires using nursing knowledge about the clinical event encountered, thinking about generated solutions, determining necessary actions to meet goals, understanding the rationale for such actions, and implementing these actions. As a nurse, you need to ask yourself: *What will I do? Why do I need to do this? What support do I need?* and *How do I accomplish this?* Sometimes you need to think and make quick decisions about immediate actions to take, and that is why nursing knowledge is so important. You need to know what action(s) are appropriate and necessary, which address the highest priorities of care, and how the actions will be performed. Therefore the cognitive skill *Take Action* is essential to meet the client's needs and ensure client safety and high-quality care. This ability will be measured both on the NGN and by your instructors on course exams and in the laboratory and clinical settings.

How Do You Know What Actions to Take?

Implementing care after deciding what actions to take is the focus of the clinical judgment cognitive skill *Take Action*. Once you have generated a list of possible interventions that will resolve or manage the client's priority health problems, think about other factors that may have an impact on the actions you take. Some factors are as follows, along with questions to ask yourself.

Clinical scenario: What is happening to the client? What are the priority needs? What must I do to address and meet these needs? What are the goals of care? What do I need to do to prevent complications and clinical deterioration in the client?
Nursing knowledge: What have I learned about these assessment findings and clinical scenario? What nursing interventions have I learned are necessary in the care of a client with these assessment findings?
Clinical experiences: Have I cared for a client in the past with similar health problems or client needs? What actions did I take in caring for a client with similar needs?
Scope of practice: What necessary actions must I take? What necessary actions can be done by another health care provider?

How Will Nursing Actions Be Tested?

Taking a nursing action is the same as implementing nursing care. Much of what you will do as a nurse involves taking actions to care for a client and meet that client's needs. Therefore you can expect to be frequently tested on nursing actions. Beginning with

THINKING SPACE

NGN TIP

Remember: Focus on the needs of the client and think about what you will do to meet these needs. Ask yourself: *What action(s) will I take?*

NGN TIP

Remember: A Drop-Down Rationale item provides you with a scenario and data about the client and includes a *Take Action* sentence in which you need to select the correct action to take and the rationale for that action from the drop-down menus.

 THINKING SPACE

your first nursing course, you have been tested on actions you would take in a variety of clinical scenarios. Sometimes testing required you to identify the actions you need to take; other times you were tested on how the actions would be performed. As a basic example, you may have been presented with a scenario in which a client is experiencing constipation and been asked what actions you would take to alleviate this health problem. Or you may have been asked about actions you would take if a client experienced cramping during administration of an enema to alleviate constipation. As a more complex example, you may have been presented with a scenario in which a client with heart failure is experiencing dyspnea and been asked what actions you would take. Or you may have been asked what actions you would take if a client with heart failure were to develop signs and symptoms of pulmonary edema.

What NGN Item Types Optimally Measure *Take Action*?

As noted in Chapter 2, NGN questions will begin with a clinical scenario presented as either a Stand-alone item or an Unfolding Case Study. The types of test items and the variations that may be used to measure the cognitive skill *Take Action* are presented in Table 7.1. Some of these types are presented in the Sample Questions through this chapter. These test item types are discussed in Chapter 2 with additional examples. Also, refer to the Evolve site for additional practice with these item types.

TABLE 7.1 Test Items and Variations That Optimally Measure *Take Action*	
Type of Test Item	**Variations**
Drop Down	Drop-Down Cloze Drop-Down Rationale Drop-Down in Table
Multiple Response	Multiple Response Select All That Apply Multiple Response Select N Multiple Response Grouping Matrix Multiple Response
Multiple Choice	Multiple Choice Single Response Matrix Multiple Choice
Drag-and-Drop	Drag-and-Drop Cloze Drag-and-Drop Rationale Drag-and-Drop in Table (may replace Drop-Down in Table)

Sample Question 7.1	Drop-Down Rationale: Take Action

The home care nurse visits a 79-year-old client who was discharged from the hospital 1 week ago for treatment of heart failure. The client tells the nurse that the exercise regimen of walking 3 times weekly was started but feels extremely fatigued the day after walking. The client has avoided walking this week because of feeling so tired. The nurse gathers additional data and documents the following:

Health History	Nurses' Notes	Diagnostic Studies	Laboratory Results

1100: VS: T = 98.6°F (37°C); HR = 68 BPM; RR = 20 bpm; SpO$_2$ = 92% on RA; BP = 112/68 mm Hg
Lung sounds clear bilaterally, no peripheral edema. Sleeping well with 2 pillows for head elevation. Up to bathroom to void once nightly.

Complete the following sentence by choosing from the list of options.

The nurse would **advise the client to slow down on the exercising** because **tolerance to increased activity needs to be built up and takes time**.

Options for 1	Options for 2
Advise the client to slow down on the exercising	The heart needs to contract efficiently, and exercise is one treatment measure to accomplish this
Inform the client to maintain the same exercise regimen	An additional dose of the prescribed diuretic needs to be taken before exercising
Instruct the client to check the amount of ankle edema before exercising	Tolerance to increased activity needs to be built up and takes time

Rationale: The client with heart failure would be encouraged to stay as active as possible and to develop a regular exercise program such as a home walking program. However, the client needs to be taught not to overexert. The client should try to walk at least 3 times a week and should slowly increase the time walked over several months. Tolerance to the increased activity needs to be built up and takes time. If chest pain or severe dyspnea occurs while exercising or the client is fatigued the next day, the client is probably advancing the activity too quickly and should slow down. Telling the client to maintain the same exercise regimen is incorrect and could actually be harmful. Checking the amount of ankle edema before exercising may be a helpful action but is not related to the exercise and the fatigue. The nurse would not advise a client to take an additional dose of the prescribed diuretic because prescribing medications is not part of a nurse's scope of practice and because this action does not specifically address the problem or concern. The heart does need to contract efficiently, and exercise is one component of the treatment program, but this is not related to the action the nurse would take to assist the client with alleviating the extreme fatigue experienced. The client's VS and other findings are not abnormal for this client. The HR and BP may be lower than normal range, but this is expected owing to medication usually prescribed to treat heart failure. The need to void during the night is expected because of the diuretic therapy normally prescribed to treat heart failure.

Test-Taking Strategy: Focus on the information in the scenario and note that the client feels extremely fatigued the day after walking. Think about the pathophysiology associated with heart failure and the healing process of the heart in this condition. Use your knowledge about heart failure to determine that the findings noted in the Nurses' Notes are expected. Organize your thinking process as illustrated in the table and think about the possible effect on the heart and subsequently the fatigue, with each action.

Nursing Action	Possible Effect on Heart and Fatigue
Advise the client to slow down on the exercising	Allow the heart to recover while also still benefiting from exercise, which should help with fatigue
Inform the client to maintain the same exercise regimen	May cause overexertion of the heart, worsening fatigue
Instruct the client to check the amount of ankle edema before exercising	May help to promote early detection of problems, but not specifically related to fatigue

Think about what the nurse would do. Once you have determined the action to take, think about the reason for that action. Maintaining the same exercise regimen could be harmful, so eliminate that option. Checking the amount of edema in the ankles is not an incorrect measure, but it is unrelated to the information in the scenario. Therefore your action would be to advise the client to slow down on exercising. Next, think about why you are taking this action. Remember that the heart needs to heal and this takes time and building up tolerance.

Content Area: Medical-Surgical Nursing
Priority Concept: Perfusion
Reference(s): Ignatavicius et al., 2021, p. 680

NGN TIP

Remember: Before taking a nursing action, you need to consider what is relevant in the client scenario, what is happening to the client, what the priority client needs are, and the goals of care.

THINKING SPACE

Test-Taking Strategy

Sample Question 7.2 | Multiple Response Select N: Take Action

A 25-year-old client hospitalized in a mental health unit is restless and pacing in the hallway. The client begins yelling at other clients who are in the day room and then runs down the hallway slamming doors of other clients' rooms, yelling and arguing with the nurse about the need to take prescribed medication.

Select five actions that the nurse would take to de-escalate the client's behavior. **Click in the box to select the five actions.**

- ☒ Maintain a calm and in-control approach.
- ☒ Listen closely to what the client is saying.
- ☒ Set clear and enforceable limits for the client.
- ☐ Face the client and maintain consistent eye contact.
- ☒ Provide the client with options that deal with the behavior.
- ☐ Talk to the client when the client is yelling, in order to stop the behavior.
- ☒ Describe the consequences of the behavior for the client and others.

NGN TIP

Remember: A Multiple Response Select N item provides you with a scenario and data about the client and includes answer options. The item will tell you the number of options (N) that need to be selected. You will not be allowed to select more options than the N specifies. You can select fewer options than the N specifies, but then you will lose some credit. So be sure to follow the directions for these item types.

Test-Taking Strategy

THINKING SPACE

Rationale: Signs and symptoms that can precede violence include an angry, aggressive, and irritable affect; hyperactivity such as restlessness or pacing; slamming doors; yelling; and argumentativeness. Other signs include verbal abuse and profanity. The nurse needs to implement de-escalation techniques in order to protect other clients, self and staff, and the individual who is losing control. The nurse would maintain a calm and in-control approach; the perception that someone is in control can be comforting and calming to someone who is losing control. Listening closely allows the client to feel heard and understood and helps build rapport, and thus energy can be channeled productively. Setting clear and enforceable limits and describing the consequences of the behavior provides the client with an understanding of expectations and consequences of not adhering to those behaviors. Providing the client with options assists and involves the client in problem solving. Facing the client and maintaining consistent eye contact can be threatening to the client. The nurse would not try to speak when the aggressive person is yelling because the client will view this as arguing, and this will escalate the anger and can lead to violence.

Test-Taking Strategy: The focus of the question is on nursing actions to take to de-escalate the client's angry and aggressive behavior. Note also that you need to select five actions. Read each option and think about what its effect would be on a client who is already angry and showing aggression. Avoid any actions that will make the client feel angrier or threatened. You need to remember that the client is out of control, and your actions need to focus on safety and providing control of the situation. Using the table, think about each nursing action, whether it would promote safety, and the possible outcome to assist in answering the question correctly. The correct options in this question promote safety and de-escalation; the incorrect options could result in further escalation.

Nursing Action	Safety	Possible Outcomes
Maintain a calm and in-control approach.	Promotes	De-escalation
Listen closely to what the client is saying.	Promotes	De-escalation
Set clear and enforceable limits for the client.	Promotes	De-escalation
Face the client and maintain consistent eye contact.	Does not promote	Escalation
Provide the client with options that deal with the behavior.	Promotes	De-escalation
Talk to the client when the client is yelling, in order to stop the behavior.	Does not promote	Escalation
Describe the consequences of the behavior for the client and others.	Promotes	De-escalation

Content Area: Mental Health Nursing
Priority Concept: Mood and Affect
Reference(s): Varcarolis & Fosbre, 2021, pp. 380–383

Sample Question 7.3 — Matrix Multiple Choice: Take Action

A 28-year-old client in labor who is receiving an oxytocin infusion reports, "My water broke, and I feel like something is coming through my vagina." The nurse performs a vaginal assessment and finds that the umbilical cord is protruding from the vagina.

For each nursing action, click in the box to indicate whether the nursing action is indicated (appropriate or necessary) or contraindicated (could be harmful).

Nursing Action	Indicated	Contraindicated
Administer oxygen to the client.	☒	☐
Notify the obstetric health care provider.	☒	☐
Monitor the FHR continuously.	☒	☐
Increase the flow rate of the oxytocin infusion.	☐	☒
Gently push the cord into the vagina toward the cervix.	☐	☒
Position the client with the head of the bed elevated at 30 degrees.	☐	☒
Wrap the cord in a sterile towel saturated with warm normal saline.	☒	☐
Glove the hands and insert two fingers into the vagina and exert upward pressure against the presenting part.	☒	☐

THINKING SPACE

NGN TIP

Remember: A Matrix Multiple Choice item provides you with a scenario and data about the client and includes two or three options columns. There will be at least four rows that present the nursing actions. You need to select one response for each nursing action.

Rationale: In cord prolapse, the nurse stays with the client and asks someone to notify the obstetric health care provider. The client is placed into the extreme Trendelenburg or modified left-lateral position or a knee-chest position to relieve pressure of the presenting part on the cord. A supine or Fowler or upright position is contraindicated because these positions exert pressure on the presenting part, further compressing the cord. Oxygen is administered by a nonrebreather face mask at 8 to 10 L/min. If oxytocin is infusing, it would be immediately stopped, and IV fluids such as lactated Ringer's or another prescribed solution are infused. With a gloved hand, the nurse inserts two fingers into the vagina and exerts upward pressure against the presenting part to relieve pressure on the cord. If the cord is protruding from the vagina, it is wrapped in a sterile towel saturated with warm normal saline. The nurse would not attempt to replace the cord into the vagina because this could cause damage to the cord and disrupt circulation to the fetus. The fetal status is monitored continuously and the client is prepared for immediate birth.

Test-Taking Strategy: Focus on the data in the scenario and visualize this event. Think about the purpose of the umbilical cord and that it delivers oxygen to the fetus. Next, thinking about what would happen if the cord were compressed and thinking about what needs to be done to alleviate cord compression will assist in answering correctly. Also, recalling that this is an emergency situation and recalling the effect of oxytocin on uterine contractions will assist in selecting the indicated and contraindicated actions. Thinking about the effects of the actions on the fetus by using the table may assist in answering the question correctly.

⚡ THINKING SPACE

Nursing Action	Promotes Fetal Well-Being	May Cause Fetal Harm
Administer oxygen to the client.	☒	☐
Notify the obstetric health care provider.	☒	☐
Monitor the FHR continuously.	☒	☐
Increase the flow rate of the oxytocin infusion.	☐	☒
Gently push the cord into the vagina toward the cervix.	☐	☒
Position the client with the head of the bed elevated at 30 degrees.	☐	☒
Wrap the cord in a sterile towel saturated with warm normal saline.	☒	☐
Glove the hands and insert two fingers into the vagina and exert upward pressure against the presenting part.	☒	☐

Content Area: Maternal-Newborn Nursing
Priority Concept: Perfusion
Reference(s): Lowdermilk et al., 2020, pp. 716–717

| Sample Question 7.4 | Multiple Response Select All That Apply: Take Action |

A 5-year-old child with a history of asthma is brought to the ED by the parents, who tell the nurse that the child is having an asthma attack.

| Health History | Nurses' Notes | Diagnostic Studies | Laboratory Results |

0900: Child is dyspneic and complaining of chest tightness. Apprehensive and anxious. Wheezing heard bilaterally in lungs. Retractions noted. SpO$_2$ 90% on RA. VS: T = 98.6°F (37°C); HR = 112 BPM; RR = 24 bpm; BP = 124/82 mm Hg

Which actions would the nurse take? **Select all that apply.**

- ☒ Initiate an IV line.
- ☒ Obtain arterial blood gases.
- ☒ Administer quick relief (rescue) medications.
- ☐ Assist the child into a left lateral position.
- ☐ Administer oxygen via NC at 2 L/min.
- ☐ Ask the parents to wait in the ED waiting room.
- ☒ Place the child on continuous cardiorespiratory and pulse oximetry monitoring.
- ☒ Obtain blood specimens for electrolytes, complete blood count, and renal function tests.

Rationale: For a child with an acute asthma exacerbation the nurse would monitor airway, breathing, and circulation closely in the event that supportive measures are needed. Pulse oximetry is monitored as well, to ensure an oxygen saturation level above 90% and to ensure adequate oxygenation of tissues. Humidified oxygen via simple face mask is administered to avoid drying secretions. Oxygen via NC will dry secretions. Dyspnea, chest tightness, wheezing, and retractions are indicators of respiratory compromise. The child with acute asthma exacerbation is usually very apprehensive and anxious and needs to be comforted. It is important to reassure the child that the child will not be left alone and to allow the parents to remain with the child. The child is allowed to assume a position of comfort that will promote maximum ventilation function. A left lateral position is not a position that will enhance breathing and ventilation. An IV line is necessary for the administration of fluids and IV medications if needed. Quick relief (rescue) medications usually via inhalation are given to open constricted airways and allow air exchange and to enhance tissue oxygenation. Laboratory studies and arterial blood gases are done to obtain a baseline and to determine the need for additional and more aggressive intervention. The elevated pulse, RR, and BP are expected to return to normal range once treatment is provided.

Test-Taking Strategy: Focus on the information in the scenario and note the child's problem, an acute asthma exacerbation. You need to use knowledge about the pathophysiology of an acute asthma exacerbation to assist in answering correctly. Think about what is expected in this event to determine nursing actions. Recalling that the primary goals of care are to provide oxygenation and to implement measures that will ensure adequate ventilation will assist in answering correctly. Also recall that anxiety and apprehension exacerbate a problem with airway and oxygenation, so ensuring psychosocial support is important. You can also follow a logical path for answering this question by using the approach illustrated in the table.

NGN TIP

Remember: A Multiple Response Select All That Apply item provides you with a scenario and data about the client and a list of actions. You will need to select one or more answer options. There may be only one correct option or multiple correct options. There will be at least five options with no more than 10 options, but all 10 options could be correct.

Test-Taking Strategy

⚡ THINKING SPACE

THINKING SPACE

Nursing Action	Helpful/Likely to Address Problem	Not Helpful/Not Likely to Address Problem
Initiate an IV line.	☒	☐
Obtain arterial blood gases.	☒	☐
Administer quick relief (rescue) medications.	☒	☐
Assist the child into a left lateral position.	☐	☒
Administer oxygen via NC at 2 L/min.	☐	☒
Ask the parents to wait in the ED waiting room.	☐	☒
Place the child on continuous cardiorespiratory and pulse oximetry monitoring.	☒	☐
Obtain blood specimens for electrolytes, complete blood count, and renal function tests.	☒	☐

Content Area: Pediatric Nursing
Priority Concept: Gas Exchange
Reference(s): Hockenberry et al., 2019, pp. 939–940; Ignatavicius et al., 2021, p. 541

Practice Questions

Practice Question 7.1 — Multiple Response Select All That Apply

An occupational nurse is called for emergency assistance to a 42-year-old victim of an accident in which the victim's index and middle finger were completely severed by a machine saw. The victim is sitting on the floor leaning against a wall and the fingers are seen on the floor 2 feet away from the client.

Health History	Nurses' Notes	Vital Signs	Laboratory Results

0800:
VS: T = 98.2°F (36.7°C); HR = 120 BPM; RR = 22 bpm; BP = 132/84 mm Hg

What actions would the nurse take? **Select all that apply.**

☐ Call 911 (EMS).

☐ Elevate the affected hand above heart level.

☐ Place the fingers in a waterproof sealed plastic bag.

☐ Check the victim for airway or breathing problems.

☐ Place the waterproof sealed bag containing the fingers on ice.

☐ Apply direct pressure to the amputation sites with layers of dry gauze.

☐ Remove the dry gauze after 10 minutes to check the status of the bleeding.

☐ Ensure that the amputated fingers are transported to the hospital with the victim.

Practice Question 7.2   Drag-and-Drop Cloze

The nurse is preparing to administer medications to a hospitalized 82-year-old client recovering from an acute exacerbation of heart failure. The client was taking eight different routine medications at home and is started on three additional medications to be taken while in the hospital. Recognizing the safety risks of polypharmacy and the importance of safe medication administration, the nurse takes steps to prevent medication errors.

Complete the following sentence. Drag or select words from the options below to fill in each blank.

To promote medication administration safety and to prevent medication errors, the nurse checks at least _____1 [Select] _____ client identifier(s), reads medication labels at least _____2 [Select] _____ time(s), and documents medication administration _____3 [Select] _____.

Options for 1	Options for 2	Options for 3
One	One	As soon as medications are given
Two	Two	Immediately before medications are given
Three	Three	After medications are given and after leaving the room
Four	Four	Before removing the medications from the dispensing system

Practice Question 7.3   Matrix Multiple Response

A 65-year-old client was hospitalized and treated for symptoms of heart palpitations and extreme shortness of breath. On admission, diagnostic studies showed the following:

Health History	Nurses' Notes	Vital Signs	Diagnostic Studies

- ECG: atrial fibrillation
- CT of the lungs: negative for embolism
- Chest x-ray: enlarged left ventricle

The nurse is preparing the client for discharge and provides teaching about prescribed medications.

For each medication listed, click in the box to specify the teaching point the nurse would provide to the client. Each teaching point may support more than one medication.

Teaching Point	Amiodarone	Metoprolol	Warfarin
Routine laboratory monitoring	☐	☐	☐
Monitor and report signs of bleeding	☐	☐	☐
Monitor and report shortness of breath	☐	☐	☐
Monitor BP and HR	☐	☐	☐
Consume consistent amounts of green leafy vegetables	☐	☐	☐

Practice Question 7.4　　**Matrix Multiple Choice**

The nurse is caring for an 80-year-old client on the medical-surgical unit admitted with complicated UTI. The client takes lisinopril and metformin at home and is started on antibiotics for infection and antipyretics as needed. The physician ordered the Modified Early Warning Score (MEWS) to be calculated every 4 hours to monitor for signs of septic shock. Assessment findings include RR, 12 bpm; HR, 110 BPM; systolic BP, 92 mm Hg; temperature, 100.5°F (38.1°C); and the client is currently alert and responsive. The client's MEWS is currently a 2 and is documented as follows:

	+3	+2	+1	o	+1	+2	+3
RR				X			
HR					X		
Systolic BP		X					
T				X			
Mental status				X			

MEWS Scoring Key

RR (bpm)		Systolic BP (mm Hg)	
<9	+2	≤70	+3
9–14	o	71–80	+2
15–20	+1	81–100	+1
21–29	+2	101–199	o
≥30	+3	≥200	+2
HR (BPM)		**T**	
<40	+2	<35°C / 95°F	+2
41–50	+1	35-38.4°C / 95–101.1°F	o
51–100	o	≥38.5°C / 101.3°F	+2
101–110	+1	**Mental Status**	
111–129	+2	Alert	o
≥130	+3	Reacts to voice	+1
		Reacts to pain	+2
		Unresponsive	+3

*Based on this assessment, click in the box to specify nursing actions that are **Indicated** (appropriate or necessary) and those that are **Contraindicated** (could be harmful).*

Nursing Action	Indicated	Contraindicated
Perform hourly VS, urine output, neurologic, and cardiopulmonary measurements	☐	☐
Administer prescribed daily BP medication	☐	☐
Administer ibuprofen for fever	☐	☐
Administer prescribed antibiotics	☐	☐
Notify the physician of an increase in the MEWS	☐	☐

Practice Question 7.5 — Multiple Response Select All That Apply

A 48-year-old client underwent laparoscopic cholecystectomy and is transferred to the surgical outpatient unit. The nurse performs a postoperative assessment and documents in the Nurses' Notes.

| Health History | Nurses' Notes | Diagnostic Studies | Laboratory Results |

1100:
VS: T = 99.2°F (37.3°C); HR = 92 BPM; RR = 16 bpm; BP = 118/72 mm Hg; SpO$_2$ = 97% on RA
Alert and oriented. Dressing dry and intact. IV 5% dextrose/lactated Ringer's infusing at 100 mL/hr. Has not voided. Pain 4/10.

The nurse would take which actions in managing this client's care in the immediate postoperative period? **Select all that apply.**

☐ Keep the head of the bed flat.

☐ Assist to the bathroom to void.

☐ Assess incision sites frequently.

☐ Administer antiemetics as needed.

☐ Maintain strict NPO status.

☐ Administer pain medication.

☐ Encourage use of the incentive spirometer.

Practice Question 7.6 — Drop-Down Rationale

The nurse is caring for a 70-year-old client with cellulitis on both lower extremities caused by methicillin-resistant *Staphylococcus aureus (MRSA)* and who is being treated with IV vancomycin. The next dose of vancomycin is due now, and the nurse checks the laboratory results.

| Health History | Nurses' Notes | Vital Signs | Laboratory Results |

Test	Result	Normal Reference Range
Vancomycin trough level	16 mcg/mL (11.3981 mcmol/L)	10–20 mcg/mL (10.3498–13.7998 mcmol/L)
White blood cells (WBCs)	10,000/mm³ (10 × 10⁹ /L)	5000–10,000/mm³ (5–10 × 10⁹ /L)
Blood urea nitrogen (BUN)	20 mg/dL (7.1 mmol/L)	10–20 mg/dL (3.6–7.1 mmol/L)
Creatinine	0.6 mg/dL (53 mcmol/L)	0.5–1.2 mg/dL (44–106 mcmol/L)

Based on this information, which action would the nurse take? Complete the following sentence by choosing from the list of options.

The nurse would _____ 1 [Select] _____ because _____ 2 [Select] _____.

Options for 1	Options for 2
Hold the next dose	The WBC count is high
Administer a lower dose	The trough level is normal
Administer the next dose orally	The creatinine level indicates toxicity
Administer the next dose as prescribed	The BUN level is high but not toxic

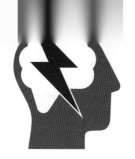

CHAPTER **8**

Strategies for Answering NGN Questions: Evaluate Outcomes

Evaluate Outcomes is a CJ cognitive skill that involves examining outcomes and measuring client progress toward meeting those outcomes in the plan of care. It is an ongoing and continuous process that compares actual client outcomes with the expected outcomes in a clinical scenario. It provides a basis for determining the need to modify the plan of care. As an iterative process, this skill involves revisiting the clinical scenario and examining the application of the cognitive skills *Recognize Cues, Analyze Cues, Prioritize Hypotheses, Generate Solutions,* and *Take Action.* Thus the cognitive skill *Evaluate Outcomes* involves looking back and making necessary revisions or modifications to provide safe and effective client care.

A nurse always needs to determine the effectiveness of the plan of care. In addition to determining effectiveness of the plan of care, the cognitive skill *Evaluate Outcomes* requires communication of client findings, as well as documenting and reporting the client's response to treatment and care. As a nurse, you need to ask yourself: *Did my actions help? Are things improved? Are things worse; has the client's condition declined?* and *Are things unchanged?* Based on your evaluation findings, you will need to think about how to move forward and what changes may be necessary in order to achieve the outcomes of care. Therefore the cognitive skill *Evaluate Outcomes* is essential to meet the client's needs and ensure client safety and high-quality care. This ability will be measured both on the NGN and by your instructors on course exams and in the laboratory and clinical settings.

How Do You Evaluate Outcomes?

Determining the effectiveness of the care provided is the focus of the CJ thinking skill *Evaluate Outcomes.* Once you have completed a phase of care or an aspect of care, think about what information you need to determine if the care was effective and to what degree. You may determine that expected outcomes have been met, unmet, or partially met. You will likely need to think about factors influencing the care and subsequent outcomes so that you can decide what needs to happen next to move toward the outcomes. Questions to ask yourself as you apply this cognitive skill may include:

- Based on previous assessments and interventions, what is happening to the client now?
- Are there ongoing or new client needs? If so, which ones are the priority?
- What must I do to address and meet these needs?
- Are the outcomes of care the same, or do they need to be revised?
- What else do I need to do to promote achievement of client outcomes?

NGN TIP

Remember: Focus on the outcomes of client care and think about what you need to consider as possible revisions to the plan of care. Ask yourself: *What else needs to be done and what needs to change to meet the expected outcomes?*

How Will *Evaluate Outcomes* Be Tested?

In every client interaction, you will evaluate outcomes of the plan of care. Therefore you can expect that you will be tested on your ability to accurately evaluate the outcomes of care provided, and the necessary follow-up based on that evaluation. Beginning with your first nursing course, you were asked about interpreting the outcomes of care in a variety of clinical scenarios. Sometimes testing required you to determine follow-up assessments you need to take; at other times you were tested on follow-up nursing actions that are needed to meet established outcomes. For example, you may have been presented with a clinical scenario in which a client was administered a unit of PRBCs because of a GI hemorrhage. In this scenario, evaluating assessment findings after administration of the blood product to determine the outcome of that intervention was likely a focus of the question or questions. Or maybe you were asked about interpreting VS and conducting a follow-up pain assessment after administering pain medication to a postoperative client.

NGN Question Stems Addressing *Evaluate Outcomes*

Test question stems will give you clues in the wording if the aim is to determine your ability to *Evaluate Outcomes.* Box 8.1 provides a list of examples of NGN question stems that will help you know that this thinking process is being addressed.

BOX 8.1   NGN Question Stems Addressing *Evaluate Outcomes*

- Click to specify which client/caregiver statement indicates the *need for further teaching.*
- Click to highlight the findings that would indicate the client is *not progressing as expected.*
- Drag one complication and one associated client finding that indicates the client's *condition has worsened.*
- Click to highlight the findings that indicate the client's health problem is *not yet resolved.*
- Click in the appropriate column to specify which client/caregiver statement/observation indicates that the home care instruction is either *understood* or *requires further teaching.*
- For each factor, click to specify if the finding *indicates readiness for discharge.*
- For each body system, click to specify the finding that indicates *progression toward expected outcomes.*
- Which findings following assessment and teaching are *unexpected and therefore require additional follow-up?*
- Click to specify if the finding is *consistent with a therapeutic outcome or an adverse outcome* of the prescribed medication.
- For each client statement, click to specify if the statement indicates that the *treatment plan is effective or ineffective.*
- Select the four findings that indicate a *therapeutic outcome* of medication therapy.
- The nurse determines that *interventions were effective* because of the _____1 [Select]_____ as evidenced by the _____2 [Select]_____ and the _____3 [Select]_____.

 NGN TIP

Remember: When you *Evaluate Outcomes*, you need to determine if expected outcomes have been met, unmet, or partially met. If outcomes are unmet or partially met, then you need to examine the application of the cognitive skills *Recognize Cues, Analyze Cues, Prioritize Hypotheses, Generate Solutions,* and *Take Action.* Then you need to determine what needs to be changed, revised, or added to the plan of care in order for outcomes to be met.

What NGN Item Types Optimally Measure *Evaluate Outcomes?*

Four types of test items optimally measure the cognitive skill *Evaluate Outcomes*. Variations of each of these types will most likely be presented on the NGN. Table 8.1 presents these item types and their variations. Sample Question 8.1 illustrates a Matrix Multiple Choice item type. Sample Question 8.2 illustrates a Highlight In Table, and Sample Question 8.3 illustrates a Multiple Response Select All that Apply item type. Sample Question 8.4 illustrates a Multiple Response Grouping type of item. The rationale and test-taking strategy to help you derive the correct responses are also provided.

TABLE 8.1 Test Items and Variations That Optimally Measure *Evaluate Outcomes*	
Type of Test Item	**Variations**
Highlight	Highlight in Text Highlight in Table
Multiple Response	Multiple Response Select All That Apply Multiple Response Select N Multiple Response Grouping Matrix Multiple Response
Multiple Choice	Multiple Choice Single Response Matrix Multiple Choice
Drag-and-Drop	Drag-and-Drop Cloze Drag-and-Drop Rationale Drag-and-Drop in Table (may replace Drop-Down in Table)
Drop Down	Drop-Down Cloze Drop-Down Rationale Drop-Down in Table

Sample Question 8.1	Matrix Multiple Choice: Evaluate Outcomes

A 38-year-old client (gravida 6, para 6) at 40 weeks of gestation is admitted to the labor and delivery unit for a scheduled induction of labor. A vaginal examination is done, and it is determined that the cervix is 80% effaced and 4 cm dilated. The client is not experiencing contractions. The obstetrician prescribes IV oxytocin. The nurse starts the oxytocin infusion per agency protocol and monitors the client and the fetus on the fetal monitor to determine effectiveness of the oxytocin.

For each assessment finding, click to specify if the finding is consistent with a therapeutic outcome or an adverse outcome of oxytocin. **Each row must have one response option selected.**

Assessment Finding	Therapeutic Outcome	Adverse Outcome
Altered mental status	☐	☒
Adventitious lung sounds	☐	☒
Contractions every 3–5 minutes lasting 45 seconds each	☒	☐
Sudden pain between contractions	☐	☒
Decelerations on the fetal monitor	☐	☒
Pain intensifying gradually with contractions	☒	☐

Rationale: Oxytocin is a hormone that is produced naturally by the posterior pituitary gland. Oxytocin produces uterine contractions during pregnancy and can be administered to induce labor for a term pregnancy. Additional therapeutic outcomes include milk ejection and control of postpartum hemorrhage. When given for labor, the client will experience intensifying contractions, including intensifying pain as the labor progresses, until eventually the contractions are occurring every 3 to 5 minutes and lasting 45 seconds each. Because oxytocin exerts an antidiuretic effect, water intoxication is an adverse outcome of oxytocin. Assessment findings related to water retention may be noted, such as altered mental status, adventitious lung sounds, and peripheral swelling. Another adverse outcome that can occur is uterine rupture. Sudden pain between contractions, excessive vaginal bleeding, and decelerations on the fetal monitor would be noted with this complication. The client with higher parity, specifically more than five pregnancies, is at higher risk for uterine rupture when given oxytocin.

Test-Taking Strategy: Note that this question is asking you to evaluate assessment findings and decide whether they are consistent with a therapeutic or adverse outcome of oxytocin. The question is asking about the use of oxytocin for the induction of labor; therefore you need to think about the findings in the context of normal labor progression. Any finding that is not specifically related to or associated with normal labor progression should be classified as an adverse outcome. Using a table format to organize your thoughts may be helpful.

NGN TIP

Remember: In a Matrix Multiple Choice question, each row must have one response item selected. If you don't select a response item for each row, you won't be able to move on to the next item on the exam.

Test-Taking Strategy

Assessment Finding	Associated With Normal Labor Progression	Not Associated With Normal Labor Progression
Altered mental status	☐	☒
Adventitious lung sounds	☐	☒
Contractions every 3–5 minutes lasting 45 seconds each	☒	☐
Sudden pain between contractions	☐	☒
Decelerations on the fetal monitor	☐	☒
Pain intensifying gradually with contractions	☒	☐

Altered mental status, adventitious lung sounds, sudden pain *between* contractions, and decelerations on the fetal monitor are not normal findings and are not specifically related to normal labor progression.

Content Area: Maternal-Newborn Nursing
Priority Concept: Perfusion
Reference(s): Burchum & Rosenthal, 2022, p. 783

Sample Question 8.2 | **Highlight in Table: Evaluate Outcomes**

An 86-year-old client was hospitalized 4 days ago because of multiple episodes of severe watery diarrhea, anorexia, and weakness. The client's spouse reports that the client had not eaten much for 4 days prior to admission and complained of thirst but hadn't been able to "hold anything down." On admission, the physician prescribed IV fluids with potassium chloride, antiemetic and antidiarrheal medication, laboratory studies, and stool and blood cultures. The stool culture and blood culture were negative, but laboratory findings and VS measurements indicated severe dehydration.

On day 4 of hospitalization, the daytime nurse assesses the client, reviews the laboratory results drawn in the morning, and documents the findings.

Click to highlight below the findings that indicate that the client's health problem is not yet resolved.

Health History	Nurses' Notes	Vital Signs	Lab Results

Assessment	Findings
GI	Tolerating clear liquids and soft foods. States has an appetite. Had two episodes of brown watery diarrhea at 0700 and 0800. Reports cramping abdominal pain rated currently as 4/10.
Genitourinary	Urine output 240 mL during the night. Voided 100 mL at 0800, yellow and concentrated.
VS	T = 100.8°F (38.2°C); HR = 98 BPM; BP = 118/80 mm Hg; RR = 20 bpm; SpO$_2$ = 95% on RA

Laboratory Results

Test	Result	Normal Reference Range
White blood cells (WBCs)	10,000/mm³ (10 × 10⁹/L)	5000–10,000/mm³ (5–10 × 10⁹/L)
Blood urea nitrogen (BUN)	22 mg/dL (7.92 mmol/L) H	10–20 mg/dL (3.6–7.1 mmol/L)
Creatinine	0.9 mg/dL (79.5 mcmol/L)	0.6–1.2 mg/dL (53–106 mcmol/L)
Potassium	3.3 mEq/L (3.3 mmol/L) L	3.5–5.0 mEq/L (3.5–5.0 mmol/L)
Sodium	148 mEq/L (148 mmol/L) H	135–145 mEq/L (135–145 mmol/L)

Rationale: The client has been treated for severe dehydration. Although the nurse is not provided with baseline information about the client, there are abnormal data that indicate that the client's health problem has not resolved. The client had multiple episodes of diarrhea, and although the cause of the diarrhea is unknown, it has led to severe dehydration. The client had two episodes of brown watery diarrhea at 0700 and 0800 on day 4 of hospitalization, 1 hour apart, and also reports cramping abdominal pain rated as 4/10. This indicates that the client is still experiencing the health problem. Although the urine output is minimally adequate, the urine is concentrated, indicating insufficient body fluid. In addition, a deficit of normal body fluid can cause hyperthermia, and this client is exhibiting an elevated temperature at 100.8°F (38.2°C). Because the stool and blood cultures are negative and the WBC count is within the normal range (5000/mm³ to 10,000/mm³ [5–10 × 10⁹/L]), infection is not likely, and the temperature elevation is probably associated with dehydration. In dehydration, some electrolytes are lost, specifically potassium. The client's potassium level is low at 3.3 mEq/L (3.3 mmol/L), known as hypokalemia; normal potassium level is 3.5 to 5.0 mEq/L (3.5–5.0 mmol/L). The sodium level is elevated (known as hypernatremia), and this is an indicator of dehydration and that the health problem is not resolved. Normal sodium level is 135 to 145 mEq/L (135–145 mmol/L). In hypernatremia, the body contains too little water for the amount of sodium; therefore the sodium level in the blood becomes abnormally high when water loss exceeds sodium loss. The BUN is slightly elevated at 22 mg/dL (7.92 mmol/L), and in the setting of a normal creatinine level, this indicates dehydration. The normal BUN level is 10 to 20 mg/dL (3.6–7.1 mmol/L). The normal creatinine level ranges from 0.6 to 1.2 mg/dL (53–106 mcmol/L).

Test-Taking Strategy: Note that the question is asking you to evaluate assessment findings that indicate that the client's health problem has not yet resolved. Focus on the information in the scenario and note that the client is severely dehydrated. Use knowledge of the pathophysiology associated with dehydration and its manifestations. Look for abnormal data in the findings that indicate a dehydrated state. Using a table format to organize your thoughts may be helpful.

NGN TIP

Remember: In a Highlight in Table question, you will select from a table pieces of information that are significant to the question being asked. The table may display part of a medical record, such as Nurses' Notes, flow sheet data, Physician's Orders, or Laboratory Results.

Test-Taking Strategy

Related to or Consistent With Dehydration	Unrelated to or Inconsistent With Dehydration
• Had two episodes of brown watery diarrhea at 0700 and 0800 • Reports cramping abdominal pain rated currently as 4/10 • Concentrated urine • Temperature 100.8°F (38.2°C) • BUN: 22 mg/dL (7.92 mmol/L) • Creatinine: 0.9 mg/dL (79.5 mcmol/L) • Potassium: 3.3 mEq/L (3.3 mmol/L) • Sodium: 148 mEq/L (148 mmol/L)	• Tolerating clear liquids and soft foods • States has an appetite • Urine output 240 mL during the night • Yellow urine • HR 98 BPM • BP 118/80 mm Hg • RR 20 bpm • SpO₂ 95% on RA • WBCs: 10,000/mm³ (10 × 10⁹/L)

Note that questions requiring you to evaluate assessment findings specific to such things as body systems, VS, or laboratory results may ask about those indicating that the problem has resolved or has not yet resolved. Some findings listed, may be normal but are related to the health problem, such as the creatinine level. You need to decide which findings are related and which are not. For example, in the case of dehydration, yellow urine would be noted in an improved state, as well as in an unchanged state. However, concentrated urine indicates lack of improvement in the client condition. Be sure to consider all findings in the assessment when evaluating outcomes.

Content Area: Medical-Surgical Nursing
Priority Concept: Fluid and Electrolyte Balance
Reference(s): Ignatavicius et al., 2021, pp. 247–248, 253, 925, 1135–1137

Sample Question 8.3	Multiple Response Select All That Apply: Evaluate Outcomes

A hospitalized 68-year-old client has a biventricular pacemaker placed in the right subclavicular area. The nurse is providing care following the procedure and is initiating postprocedure teaching.

Which findings following postprocedure assessment and teaching are unexpected and therefore require additional follow-up? **Select all that apply.**

- ☒ The client reports pain at the level of the diaphragm.
- ☒ The client reports hiccupping that lasts longer than usual.
- ☐ The dressing over the pacemaker site is clean, dry, and intact.
- ☐ The client uses the left ear when talking on the cell phone.
- ☒ The client performs right-shoulder range-of-motion exercises.
- ☐ The client avoids lifting more than 10 lb on the affected side.
- ☐ The implantation site is free of redness, swelling, and drainage.
- ☒ Muscle contractions are noted over the diaphragm that correspond to the HR.

NGN TIP

Remember: In a Multiple Response Select All That Apply question, you will need to select all options that are correct. There will be at least five options to select from and no more than 10 options for selection. There may be only one correct response or multiple correct responses, or all options listed could be correct. With a Multiple Response Select N item, you need to select the exact number of options that the instructions indicate. You can select fewer than the number of options provided, but not more. However, if you do select fewer than the number (N) indicated in the question, you will not receive full credit.

Test-Taking Strategy

Rationale: A permanent pacemaker may be needed for a client who experiences cardiac conduction disorders that do not improve with other measures. The pacemaker is placed in a subcutaneous pocket at the shoulder in the right or left subclavicular area. Complications of pacemaker placement include pericardial effusion, pericardial tamponade, and diaphragmatic pacing. Client reports of pain at the level of the diaphragm and muscle contractions noted over the diaphragm that correspond to the HR may indicate diaphragmatic pacing, which occurs when the pacemaker is malpositioned or one of the leads is dislodged, and would require additional follow-up. Although some shoulder movement should be encouraged to prevent stiffness, the client needs to avoid lifting the arms over the head; therefore if the client is performing range-of-motion shoulder exercises, additional follow-up is needed. In addition, the client should avoid lifting anything more than 10 lb on the affected side because this could dislodge the pacemaker wire. Signs of pacemaker malfunction need to be reported to the primary health care provider, including difficulty breathing, dizziness, fainting, chest pain, weight gain, and prolonged hiccupping. The dressing should be clean, dry, and intact, and the pacemaker implantation site should be free of redness, swelling, and drainage. The client needs to avoid sources of electromagnetic fields and telecommunications transmitters because these could cause a disruption in the pacemaker settings; therefore the client should use the left ear to talk on the cell phone if the pacemaker site is on the right side.

Test-Taking Strategy: Note that this question is asking you to determine which assessment findings require additional follow-up. Using a thinking process as illustrated in the table, consider whether each option is normal or expected and therefore not likely to cause harm, or whether it is abnormal and unexpected and has the potential for harm. Any option that has the potential for harm would be selected because this would require additional follow-up.

Assessment Finding	Normal/Expected/Not Likely to Cause Harm	Abnormal/Unexpected/Potential for Harm
The client reports pain at the level of the diaphragm.	☐	☒
The client reports hiccupping that lasts longer than usual.	☐	☒
The dressing over the pacemaker site is clean, dry, and intact.	☒	☐
The client uses the left ear when talking on her cell phone.	☒	☐

Assessment Finding	Normal/Expected/Not Likely to Cause Harm	Abnormal/Unexpected/ Potential for Harm
The client performs right-shoulder range-of-motion exercises.	☐	☒
The client avoids lifting more than 10 lb on the affected side.	☒	☐
The implantation site is free of redness, swelling, and drainage.	☒	☐
Muscle contractions are noted over the diaphragm that correspond to the HR.	☐	☒

THINKING SPACE

The client reporting pain at the level of the diaphragm, the client performing right-shoulder range-of-motion exercises, the client reporting hiccupping lasting longer than usual, and muscle contractions noted over the diaphragm that correspond to the HR are all abnormal, are unexpected, and/or have the potential to cause harm and therefore require additional follow-up. Therefore these are the correct answers to the question.

Content Area: Medical-Surgical Nursing
Priority Concept: Perfusion
Reference(s): Ignatavicius et al., 2021, pp. 648–649

Sample Question 8.4   **Multiple Response Grouping: Evaluate Outcomes**

A hospitalized 65-year-old client is recovering on the postoperative unit following open reduction with internal fixation of the left hip. The nurse is performing the first assessment after having received the client from the PACU 15 minutes ago.

For each body system below, click to specify the assessment finding(s) consistent with expected post-operative outcomes. Each body system may support more than one assessment finding.

Body System	Assessment Finding
Respiratory	☐ RR 8 bpm
	☒ SpO$_2$ 93% on 3 L/min per NC
	☒ Lung sounds clear to auscultation bilaterally
Cardiovascular	☐ BP 90/56 mm Hg
	☐ HR 120 BPM
	☒ Peripheral pulses 2+ bilaterally
Neurological	☒ Drowsy, arousable and responsive to stimuli
	☒ Pupils equal, round, and reactive to light
	☒ Sensation intact in bilateral lower extremities
GI/Genitourinary	☒ Bowel sounds hypoactive × 4 quadrants
	☐ Urine output 20 mL/hr
	☒ Urine yellow, clear, no odor
Integumentary	☐ Surgical dressing saturated with bright red blood
	☒ No redness over pressure point areas
	☒ No petechiae or rashes throughout the skin

Rationale: An RR of 8 bpm indicates a problem with the airway or respiratory system and is not consistent with an expected postoperative finding. The normal pulse oximetry range in the postoperative period is 92% to 100%, so an SpO$_2$ of 93% is acceptable; in addition, the client will likely be on supplemental oxygen at this time. Lung sounds should be clear. BP should be at or above baseline and may be elevated owing to pain. This client's BP is low, which is an unexpected postoperative finding and could indicate a problem with perfusion or bleeding. The HR may be elevated above baseline because of pain; however, if it is substantially elevated, such as a HR of 120 BPM, this may be due to a problem with perfusion or bleeding. Peripheral pulses 2+ bilaterally is normal and expected progression. In the postoperative period, it is expected for the client to be drowsy but arousable and responding to stimuli. Pupils should be round, equal, and reactive to light. Sensation should be intact in the extremities. Hypoactive bowel sounds in all four quadrants are expected in the postoperative period because of the effects of anesthesia. Clear, yellow urine without odor is normal and expected. Urine output of 20 mL/hr may indicate renal impairment and could be associated with perfusion problems; this is not an expected outcome. A surgical dressing saturated with bright red blood likely indicates bleeding from the incision site and is not an expected outcome. No redness over pressure point areas is important to note as the operating room table can cause pressure injuries; this finding is normal and expected. No petechiae or rashes throughout the skin is also normal and expected progression for the client in the postoperative period.

Test-Taking Strategy

Test-Taking Strategy: Begin to answer this question by looking at each assessment finding, and consider whether it would require continued monitoring versus additional or immediate action or follow-up. If the evaluation necessitates additional or immediate action or follow-up, then it would not be consistent with expected or normal outcomes in the postoperative period. Organize your thinking process as illustrated in the table.

Assessment Finding	Continue to Monitor	Requires Additional or Immediate Action/ Follow-up
RR 8 bpm	☐	☒
SpO$_2$ 93% on 3 L/min per NC	☒	☐
Lung sounds clear to auscultation bilaterally	☒	☐
BP 90/56 mm Hg	☐	☒
HR 120 BPM	☐	☒
Peripheral pulses 2+ bilaterally	☒	☐
Drowsy, arousable and responsive to stimuli	☒	☐
Pupils equal, round, and reactive to light	☒	☐
Sensation intact in bilateral lower extremities	☒	☐
Bowel sounds hypoactive × 4 quadrants	☒	☐
Urine output 20 mL/hr	☐	☒
Urine yellow, clear, no odor	☒	
Surgical dressing saturated with bright red blood	☐	☒
No redness over pressure point areas	☒	☐
No petechiae or rashes throughout the skin	☒	☐

Recall that evaluating outcomes questions will require that you examine outcome data provided. Depending on what the question is asking, you need to determine whether the data are expected, unexpected, or unrelated. Then you need to think about additional actions or follow-up that may be necessary based on the conclusions you have made.

Content Area: Foundations of Nursing
Priority Concept: Perfusion
Reference(s): Potter et al., 2021, pp. 1348–1350

 Practice Questions

Practice Question 8.1	**Matrix Multiple Choice**

The nurse is preparing a 68-year-old client in a rehabilitation center for discharge to home. The client was transferred from the hospital 2 weeks ago following treatment for a right cerebral stroke. On admission to the rehabilitation center, the following findings were documented.

Health History	Nurses' Notes	Vital Signs	Physician's Orders

T = 98.6°F (36.0°C); HR = 92 BPM; BP = 132/78 mm Hg; RR = 20 bpm; SpO$_2$ = 95% on RA

Health History	Nurses' Notes	Vital Signs	Physician's Orders

Client is accompanied by spouse, who will be the primary caregiver when the client returns home.

Alert and oriented and understands about receiving rehabilitative therapy before returning to home. States doesn't really have "much to rehab" and is fine but will do what the doctor says to get home.

Has left-side weakness and seems impulsive with movements. Able to move right arm and leg with adequate strength noted.

Has difficulty focusing and attention span is short; spouse is assisting in answering questions.

Spouse notes that the client's judgment is impaired and is concerned about the client's safety because of the client's impulsivity.

Client also exhibits left-sided neglect; lacks proprioception.

Has homonymous hemianopsia.

Health History	Nurses' Notes	Vital Signs	Physician's Orders

PT and OT evaluation and initiate a treatment plan as needed
Low-fat diet
Out of bed as much as tolerated
Begin to prepare client and spouse for discharge to home
Referral to case manager to plan discharge
Clopidogrel 75 mg oral daily
Carvedilol 3.125 mg oral twice daily
Docusate 100 mg oral daily
Simvastatin 20 mg oral daily

The nurse consults with the case manager about the plan for home care. Collaboration with the client and spouse and the case manager reveals that the spouse will need assistance with the client's personal needs and ADLs and with ambulation and PT. A home care aide is scheduled to visit the client daily for 3 hours a day. In addition, PT is planned for home visits 3 times weekly. The nurse implements a teaching plan for the client and spouse and monitors the client's readiness for discharge.

Which client or spouse statement/observation indicates that the home care instruction is either understood or requires further teaching? **Place an X in either the Understood column or the Requires Further Teaching column.**

Client or Spouse Statement/Observation	Understood	Requires Further Teaching
Client places the right arm into the shirt sleeve first when putting the shirt on.	☐	☐
Spouse states: "It will help vision if I approach my spouse from the right side."	☐	☐
Spouse states: "I will talk to the home care aides when they come, to be sure they get all of the care done during the first hour after they arrive."	☐	☐
Client turns the head to the right and then to the left before taking on an activity.	☐	☐
Client states: "I know that I need to call for help if I need to use the bathroom."	☐	☐
Client states: "I can skip the stool softener medication if I have a bowel movement."	☐	☐
Client picks up a washcloth with the left hand to wash the face.	☐	☐

A 16-year-old client was admitted to the mental health residential treatment center. The nurse performs an admission assessment and documents the following findings.

Health History	Nurses' Notes	Vital Signs	Lab Results

T = 96.4°F (35.7°C); HR = 40 BPM; BP = 88/48 mm Hg;
   RR = 16 bpm; SpO$_2$ = 92% on RA
Height: 5 ft 6 inches
Weight: 88 lb (40 kg)
BMI: 15.99 kg/m^2

Health History	Nurses' Notes	Vital Signs	Lab Results

Client is accompanied by a parent. The parent consistently interrupts the client during the interview.

Parent states that the client is compulsive and always has to have everything in perfect order otherwise becomes anxious.

Parent states, "I was just like my child when I was that age and always had to look perfect and be perfect with everything that I did. I know my child is very skinny, but that is how I was when I was a teenager and I had to starve myself like my child does in order to keep my hourglass figure."

Client reports not socializing much because of being too busy exercising and reports constant exercising all day long, at least 10 times a day for an hour each session. Reports the need to burn off calories and stay in control of weight.

States hardly eats because of feeling fat and feeling appearance is fat. Is very fearful of gaining weight; describes restrictive eating patterns.

Loves to collect food recipes and cookbooks and prepare huge meals for other people but doesn't eat with them.

Denies alcohol or drug misuse.

Denies suicidal thoughts.

Denies food binging and purging, or use of laxatives or enemas.

Reports amenorrhea for the past 3 months.

Face is hollowed with sunken eyes.

Skin is pale, hair dry and thin.

Growth of lanugo on skin, skin is yellow tinged.

Complains of dizziness and skipped heart beats.

An interdisciplinary treatment approach was instituted to treat the client's eating disorder and included nutritional consultation, weight restoration therapy, and intensive psychotherapy and counseling. In addition, family therapy was planned. After 70 days of treatment, the interdisciplinary team meets to discuss the client's readiness for discharge to home and use of outpatient support services.

The nurse evaluates the client for acceptable outcome criteria indicating readiness for discharge. For each factor below, click to specify if the finding indicates readiness for discharge. **Each factor may support more than one finding.**

Factor	Finding
Physiological	☐ Weight: 102 lb (46.3 kg)
	☐ Eating 80% of each of the 3 meals delivered by the dietary department and 2 snacks
	☐ Electrolyte results indicate:
	• **Potassium:** 3.2 mEq/L (3.2 mmol/L) **L** (normal reference range: 3.5–5.0 mEq/L [3.5–5.0 mmol/L])
	• **Sodium:** 130 mEq/L (130 mmol/L) **L** (normal reference range: 135–145 mEq/L [135–145 mmol/L])
	• **Chloride:** 95 mEq/L (95 mmol/L) **L** (normal reference range: 98–106 mEq/L [98–106 mmol/L])
Psychological	Client states:
	☐ "I really need to walk around the nursing unit 10 times a day and do 45 laps each time. I was doing 50 laps each time but cut down to 45."
	☐ "I counted my calories that I ate for the day and it came to 950. I think that's more than enough but I need to keep counting the calories to be sure."
	☐ "I am clear about what triggers my disruptive eating patterns and I know what alternative behaviors I need to take to help this."
Social	Client states:
	☐ "My best friend asked if I would go to lunch with some of our friends but I'm not going to go because I have nothing to wear that makes me look good. All my clothes are too tight."
	☐ "My parent is taking me and my siblings to that new movie that just came out; it'll be fun. I'm really looking forward to sharing a big box of popcorn and drinking a cola!"
	☐ "I have no interest in going to my prom this year. I've gained this weight and people in my class are definitely going to notice that."
Family Support	☐ Parent states will be sure that the child eats at least 3 full meals a day and 2 snacks and will remove and throw away any "teen magazines" or other distracting books or magazines that are in the child's bedroom.
	☐ Parent states that all of the children are going to take a 15-minute walk every evening after dinner.
	☐ Parent states, "My child seems to want to stay close to home, but I'm encouraging my child to spend some time with friends from school. I think these peer relationships are important."
Follow-up	☐ Parent states that family therapy sessions are not necessary since the problem is with the one child "and not the family."
	Client states:
	☐ "I have an appointment with the nutrition person in 2 weeks, but I'm thinking that if I maintain my weight and eat like I'm supposed to, then I can cancel it."
	☐ "The nurse at my school says there is a support group for students with eating problems and that they meet weekly. Do you think that this will help me?"

Practice Question 8.3 — Multiple Response Select N

A 68-year-old client is admitted to the ED with a diagnosis of atrial fibrillation and rapid ventricular response. The ED physician completes the history and physical, and prescribes IV amiodarone to treat the dysrhythmia.

Health History	Nurses' Notes	Vital Signs	Lab Results

A 68-year-old client presents to the ED at 1215 with complaints of "heart fluttering" and shortness of breath that started 2 hours ago. Associated with fatigue and dizziness, worsened by activity. No alleviating factors, symptoms are constant. Denies chest pain, losing consciousness, and difficulty breathing while lying down. Reports past medical history of hypertension, hyperlipidemia, and type 2 DM. Family history is negative for cardiac events.

Speaks in short sentences, appears short of breath while talking. Skin is warm, dry, and intact throughout. Rapid, irregular HR, 120–140 BPM on auscultation. Lung sounds clear to auscultation in all fields. No peripheral edema.

Health History	Nurses' Notes	Vital Signs	Lab Results

12:15: T = 98.8°F (37.1°C); apical HR = 120–140 BPM and irregular; RR = 22 bpm; BP = 128/76 mm Hg; SpO$_2$ = 95% on RA

Health History	Nurses' Notes	Vital Signs	Lab Results

1215: Client admitted to ED. Received orders for IV amiodarone.

1230: Admission assessment completed. Amiodarone started. Continuous VS monitoring and cardiac monitor in place. Cardiac monitor shows shortened PR interval, narrowed QRS complex, atrial fibrillation with an irregular rate of 120–140 BPM.

1300: Follow-up VS and assessment completed. Client reports tremors, light sensitivity, lack of appetite with nausea, vomiting × 1 undigested food, no hematemesis. BP 90/56 mm Hg, HR 102 BPM. Cardiac monitor shows prolongation of previously shortened PR interval, widening of previously narrowed QRS complex, atrial fibrillation converted to sinus rhythm. HR regular at 102 BPM. 2+ pitting peripheral edema.

Select the four findings that indicate a therapeutic outcome of medication therapy.

- ☐ Reports of tremors
- ☐ Reports of photosensitivity
- ☐ BP 90/56 mm Hg
- ☐ HR regular at 102 BPM
- ☐ Prolongation of the PR interval
- ☐ Widening of the QRS complex
- ☐ Peripheral edema 2+ pitting bilaterally
- ☐ Reports of anorexia, nausea, and vomiting
- ☐ Atrial fibrillation converted to sinus rhythm

Practice Question 8.4   **Matrix Multiple Choice**

A 39-year-old client is being seen in the outpatient pain management clinic. The client was in a motor vehicle accident 1 year ago and sustained an injury to the cervical and lumbar spine and has been experiencing neck and back pain since the injury. The client has tried conservative measures, including ice and heat, massage, and PT. The client has also tried acetaminophen, NSAIDs, muscle relaxants, and opioid analgesics, and the pain has become intolerable again even with these measures. The pain management specialist has added amitriptyline to the treatment plan, and the nurse provides teaching to the client about the plan. The client returns to the clinic 1 month later for follow-up evaluation.

Which observations indicate that the treatment plan is effective? **For each client statement/observation, click to specify if the statement indicates that the treatment plan is *Effective* or *Ineffective*.**

Statement/Observation	Effective	Ineffective
Client states: "My back and neck are sore after PT."	☐	☐
Client states: "I have been walking a mile each day before going to work."	☐	☐
Client states: "I need to wear my neck collar all the time because I need it for added support."	☐	☐
Client ambulates to the examination room and is limping and leaning the hand on the wall while walking.	☐	☐
Client states: "I know that new medication is used for depression but it has helped my pain too."	☐	☐

Practice Question 8.5 — Drop-Down Cloze

A 58-year-old client is admitted to the medical-surgical unit at 0600 from the ED with abdominal pain, fatigue, dizziness, and bright red blood in the stool, and is diagnosed with GI hemorrhage. The nurse reviews the medical record on admission.

| Health History | Nurses' Notes | Physician's Orders | Lab Results |

Past medical history: DM, osteoarthritis, depression
Social history: Smokes cigarettes 1 pack per day for 10 years, drinks 3 glasses of wine nightly, denies other recreational drug use
Medications: Metformin 500 mg twice daily, ibuprofen 800 mg three times daily for joint pain, citalopram 10 mg daily

| Health History | Nurses' Notes | Physician's Orders | Lab Results |

Complete blood count (CBC)
Prothrombin time (PT)
Partial thromboplastin time (aPTT)
International normalized ratio (INR)
Type and crossmatch
1 unit PRBCs if hemoglobin is less than 8.0 g/dL (80 g/L), repeat hemoglobin and hematocrit level 2 hours after transfusion is complete
Bowel preparation (polyethylene glycol as directed) for colonoscopy
Obtain consent for colonoscopy
Pantoprazole 40 mg intravenously every 8 hours
Bowel rest, NPO
Normal saline IV maintenance fluids at 125 mL/hr
Hydromorphone 1 mg IV push every 3 hr as needed for pain
GI specialist consultation

| Health History | Nurses' Notes | Physician's Orders | Lab Results |

0800: Received and reviewed laboratory results. Started blood transfusion per protocol. Administering 1 unit PRBCs. Client reports continued abdominal pain, fatigue, dizziness. VS stable.
1200: 1 unit PRBCs completed. VS stable throughout transfusion. Client reports abdominal pain is unchanged. States no longer feels dizzy and feels less fatigued.
1400: Hemoglobin and hematocrit result updated. T = 98.8°F (37.1°C); apical HR = 82 BPM and regular; RR = 18 bpm; BP = 122/74 mm Hg; SpO$_2$ = 95% on RA.

| Health History | Nurses' Notes | Physician's Orders | Lab Results |

0800:

Test	Result	Normal Reference Range
Complete Blood Count		
Red blood cells (RBCs)	4.5 (4.5 × 10^{12})	4.2–6.2 × 10^{12}/L (4.2–6.2 × 10^{12}/L)
White blood cells (WBCs)	8000/mm^3 (8 × 10^9/L)	5000–10,000/mm^3 (5–10 × 10^9/L)
Platelets	180,000/mm^3 (180 × 10^9/L)	150,000–400,000/mm^3 (150–400 × 10^9/L)
Hemoglobin (Hgb)	7.6 g/dL (76 g/L) **L**	12–18 g/dL (120–180 g/L)
Hematocrit (Hct)	32% (0.32) **L**	37%–52% (0.37–0.52)
Coagulation Studies		
aPTT	32 seconds	30–40 sec
PT	12.5 seconds	11–12.5 sec
INR	1.0	0.81–1.2
Fecal Occult Blood Test		
Occult blood	Detected	Negative
Type and Crossmatch		
Type and crossmatch	O positive No antibodies detected	

1400:

Test	Result	Normal Reference Range
Hemoglobin (Hgb)	9.0 g/dL (90 g/L) **L**	12–18 g/dL (120–180 g/L)
Hematocrit (Hct)	39% (0.39)	37%–52% (0.37–0.52)

Based on the client findings, complete the following sentence by choosing from the lists of options provided.

The nurse determines that the _____1 [Select]_____ was effective, as evidenced by the _____2 [Select]_____ and the _____3 [Select]_____.

Options for 1	Options for 2	Options for 3
Pantoprazole	Hemoglobin level	VS
Hydromorphone	Coagulation studies result	Abdominal pain
Blood transfusion	Fecal occult blood test result	Report about fatigue and dizziness

Practice Question 8.6   Highlight in Text

A 3-day-old newborn is seen in the outpatient pediatric clinic for a post-hospital follow-up appointment. The nurse reviews the health history and notes the following.

Health History	Nurses' Notes	Vital Signs	Lab Results

Infant born full-term via vaginal delivery. No labor or birth complications.
Birth weight: 7 lb 3 oz (3.3 kg)
Birth length: 19 inches

Test	Result	Normal Reference Range
Bilirubin	3.1 mg/dL (52.7 mcmol/L) H	0.2–1.4 mg/dL (3.4–23.8 mcmol/L)

The nurse performs an assessment on the newborn and obtains a blood specimen for evaluation of the bilirubin level. The following notes are documented.

Click to highlight the findings that indicate the need for follow-up in the 3-day-old newborn.

Health History	Nurses' Notes	Vital Signs	Lab Results

Breast-feeding/chest-feeding every 2 to 3 hours without difficulty. Parents report infant urinates 12 to 15 times per day and has a bowel movement 5 to 6 times per day. They report that stool is greenish brown to yellowish brown, thin and less sticky in consistency than it has been. They have noticed the skin looks tan and the eyes look yellow.

Health History	Nurses' Notes	Vital Signs	Lab Results

T = 99.6°F (37.5°C) axillary; apical HR = 180 BPM and regular; RR = 70 bpm; weight = 7 lb 5 oz (3.4 kg)

Health History	Nurses' Notes	Vital Signs	Lab Results

Test	Result	Normal Reference Range
Bilirubin	4.8 mg/dL (81.6 mcmol/L) H	0.2 –1.4 mg/dL (3.4–23.8 mcmol/L)

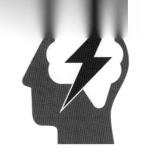

CHAPTER 9

Strategies for Answering NGN Stand-alone Items and Unfolding Case Studies

Case studies provide the foundation for the NGN test items. There are two types of case studies used on the NGN: the Stand-alone items and the Unfolding Case Study. Although there are some differences between the two types of cases, both types present a realistic clinical situation commonly encountered in practice by the new nursing graduate. This chapter describes the differences between the Stand-alone items and the Unfolding Case Study. Samples of each type of case and accompanying NGN items are illustrated throughout the chapter along with rationales and test-taking strategies.

The NCSBN NCJMM identifies the six clinical judgment cognitive (thinking) skills that the nurse applies when caring for a client and making a clinical decision to ensure safety and high-quality care (Box 9.1). The model also identifies factors that influence the ability of the nurse to make appropriate clinical judgments; these are known as *Environmental Factors* and *Individual Factors* and are the external factors considered in the daily care of a client. *Environmental Factors* focus on the client and the environment. *Individual Factors* are those related to the nurse caring for the client. Table 9.1 provides a list of these environmental and individual factors. As case studies are presented throughout this chapter, these environmental and individual factors are identified with color shading to distinguish them and illustrate how they are represented in a case study. Also, refer to Chapter 5 for a description and examples of how each external factor affects your thinking process in making clinical judgments.

> **NGN TIP**
>
> **Remember:** *Environmental Factors* and *Individual Factors* are the external factors considered in the daily care of a client. *Environmental Factors* focus on the client and the environment, and *Individual Factors* are those related to the nurse caring for the client. These factors influence your thinking process in making clinical judgments.

What Are Stand-alone Items?

Stand-alone items present a short paragraph of client information. These item types present a stated diagnosis or an implied diagnosis and include clinical information for a specific client. The client information may be presented in paragraph form or in the form of a medical record such as Nurses' Notes, medical history, physician orders, VS, I&O, or laboratory and diagnostic tests, for example. There are two types of Stand-alone items used on the NGN: the Bow-tie item and the Trend item. Both item types provide information that require you to make one or more clinical decisions. Thus these item types can measure more than one CJ cognitive skill.

BOX 9.1 Cognitive Skills of the NCJMM
Recognize Cues
Analyze Cues
Prioritize Hypotheses
Generate Solutions
Take Action
Evaluate Outcomes

TABLE 9.1	Environmental and Individual Factors That Influence Clinical Judgment	
Environmental Factors		**Individual Factors**
Client observation		Candidate (test-taker) characteristics
Consequences and risks		Knowledge
Cultural considerations		Level of experience
Environment		Prior experience
Medical records		Skills
Resources		Specialty
Task complexity		
Time pressure		

From National Council of State Boards of Nursing (NCSBN). (2019). *Next Generation NCLEX® News*, Winter 2019. https://www.ncsbn.org/NGN_Winter19.pdf

Bow-tie Item

The Bow-tie item can address all six cognitive skills in the NCJMM and provides a clinical scenario that includes client data at *one point in time.* Using drag-and-drop technology, the responses to the item are dragged and placed into three areas (categories) of a "figure" that looks like a bow-tie. The Bow-tie item has headers identifying each of the three areas. The options are provided, in addition to specific directions as to how to answer the item. Samples of Bow-tie items are presented in Sample Question 9.1 and Sample Question 9.2. These samples provide client data in the form of a medical record.

NGN TIP

Remember: According to the NCSBN, in a Bow-tie item the response options are known as the *tokens* and the placeholders for the response items are known as the *targets.* In order to move forward in the exam, all targets must be filled with the tokens, which are found directly below the Bow-tie in labeled columns.

NGN TIP

Remember: For the Bow-tie item in Sample Question 9.1, you need to read the information in the scenario and recognize which findings are relevant *(Recognize Cues)*, make connections to determine what these relevant findings mean and what condition the client may be experiencing *(Analyze Cues)*, and identify the client's immediate problem(s) *(Prioritize Hypotheses)*. Then you need to identify possible solutions to address the client's needs *(Generate Solutions)*, the appropriate actions to take *(Take Action)*, and parameters to monitor once actions have been taken *(Evaluate Outcomes)*.

NGN TIP

Remember: To answer a Bow-tie item, select from the middle well first, which in Sample Question 9.1 is the *Potential Condition*. To make the correct selection, identify relevant data and organize those data to determine what the client's condition is in the clinical scenario. Then review the choices under *Potential Conditions* and select the one that best matches your analysis. After selecting or dragging the client condition into the middle section of the Bow-tie figure, decide on the Nursing Actions that would be appropriate to manage the client condition and the Parameters that a nurse would need to monitor to determine if those actions were effective.

Sample Question 9.1 — Sample Bow-tie Item

Health History | Nurses' Notes | Vital Signs | Lab Results

A 53-year-old client undergoes a right lung wedge resection to remove a tumor. Biopsy results are pending but the tumor has caused moderate to severe pain in the right lung area. The client has no history of cancer and reports no history of cancer in the family. The client reports being a nurse and works at a home health agency as a visiting nurse. The medical history includes hyperlipidemia and taking atorvastatin 40 mg daily. No other medical or surgical history reported.

Health History | Nurses' Notes | Vital Signs | Lab Results

1100: Client was admitted to medical-surgical unit from the recovery unit following right wedge resection with one chest tube attached to a 3-chamber closed chest tube drainage system. Dressing covering the chest tube insertion site is occlusive, dry, and intact. 50 mL bloody drainage in the collection chamber, intermittent bubbling in the water seal chamber, gentle bubbling in the suction control chamber. Arousable and oriented, oxygen via NC at 2 L/min, HOB at 30 degrees.

VS: T = 98.6°F (37.0°C); HR = 80 BPM; RR = 20 bpm; BP = 118/70 mm Hg.

SpO_2 95% on 2 L oxygen. Pain 3/10 right chest tube insertion site, increases with deep breathing and coughing.

1200: The nurse notes that the client has dyspnea and reports an increase in pain to 5/10. Drainage in the collection control chamber is at 100 mL bloody drainage; there is continuous vigorous bubbling in the water seal chamber and gentle bubbling in the suction control chamber.

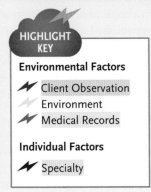

HIGHLIGHT KEY

Environmental Factors

⚡ Client Observation
⚡ Environment
⚡ Medical Records

Individual Factors

⚡ Specialty

Complete the diagram by dragging (or selecting) from the choices below one potential condition, two actions the nurse would **immediately** take to address the condition, and two parameters the nurse would monitor to assess the client's progress.

```
Action to Take ──┐                      ┌── Parameter to Monitor
                 ├── Potential Condition ┤
Action to Take ──┘                      └── Parameter to Monitor
```

Action to Take	Potential Condition	Parameter to Monitor
Clamp the tubing and determine location of the problem.	Bleeding	Chest x-ray
Apply pressure to the chest tube insertion site.	Air leak in the drainage system	Hemoglobin, hematocrit, platelets, red blood cells
Check for subcutaneous emphysema.	Displacement of the chest tube in the pleural space	Respiratory status, HR, BP, RR, SpO_2
Disconnect and submerge the chest tube in a bottle of sterile water.	Lung has re-expanded	Fluctuation and bubbling in the water seal chamber
Notify the surgeon.		Drainage amount in the collection chamber

Answers

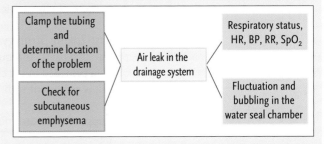

Rationale: A chest tube is a catheter inserted through the rib cage into the pleural space to remove air, fluid, or blood; to prevent air, or fluid from re-entering the pleural space; or to re-establish normal intrapleural pressure after trauma or surgery to promote lung re-expansion. After a chest tube is inserted, it is attached to a drainage system.

⚡THINKING SPACE

A traditional chest drainage system has three chambers: one for collection of drainage, one for maintaining a water seal, and one for suction control. The fluid in the collection chamber needs to be measured hourly for the first 24 hours after insertion by marking the drainage level in the collection chamber with a piece of tape or per agency procedure. Unless otherwise specified by the surgeon, drainage amounts greater than 70 to 100 mL per hour are a concern. Following lung resection, bloody drainage would be expected; but if the drainage changes to bright red or increases suddenly, bleeding is suspected and the surgeon is notified immediately. The water seal chamber prevents air from re-entering the client's pleural space. Fluctuation of the water (moves up as the client inhales and moves down as the client exhales) is expected. Intermittent bubbling in this chamber may be noted and indicates air leaving the pleural space.

If the lung has re-expanded the nurse would note that the fluctuation has stopped. A sign of a displaced chest tube is also absence of fluctuation. A chest x-ray would confirm either situation. However, continuous and vigorous bubbling indicates a leak in the drainage system or the presence of a pneumothorax. If this occurs, the nurse immediately assesses the system and the client to determine the location and extent of the leak. Leaks can occur outside the client's body (such as within the drain or tubing connections) or within the body (for instance, at the tube insertion site or inside the chest cavity). To determine the location of the leak, the nurse would clamp the tubing as close as possible to the client. If bubbling continues, the leak is in the tubing or there could be damage to the drainage device. If bubbling disappears when the tube is clamped, the air leak is likely at the insertion site or within the chest wall. With a significant internal air leak, the nurse would palpate subcutaneous emphysema or "crackling" (also known as crepitus) under the skin around the insertion site. If the leak is at the insertion site the nurse would apply petroleum gauze and a sterile occlusive dressing to seal it off. If the air leak is due to a cracked drainage system, the nurse would replace the system following agency procedure.

Whatever its source, an air leak needs to be addressed and resolved because of the risk of tension pneumothorax; this can result in cardiac tamponade—a life-threatening emergency. Once the nurse locates the air leak and takes actions to resolve it, the surgeon is notified. The nurse monitors the client's respiratory status, HR, BP, RR, and SpO$_2$ level. The nurse would also closely monitor the status of the water seal chamber, looking for fluctuations and the absence of continuous vigorous bubbling. If bleeding is suspected, depending on its location, pressure may need to be applied to the insertion site and the drainage amount will be monitored. In addition, laboratory values such as the hemoglobin, hematocrit, platelets, and red blood cells would be monitored to assess blood loss and the need for blood administration or surgical intervention. If a chest tube disconnected from the system, it would be submerged in a bottle of sterile water in order to maintain the water seal until the system could be re-established.

Test-Taking Strategy: To begin answering this question, organize your thought process into two parts. This question is asking you to decide on the potential condition based on data provided in the clinical scenario. Think about each assessment finding, and decide if it is consistent with the condition listed, as illustrated in the table.

Supportive Assessment Finding	Potential Condition
VS	N/A, WNL
Dyspnea	Bleeding, air leak in the drainage system, displacement of the chest tube in the pleural space
Increased pain	Bleeding, air leak in the drainage system, displacement of the chest tube in the pleural space
100 mL bloody drainage in collection control chamber	N/A, expected
Vigorous bubbling in the water seal chamber	Air leak in the drainage system
Gentle bubbling in suction control chamber	N/A, expected

N/A, Not applicable; *WNL,* within normal limits.

THINKING SPACE

The VS are within normal limits and therefore are not related to any of the potential conditions. The dyspnea could be related to bleeding, an air leak in the drainage system, or displacement of the chest tube in the pleural space. Increased pain could be related to bleeding, an air leak in the drainage system, and displacement of the chest tube in the pleural space. The 100 mL of bloody drainage in the collection control chamber is an expected finding, as is gentle bubbling in the suction control chamber. Vigorous bubbling in the water seal chamber is consistent with an air leak in the drainage system. Considering that most of the supportive assessment findings relate to an air leak in the drainage system, you should choose this as the potential condition. After you have identified the most likely potential condition, the second part of your thought process will be to decide on the most appropriate nursing actions for the care of the client with an air leak. To decide on the two interventions the nurse would immediately take, think about whether there are data to support performing each intervention, as illustrated in the table.

Immediate Action to Take	Supporting Data
Clamp the tubing.	Yes
Apply pressure to the chest tube insertion site.	No
Check for subcutaneous emphysema.	Yes
Disconnect and submerge the chest tube in a bottle of sterile water.	No
Notify the surgeon.	No

The dyspnea, increased pain, and vigorous bubbling in the water seal chamber are the data that support clamping the tubing to further assess for an air leak in the drainage system. There are no data supporting applying pressure to the chest tube insertion site. Because an air leak is suspected based on the assessment, there are data to support checking for subcutaneous emphysema. There are no data to support disconnecting and submerging the chest tube in a bottle of sterile water because the chest tube has not been dislodged from the chest. There are no data to support contacting the surgeon yet, until further assessment data are gathered. Next, you need to decide on additional parameters to monitor based on the actions you decided on. To help you with this, decide whether each listed parameter is directly related to either the condition or the nursing actions to assist in selecting the correct options, as illustrated in the table.

Parameter to Monitor	Related to Condition or Action
Chest x-ray	No—displacement of the chest tube in the pleural space and lung has re-expanded
Hemoglobin, hematocrit, platelets, red blood cells	No—bleeding
Respiratory status, HR, BP, RR, SpO$_2$	Yes
Fluctuation and bubbling in the water seal chamber	Yes
Drainage amount in the collection chamber	No—expected finding

The chest x-ray is not specifically related to an air leak in the chest drainage system, and is a distractor because this would be useful in assessing for displacement of the chest tube in the pleural space and also in assessing if the lung has re-expanded. The hemoglobin, hematocrit, platelets, and red blood cells are also a distractor because this would be useful in assessing for bleeding. The respiratory status, HR, BP, RR , and SpO$_2$ are important parameters to monitor for an air leak, as this information would enable the nurse to detect any complications of this problem. Fluctuation and bubbling in the water seal chamber is directly related, as this provides information about the functionality of the chest drainage system. The drainage amount in the collection chamber is an expected finding in this clinical scenario and therefore is not a parameter that needs to be monitored specific to the air leak.

Content Area: Medical-Surgical Nursing
Priority Concept: Gas Exchange
Reference(s): Ignatavicius et al., 2021, pp. 559–562; Potter et al., 2021, pp. 939–940; 965–971

Sample Question 9.2   Sample Bow-tie Item

| Health History | Nurses' Notes | Physician's Orders | Lab Results |

0800: A 52-year-old client arrived at the ED accompanied by the spouse and reports loss of appetite, weight loss, weakness, fatigue, and frequent nosebleeds. The client also reports occasional upper right abdominal discomfort. Past medical history includes type 2 DM, atrial fibrillation, and hypothyroidism. Client reports that the physician suspects nonalcoholic fatty liver disease (NAFLD). The client denies alcohol or drug use. States takes levothyroxine 112 mcg daily, apixaban 5 mg twice daily, and semaglutide 1 mg weekly. Reports that the recent HbA1c was 5.7.

1000: Client was admitted to medical-surgical unit. Assessment reveals yellow-colored skin and yellow sclera and the client reports itchy skin. Weblike clusters of enlarged blood vessels are noted under the skin on the face and abdomen.
VS: T = 99.2°F (37.3°C); HR = 88 BPM; RR = 22 bpm; BP = 120/68 mm Hg.
SpO_2 = 94% on RA, pain 2/10 right upper abdomen.
Weight 206 lb (93.44 kg) Height 5 ft 2 inches.

1030: The nurse is reviewing the client's admission history and Nurses' Notes to prepare the client's plan of care.

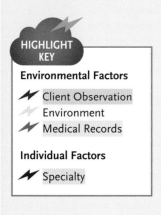

HIGHLIGHT KEY

Environmental Factors
⚡ Client Observation
⚡ Environment
⚡ Medical Records

Individual Factors
⚡ Specialty

*Complete the diagram by dragging (or selecting) from the choices below one potential complication the client is **most likely** experiencing, two **most likely** assessment findings that support that condition, and two potential interventions to treat the condition.*

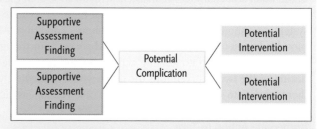

Supportive Assessment Finding	Potential Complication	Potential Intervention
Frequent nosebleeds	Variceal bleeding	Increase semaglutide dosage weekly
Jaundice	Hepatitis	Liver biopsy
Enlarged blood vessels just beneath the skin's surface	Nonalcoholic steatohepatitis (NASH)	Weight loss and exercise program
Weight 206 lb (93.44 kg)	Cirrhosis	Antihypertensive medication
Blood pressure		Medication to lower cholesterol levels

Answers

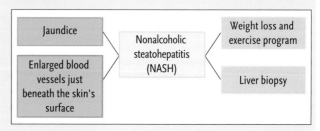

Rationale: NAFLD is a liver condition affecting individuals who drink little to no alcohol. The primary characteristic of the disorder is that in NAFLD, too much fat is stored in liver cells. The primary complication of fatty liver disease is the progression of NASH, an aggressive form of fatty liver disease, which is marked by liver inflammation and may progress to advanced scarring (cirrhosis) and liver failure. Symptoms of NASH may include severe tiredness, weakness, weight loss, yellowing of the skin or eyes (jaundice), weblike clusters of enlarged blood vessels on the skin, and itching. If NASH results in cirrhosis symptoms, fluid retention, internal bleeding, muscle wasting, and confusion occur. Cirrhosis can lead to liver failure and the need for a liver transplant. Some risk factors for fatty liver disease include obesity, diabetes or prediabetes, elevated cholesterol and triglyceride levels, and hypertension. Fatty liver disease may be suspected if liver function blood tests are abnormal and elevated.

Imaging studies such as ultrasound and magnetic resonance imaging may show fat deposits and scar tissue in the liver. However, the only way to be certain that fatty liver disease is present is with a liver biopsy. Based on analysis of the biopsy, if fat is present but no inflammation or tissue damage, the diagnosis is NAFLD. If fat, inflammation, and liver damage are present, the diagnosis is NASH. If there is scar tissue, known as fibrosis, it is probably developing cirrhosis. If the client has NASH, no medication is available to reverse the fat buildup in the liver. Although jaundice and visible blood vessels may be seen in cirrhosis, there is no evidence of fluid retention, internal bleeding, muscle wasting, or confusion; therefore cirrhosis is not a likely complication. There is also no evidence to suggest fibrosis. In some cases the liver damage stops or even reverses itself. However, in others the disease continues to progress. Therefore it is important to control any conditions that may contribute to fatty liver disease. Treatments and lifestyle changes may include weight loss, exercise, medication to reduce cholesterol or triglycerides and medications for hypertension if needed, medications to control diabetes if needed, limiting over-the-counter medications, avoiding alcohol, and consulting with a liver specialist. There is no supporting evidence that this client has variceal bleeding. Although the client has nosebleeds, these could be the result of altered coagulation studies or due to many other causes such as allergies. In addition, if the client had variceal bleeding, the client would most likely be vomiting blood. Although some of the client's symptoms are related to hepatitis, the client indicates that the physician suspects NAFLD, and hepatitis is not a complication of this health problem. The client's HbA1c was 5.7, which indicates good control of the diabetes. Therefore there is no reason to increase the semaglutide, which is an antidiabetic medication. The BP is normal, so there is no need for antihypertensive therapy. There is no evidence of hyperlipidemia, so medication to lower the cholesterol level is not indicated.

Test-Taking Strategy: To begin answering this question, organize your thought process into two parts. This question is asking you to decide on the potential complication based on the client's supportive assessment findings noted in the options. Think about each assessment finding and decide if it is consistent with the complications listed, as illustrated in the table.

Test-Taking Strategy

Supportive Assessment Finding	Potential Complication
Frequent nosebleeds	Coagulopathy
Jaundice	NASH, hepatitis, cirrhosis
Enlarged blood vessels just beneath the skin's surface	NASH, cirrhosis
Weight 206 lb (93.44 kg)	Nonspecific, although it is a risk factor for fatty liver disease
BP 120/68 mm Hg	Normal and therefore not related to a potential complication

⚡THINKING SPACE

The frequent nosebleeds are most likely related to coagulopathy from the client being on anticoagulant therapy. Jaundice could be related to NASH, hepatitis, and cirrhosis. Enlarged blood vessels beneath the skin surface could be related to NASH or cirrhosis. Weight, although nonspecific, is a risk factor for fatty liver disease. The BP is normal and therefore is not related to any potential complication. Considering that most supportive assessment findings relate to NASH and cirrhosis, you should choose NASH as the potential complication because there is no other evidence of cirrhosis, such as fluid retention, internal bleeding, muscle wasting, or confusion. After you have identified the most likely potential complication, the second part of your thought process will be to decide on the most appropriate nursing actions for the care of the client with NASH. To decide on the two interventions the nurse would perform, think about whether there are data to support performing each intervention, as illustrated in the table.

Potential Intervention	Supporting Data
Increase semaglutide dosage weekly	No
Liver biopsy	Yes
Weight loss and exercise program	Yes
Antihypertensive medication	No
Medication to lower cholesterol level	No

In NASH, a liver biopsy is needed to confirm this condition versus NAFLD; therefore there are supporting data to indicate the need for this test. Thinking about the pathophysiology and the causes of NASH, you would be able to determine that there are supporting data for the need for a weight loss and exercise program. The client's HbA1c is 5.7; therefore there are no data to support increasing the semaglutide. The client's BP is 120/68 mm Hg; therefore there are no supporting data for the need for an antihypertensive medication. There is no evidence of high cholesterol; therefore there are no data to support starting a medication for this.

Content Area: Medical-Surgical Nursing
Priority Concept: Tissue Integrity
Reference(s): Ignatavicius et al., 2021, p. 1158

Trend Item

Similar to the Bow-tie for the Stand-alone test items, the Trend item begins with a client situation that includes assessment data. The client information is presented in the form of a medical record, such as Nurses' Notes, medical history, physician orders, an I&O record, or laboratory and diagnostic tests. The difference between the Bow-tie and the Trend item is that the Trend item *presents data gathered over a period of time* rather than at one point in time. Therefore in the Trend item the candidate examines trends in data over time to determine changes in the client's condition. The Trend item can measure more than one cognitive skill in the item. In addition, any NGN item type (except a Bow-tie item) will be used in a Trend item. Samples of a Trend item are presented in Sample Question 9.3 and Sample Question 9.4.

Sample Question 9.3   Sample Trend Item

A 34-year-old G4P4 delivered their fourth baby 3 hours ago via vaginal delivery and was transferred to the postpartum unit. The postpartum nurse received hand-off report from the labor and delivery nurse.

Health History	Nurses' Notes	Physical Assessment	Lab Results

1100: Other children are 7, 5, and 2 years old. Epidural was used for pain management during labor. Labor was 8 hours, and membranes were artificially ruptured by the obstetrician. Oxytocin was administered to induce labor. Stage 2 vaginal laceration, which was repaired after delivery. Rh negative and Group B Streptococcus (GBS) negative. Last fundal assessment was firm, dark red lochia. Plans to breast-feed/chest-feed. Newborn's Apgar scores were 8, 9, and 9. Birth weight was 7 lb 12 oz (3.26 kg). First stool passed. Skin-to-skin care for 1 hour after birth, 3 feedings since birth. Erythromycin eye prophylaxis given, vitamin K injection administered.

The postpartum nurse reviews the medical record, performs a physical assessment, and documents the findings.

Health History	Nurses' Notes	Physical Assessment	Lab Results

1115:
Breast: Soft, no pain to palpation.
Breath sounds: Clear to auscultation.
Fundus: Firm, midline, at level of umbilicus.
Lochia: Lochia rubra, dark red.
Perineum: Laceration well approximated with sutures in place. Reports mild pain to the area.
Bladder: No bladder distention.
Abdomen: Soft, active bowel sounds in all quadrants.
Lower extremities: Deep tendon reflexes 1+, peripheral edema 1+ nonpitting.

1130:
Breast: Soft, no pain to palpation.
Breath sounds: Clear to auscultation.
Fundus: Firm, midline, at level of umbilicus.
Lochia: Lochia rubra, dark red.
Perineum: Laceration well approximated with sutures in place. Reports mild pain to the area.
Bladder: Has not voided, slight bladder distention.
Abdomen: Soft, active bowel sounds in all quadrants.
Lower extremities: Deep tendon reflexes 1+, peripheral edema 1+ nonpitting.

1145:
Breast: Soft, no pain to palpation.
Breath sounds: Clear to auscultation.
Fundus: Soft, boggy, deviated laterally to the left.
Lochia: Large clots, large amount of lochia rubra, dark red.
Perineum: Laceration well approximated with sutures in place. Reports mild pain to the area.
Bladder: Bladder distention noted on palpation of the abdomen.
Abdomen: Soft, active bowel sounds in all quadrants.
Lower extremities: Deep tendon reflexes 1+, peripheral edema 1+ nonpitting.

At the 1145 time point, click to specify which findings would be expected, indicating normal postpartum progression, and which findings would be unexpected, indicating a **need for follow-up.**

Assessment Finding	Expected	Indicates a Need for Follow-up
Breast	☒	☐
Breath sounds	☒	☐
Fundus	☐	☒
Lochia	☐	☒
Perineum	☒	☐
Bladder	☐	☒
Abdomen	☒	☐
Lower extremities	☒	☐

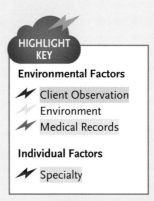

HIGHLIGHT KEY

Environmental Factors
⚡ Client Observation
⚡ Environment
⚡ Medical Records

Individual Factors
⚡ Specialty

 NGN TIP

Remember: Any NGN item type (except a Bow-tie item) is used in a Trend item. This sample Trend item provides client data in the form of a medical record presenting physical assessment data over time. The item type for this question is a Matrix Multiple Choice. In this item type, you need to select one response option for each row.

Rationale: The nurse needs to consider all assessment findings and how they relate to one another, to decide what could be happening with the client and to plan care accordingly. In comparing the findings at 1145 with previous assessment findings, the nurse would determine that there are changes, specifically with the fundus, the lochia, and the bladder assessment findings. Breasts are expected to be soft without pain to palpation during the first 1 to 2 days. On days 2 to 3 they are filling, and on days 3 to 5 they are full but soften with breast-feeding/chest-feeding. There should be no firmness, heat, pain, or engorgement of the breasts. Breath sounds should be clear to auscultation; crackles could indicate possible fluid overload, which can occur after oxytocin administration and would require follow-up. The fundus should be firm and midline and should involute approximately 1 cm or 1 finger-breadth per day. If it is soft, boggy, or higher than the expected level, this could indicate uterine atony. The lochia should be dark red, also known as lochia rubra, on days 1 to 3. On days 4 to 10 it changes to lochia serosa, which is brownish red or pink. After 10 days it changes to lochia alba, which is yellowish white. There may be a few clots, and sometimes there is a fleshy odor. Unexpected findings include a large amount of lochia, large clots, or foul odor. Any of these findings could indicate uterine atony or infection. Expected findings for the perineum would include minimal edema, and if a laceration or episiotomy is present, the edges should be approximated and any pain controlled by analgesics and nonpharmacologic interventions. Unexpected findings would be pronounced edema, bruising, hematoma, redness, warmth, or drainage, which could indicate bleeding or infection. The client should be able to void and there should not be bladder distention noted. An overdistended bladder could cause lateral fundal displacement, uterine atony, and excessive lochia. The abdomen should be soft with active bowel sounds in all quadrants. The client should expect to have a bowel movement by day 2 or 3 after birth. The lower extremities may have peripheral edema from the fluid and medications. Deep tendon reflexes should be 1+ to 2+. There should be no pain, tenderness, redness, or thrombophlebitis. The assessment findings in this scenario that are expected are the findings related to the breast, breath sounds, perineum, abdomen, and lower extremities; and the assessment findings indicating the need for follow-up are the findings related to the fundus, lochia, and bladder.

Test-Taking Strategy: Note that this question is asking you about assessment findings that are expected or indicate the need for follow-up in the postpartum period. This question is testing you on whether you can recognize signs of a complication. As illustrated in the table, categorize the assessment findings based on the complication you suspect, if any.

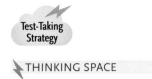

Test-Taking Strategy

THINKING SPACE

Assessment Finding	Possible Complication
Breast	N/A—expected as milk is being produced
Breath sounds	N/A—normal assessment finding
Fundus	Uterine atony
Lochia	Uterine atony/bleeding
Perineum	N/A—expected after vaginal birth
Bladder	Uterine atony due to bladder distension and lateral fundal displacement
Abdomen	N/A—normal assessment finding
Lower extremities	N/A—expected after oxytocin and fluid administration

N/A, Not applicable.

The assessment findings that would be noted with one of the complications would then be those that you select as indicating a need for follow-up, whereas the findings that are not clearly associated with a possible complication would be selected as normal or expected. Note that although an assessment finding could be abnormal, such as with the peripheral edema, it could still be expected. Peripheral edema is expected after oxytocin and fluid administration in the postpartum period and therefore does not require follow-up at this time. This thinking process can be applied to the assessment findings for the breast and perineum as well. The breath sounds and abdomen are normal assessment findings.

Content Area: Maternal-Newborn Nursing
Priority Concept: Perfusion
Reference(s): Lowdermilk et al., 2020, pp. 425–427

The nurse on the pediatric medical-surgical nursing unit is caring for a 12-year-old child admitted 2 days ago with acute post-streptococcal glomerulonephritis (APSGN). The child is being treated with medications, low-sodium diet, and close monitoring. At 0900, the nurse performs an assessment and reviews the results of the laboratory studies done early in the day and then compares findings with those done the day of admission.

Health History	Vital Signs	Nurses' Notes	Laboratory Tests

Blood Test	Normal Reference Range
Sodium	135–145 mEq/L (135–145 mmol/L)
Potassium	3.5-5.0 mEq/L (3.5–5.0 mmol/L)
Blood urea nitrogen	10–20 mg/dL (3.6–7.1 mmol/L)
Creatinine	0.5–1.2 mg/dL (44–106 mcmol/L)
ASO titer	<200; In children under the age of 5, <100

Urinalysis	Normal Reference Range
Specific gravity	1.003-1.030
Bilirubin	Negative
Glucose	Negative
Hemoglobin	Negative
pH	4.0-8.0
Protein	0-trace
Leukocytes	Negative
Nitrites	Negative
Bacteria	Negative

NGN TIP

Remember: Any NGN item type (except a Bow-tie item) is used in a Trend item. This sample Trend item provides client data in the form of a medical record presenting admission assessment data and present assessment data. This sample measures the cognitive skills *Recognize Cues* and *Evaluate Outcomes*. The item type for this question is a Highlight in Text. In this item type, you need to select parts of the text based on what the question is asking you to select. For this question, you need to select the findings that indicate improvement in the child's condition.

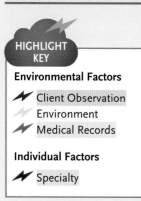

HIGHLIGHT KEY

Environmental Factors
✦ Client Observation
✦ Environment
✦ Medical Records

Individual Factors
✦ Specialty

At the **present time,** click to highlight the findings that indicate improvement in the child's condition.

	Admission	Present
VS	T: 98.7°F (37.0°C) HR: 98 BPM RR: 18 bpm BP: 158/88 mm Hg SpO₂: 99% on RA	T: 98.9°F (37.2°C) HR: 92 BPM RR: 18 bpm BP: 116/70 mm Hg SpO₂: 99% on RA
Physical assessment	Weight: 100 lb; appears lethargic Periorbital edema present Oropharynx red, erythematous, with positive exudate Neck: Anterior cervical lymphadenopathy Respiratory: Lungs clear to auscultation bilaterally Cardiovascular: Radial and pedal pulses 2+; 3+ pitting edema to bilateral lower extremities GI: Abdomen flat, nondistended; bowel sounds present × 4 quadrants Renal/urinary: Dark urine noted; urine output = 15 mL/hr	Weight: 95 lb; alert, active No periorbital edema present Oropharynx pink and moist Neck: No lymphadenopathy Respiratory: Lungs clear to auscultation bilaterally Cardiovascular: Radial and pedal pulses 2+; 1+ pitting edema to bilateral lower extremities GI: Abdomen flat, nondistended; bowel sounds present × 4 quadrants Renal/urinary: Clear yellow urine noted; urine output = 30 mL/hr
Laboratory results	Sodium: 138 mEq/L (138 mmol/L) Potassium: 3.9 mEq/L (3.9 mmol/L) Blood urea nitrogen: 32 mg/dL (11.4 mmol/L) Creatinine: 2.0 mg/dL (176.7 mcmol/L) ASO titer: 480 Todd units **Urinalysis:** Specific gravity 1.040 Bilirubin: Negative Glucose: Negative Hemoglobin: Positive pH: 6.0 Protein: 3+ Leukocytes: Negative Nitrites: Negative Bacteria: Negative	Sodium: 138 mEq/L (138 mmol/L) Potassium: 3.9 mEq/L (3.9 mmol/L) Blood urea nitrogen: 22 mg/dL (7.8 mmol/L) Creatinine: 1.6 mg/dL (141.3 mcmol/L) ASO titer: 140 Todd units **Urinalysis:** Specific gravity: 1.030 Bilirubin: Negative Glucose: Negative Hemoglobin: Negative pH: 6.0 Protein: Trace Leukocytes: Negative Nitrites: Negative Bacteria: Negative

▶THINKING SPACE

Rationale: Acute glomerulonephritis can occur on its own or can occur secondary to another disorder, and can range from mild to severe. Common features include oliguria, edema, hypertension, circulatory congestion, hematuria, and proteinuria. A common cause is streptococcal infection, resulting in APSGN. This occurs primarily in school-age children, and is uncommon in children younger than 3 years. APSGN usually occurs 1 to 2 weeks following a throat infection and 3 to 6 weeks following a skin infection. Often the association with the infection is not recognized because of the latent period between the infection and the nephritis. The infection can sometimes still be present with APSGN. Initial signs include facial puffiness with periorbital edema, anorexia, decreased urine output, and cola-colored urine. The client also exhibits paleness, irritability, lethargy, and overall unwell appearance. Facial edema is prominent in the morning and then spreads to the extremities, abdomen, and genitalia throughout the day. BP may be elevated (mildly to severely), and severe symptoms may include hypertensive encephalopathy, pulmonary and circulatory congestion, or hematuria. The initial signs of improvement in the child with APSGN are increased urinary output, decreased body weight, improved appetite, decreased BP, and decreased gross hematuria. During the acute phase, urinalysis reveals hematuria, proteinuria, and increased specific gravity. The urine is discolored and red blood cells are present, along with leukocytes, epithelial cells, and red blood cell casts. Bacteria are not present and urine cultures are negative. Throat cultures of the pharynx may be positive for streptococci. Electrolyte levels may be normal or may be out of range. Blood urea nitrogen and creatinine levels may be elevated with kidney injury. The antistreptolysin O (ASO) titer will be elevated. The chest x-ray may show cardiac enlargement, pulmonary congestion, and pleural effusion during the acute phase of the disease. Therapeutic management involves rest; improving fluid balance by monitoring VS, body weight, and I&O; and administering diuretics if fluid volume overload is present. Antihypertensives and anticonvulsants may be needed in severe disease. A decreased sodium diet is needed for clients with hypertension and edema. Antibiotic therapy is used for children with confirmed streptococcal infection.

Findings that indicate improvement in the child's condition with treatment include:

- *VS:* All VS were within normal limits at admission except the BP and are normal at present. The BP has improved with treatment.
- *Physical assessment:* The child has lost weight as the fluid balance has improved. The mental status has improved, as the child is no longer lethargic and rather is alert and active. The oropharynx is pink and moist and now without exudates, and there is no longer lymphadenopathy, indicating that the antibiotics are helping the infection. The edema in the lower extremities is decreasing, indicating that fluid balance is improving. The urine color has normalized and the urine output is increasing, which are indicators of improved fluid balance and renal function. All other findings on the physical assessment were normal at admission and are normal at present.
- *Laboratory results:* The electrolytes were normal at admission and remain normal at present. The blood urea nitrogen and creatinine levels were elevated and are improving with treatment. The ASO titer is also decreasing, an indicator of improvement. The specific gravity is improving, which indicates improved fluid balance. Hemoglobin is no longer detectable in the urine and the protein is decreasing as well, which indicate improvement in the condition. Other results on the urinalysis were normal at admission and are normal at present.

Test-Taking Strategy: Note that this question is asking you about assessment findings that indicate improvement in the child's condition. This question is testing you on whether you can recognize abnormalities and then whether you can determine trends and changes in those findings and evaluate improvement, decline, or no change. As illustrated in the table, categorize the assessment findings as an improvement, a decline, unchanged, or unrelated.

Test-Taking
Strategy

THINKING SPACE

Assessment Finding	Improvement, Decline, Unchanged/Unrelated
T: 98.9°F (37.2°C)	Unchanged/Unrelated
HR: 92 BPM	Unchanged/Unrelated
RR: 18 bpm	Unchanged/Unrelated
BP: 116/70 mm Hg	Improvement
SpO$_2$: 99% on RA	Unchanged/Unrelated
Weight: 95 lb	Improvement
No periorbital edema present	Improvement
Oropharynx pink and moist	Improvement
No lymphadenopathy	Improvement
Lungs clear to auscultation bilaterally	Unchanged/Unrelated
Radial and pedal pulses 2+	Unchanged/Unrelated
1+ pitting edema to bilateral lower extremities	Improvement
Abdomen flat, nondistended	Unchanged/Unrelated
Bowel sounds present × 4 quadrants	Unchanged/Unrelated
Clear yellow urine	Improvement
Urine output: 30 mL/hr	Improvement
Sodium: 138 mEq/L (138 mmol/L)	Unchanged/Unrelated
Potassium: 3.9 mEq/L (3.9 mmol/L)	Unchanged/Unrelated
Blood urea nitrogen: 22 mg/dL (7.8 mmol/L)	Improvement
Creatinine: 1.6 mg/dL (141.3 mcmol/L)	Improvement
ASO titer: 140 Todd units	Improvement
Specific gravity: 1.030	Improvement
Bilirubin: Negative	Unchanged/Unrelated
Glucose: Negative	Unchanged/Unrelated
Hemoglobin: Negative	Improvement
pH: 6.0	Unchanged/Unrelated
Protein: Trace	Improvement
Leukocytes: Negative	Unchanged/Unrelated
Nitrites: Negative	Unchanged/Unrelated
Bacteria: negative	Unchanged/Unrelated

The assessment findings that indicate an improvement would be the ones that you would select or highlight as the answers to this question. Note that there are not any assessment findings indicating a decline, whereas there are many findings that are unchanged or unrelated. Any findings that are unchanged or unrelated would not be highlighted.

Content Area: Pediatric Nursing
Priority Concept: Fluid and Electrolyte Balance
Reference(s): Hockenberry et al., 2019, pp. 791–795

What Are Unfolding Case Studies?

The Unfolding Case Study presents the client situation *over time* through several phases of care in the clinical scenario. It is often referred to as the NGN Case Study. The time between phases can be minutes, hours, or even days. The client may initially be evaluated in an ED, in an acute care hospital, in a clinic, at school, in an urgent care center, or at home. As the scenario changes, or "unfolds," NGN test items require you to use all of the information, including the information in the current phase of the client's care, to answer each question. On the NCLEX® you will always have access to the case study, including all of the phases as the case emerges and unfolds. Nursing candidates are expected to have three NGN Case Studies with six questions each on the NCLEX®. Each of the six questions represents one of the CJ cognitive skills.

As described in Chapter 1, the Unfolding Case Study presents a client with initial data describing the clinical situation. These data will typically be part of a client's medical record. The client will either be experiencing an urgent or emergent health problem or will be at risk for experiencing an urgent or emergent health problem. You will need the information in the initial clinical scenario to answer the first NGN test item that will measure the CJ cognitive skill *Recognize Cues*. The second NGN test item will measure your ability to *Analyze Cues,* those cues you recognized as relevant. As the clinical scenario continues, the client's condition will change over time (minutes, hours, days) through several phases of care, and new information will be presented as the case unfolds. Four additional NGN test items will follow and measure the remaining CJ cognitive skills *(Prioritize Hypotheses, Generate Solutions, Take Action, Evaluate Outcomes)* based on what client data are provided. Sample Questions 9.5, 9.6, 9.7, 9.8, 9.9, and 9.10 accompany an Unfolding Case Study in which a client's condition changes and requires immediate intervention during the home visit by the nurse.

How Are Stand-alone Items and Unfolding Case Studies Different?

There are similarities and differences between Stand-alone items and Unfolding Case Studies. According to the NCSBN, every candidate tested will be administered three Unfolding Case Studies, each with six questions testing each cognitive skill identified in the NCJMM. Not all candidates will receive Stand-alone items. The competency level determined as the test taker proceeds through the exam governs whether or not Stand-alone items will be presented. Box 9.2 illustrates these similarities and differences.

BOX 9.2 Stand-alone Items and Unfolding Case Studies: Similarities and Differences

Stand-alone Items	Unfolding Case Studies
Present a realistic clinical situation commonly encountered in practice by the new nursing graduate.	Present a realistic clinical situation commonly encountered in practice by the new nursing graduate.
The clinical situation is accompanied by one item, either a Bow-tie or a Trend item.	The case is accompanied by six NGN items.
The Bow-tie item provides a client situation at *one point in time,* and the Trend item presents client information such as VS, assessment findings, and I&O information *over time.*	Presents the client's story *over time* through several phases of care in the clinical situation. The time between phases can be minutes, hours, or even days.
Information will be presented in a medical record format.	Information will be presented in a medical record format.

Sample Question 9.5   Unfolding Case Study: Question 1: Recognize Cues—Highlight in Text

0700: The nurse plans a visit to a client who was discharged from the hospital 1 week ago. The nurse reviews the discharge summary in the medical record and the Nurses' Notes from the previous home visit done on the day after hospital discharge.

Health History	Nurses' Notes	Diagnostic Results	Discharge Summary

1 week ago: This 32-year-old client sustained a T6 spinal cord injury 3 months ago from a motor vehicle crash that caused paralysis of the lower body. The client was sideswiped by a truck, which caused the car to roll over 3 times and end up in a ditch off the roadway. The client was pinned in the car, and the front end and side of the car crushed the lower half of their body. The client was hospitalized for 3 months. During hospitalization, emergency treatment was administered, and once stabilized, the client was monitored for complications. The client received rehabilitative therapy including PT and OT, and home care services were initiated for discharge. The client is married, and the client's spouse stays at home caring for their two children, ages 7 and 10. Prior to the injury, the client was a forklift driver at an industrial manufacturing company. The client has no previous medical history, does not take any medications, does not smoke, and drinks occasionally at social gatherings.

Health History	Nurses' Notes	Diagnostic Results	Discharge Summary

One day post-discharge: Client alert and oriented. Sitting up in wheelchair. Reports using a transfer board, with spouse's assistance, to get out of bed to the wheelchair. Reports sitting in the wheelchair all day. Reports fair appetite and is drinking fluids. Complains of tiredness and falling asleep in the wheelchair during the day. Reports sweating during the night, which wakes the client; once repositioning to the side, the sweating stops but has difficulty falling back to sleep. Complains of muscle spasms in the lower body. No complaints of headache. Reports self-catheterizes every 6 hours. Last bowel movement was on the day of hospital discharge. VS: T = 98.6°F (37.0°C); HR = 86 BPM; RR = 18 bpm; BP = 120/78 mm Hg

1000: The nurse arrives at the client's home and after introductions performs a focused assessment.

*Highlight the findings in the assessment that are of **immediate** concern.*

Health History	Nurses' Notes	Diagnostic Results	Discharge Summary

VS: T = 99.2°F (37.3°C); HR = 60 BPM; RR = 18 bpm; BP = 150/90 mm Hg. Alert and oriented. Reports poor appetite over the last few days and is nauseated. Complains of tiredness and continued sweating during the night. Muscle spasms in the lower body worsening and was incontinent once during the night. Reports feeling as though is getting the flu because of nausea, nasal stuffiness, and pounding headaches. States last bowel movement was 4 days ago.

HIGHLIGHT KEY

Environmental Factors

⚡ Client Observation

⚡ Environment

⚡ Medical Records

Individual Factors

⚡ Specialty

Rationale: Spinal cord injury is caused by trauma to the spinal cord that leads to partial or complete disruption of the nerve tracts and neurons. Following the injury, spinal cord edema develops and necrosis can develop as a result of compromised capillary circulation and venous return. Loss of motor function, sensation, reflex activity, and bowel and bladder function may result. Common causes of spinal cord injury include motor vehicle crashes, falls, sporting and industrial accidents, and gunshot or stab wounds. The client's temperature is slightly elevated at 99.2°F (37.3°C), and the client is at risk for infection, specifically a UTI. The client had an episode of incontinence and is self-catheterizing, increasing this risk. The client's pulse rate is at the low level of normal and is a concern because the baseline is 86 BPM. Respirations are unchanged and not a concern. The client's BP is elevated from baseline and would be an immediate concern for the nurse. Other immediate concerns for this client would be the report of nausea, continued sweating, worsening muscle spasms, and incontinence. Other new and concerning findings are the nasal stuffiness, pounding headache, and constipation.

Test-Taking Strategy: Remember to first identify normal/usual or abnormal and expected (not relevant), and abnormal and not expected (relevant) client findings requiring follow-up. The client's findings can be categorized as shown in the table.

THINKING SPACE

Test-Taking Strategy

Client Finding	Normal/Usual or Abnormal and Expected (Not Relevant)	Abnormal and Not Expected (Relevant Requiring Follow-up)
T = 99.2°F (37.3°C)	☐	☒
HR = 60 BPM	☐	☒
RR = 18 bpm	☒	
BP = 150/90 mm Hg	☐	☒
Alert and oriented	☒	
Reports poor appetite over the last few days and is nauseated	☐	☒
Complains of tiredness and continued sweating during the night	☐	☒
Muscle spasms in the lower body worsening	☐	☒
Incontinent once during the night	☐	☒
Nausea, nasal stuffiness, and pounding headaches	☐	☒
States last bowel movement was 4 days ago.	☐	☒

Thinking about what could be happening to the client will help you determine which findings are expected versus those that are unexpected. Unexpected findings are the parts of the Nurses' Notes that should be highlighted in this question.

Content Area: Medical-Surgical Nursing
Priority Concept: Perfusion
Reference(s): Ignatavicius et al., 2021, p. 880

| Sample Question 9.6 | Unfolding Case Study: Question 2: Analyze Cues—Drop-Down Rationale |

1020: The nurse analyzes the assessment findings that are of immediate concern to make an interpretation about the client's condition.

Complete the following sentence by choosing from the list of options.

The nurse determines that the client assessment findings would *most likely* be the result of <u>noxious stimuli</u> caused by the <u>constipation</u>.

Options for 1	Options for 2
Anxiety	Infection
Noxious stimuli	Paralysis
Urinary incontinence	Constipation
Further spinal cord damage	Worsening muscle spasms

THINKING SPACE

Test-Taking Strategy

Rationale: Autonomic dysreflexia, sometimes referred to as autonomic hyperreflexia, is a potentially life-threatening condition in which noxious visceral or cutaneous stimuli cause a sudden massive, uninhibited reflex sympathetic discharge in people with high-level spinal cord injury. Some symptoms include a pounding headache; flushed face and/or red blotches on the skin above the level of spinal cord injury; sweating above the level of spinal cord injury; nasal stuffiness; nausea; a slow HR; goose bumps below the level of spinal cord injury; and cold, clammy skin below the level of spinal cord injury. The causes of autonomic dysreflexia are typically GI, gynecologic-urologic, and vascular stimulation. Specific risk factors are bladder distention, UTI, epididymitis or scrotal compression, bowel distention or impaction from constipation, or irritation from hemorrhoids. Pain; circumferential constriction of the thorax, abdomen, or an extremity (such as tight clothing); contact with hard or sharp objects; and temperature fluctuations can also cause autonomic dysreflexia. There is no information that indicates that the client has anxiety. Further spinal cord damage is unlikely unless another injury occurred; in addition, the client's assessment findings do not indicate that this is the case.

Test-Taking Strategy: Begin answering this question by noting that you have to select the correct option for the first part of the question in order to answer the question correctly. Thinking about the description in the clinical situation and assessment findings, decide whether each option could be a cause of those signs or symptoms.

Option	Possible Explanation of Signs/Symptoms
Anxiety	No
Noxious stimuli	Yes
Urinary incontinence	No
Further spinal cord damage	No

Anxiety and urinary incontinence could occur as a result of autonomic dysreflexia but are not a cause. Bladder distention, however, is a cause. Further spinal cord damage would be caused by additional injury but not by autonomic dysreflexia as a complication of an existing spinal cord injury. Next, you need to use your nursing knowledge to determine which factors precipitate autonomic dysreflexia. Remember *GGUV*—GI, gynecologic-urologic, and vascular; thus constipation is a precipitant of this complication.

Content Area: Medical-Surgical Nursing
Priority Concept: Perfusion
Reference(s): Ignatavicius et al., 2021, p. 880

Sample Question 9.7	Unfolding Case Study: Question 3: Prioritize Hypotheses—Multiple Response Select N

1030: The nurse reviews the findings from the focused assessment done on the client and identifies the potential risk conditions of concern.

*The client is at **highest risk** for developing which three conditions?*

- ☒ Infection
- ☐ Malnutrition
- ☐ Spinal shock
- ☐ Hyperthermia
- ☒ Skin breakdown
- ☐ Neurogenic shock
- ☒ Autonomic dysreflexia

Rationale: Based on the client assessment data, the client is exhibiting signs of autonomic dysreflexia, an abrupt, uncontrolled sympathetic response, elicited by stimuli below the level of injury. The client is also at risk for skin breakdown because of a report of sitting in the wheelchair all day. In addition, the client is at risk for infection, specifically a UTI. The client reports an episode of incontinence, and there is a slight increase in the temperature. Catheterization every 6 hours also places the client at risk. Although the client reports nausea and a poor appetite, there is no evidence that malnutrition is a risk. Spinal shock occurs immediately after the injury as the cord's response to the injury. This client's injury occurred 3 months ago. Clients who sustained a spinal cord injury can experience abnormal temperature control as either hypothermia or hyperthermia. Although this client is experiencing some disturbances of sweating, there are no extreme temperature fluctuations occurring; this requires monitoring but is not a high priority at this time. Neurogenic shock is a type of distributive shock, characterized by hypotension, bradycardia, and peripheral vasodilation and attributed to severe central nervous system damage such as head or cervical cord trauma, or high thoracic cord injuries. Although the client has a low pulse rate, there are no data indicating that this condition is a risk.

Test-Taking Strategy: Thinking about autonomic dysreflexia as the most likely complication occurring in this clinical scenario, consider each option and how it may or may not be pertinent. Also note that the question asks for the *highest risk,* which means that some or all of the options may be correct, but you need to decide on the three most important in this situation. Using the thinking process illustrated in the table, first determine whether the option could be a potential problem as it relates to spinal cord injury, and then from there, whether there are supporting data for that problem.

THINKING SPACE

Test-Taking Strategy

Option	Related/Unrelated	Supporting Data
Infection	Related	Yes
Malnutrition	Related	No
Spinal shock	Related	No
Hyperthermia	Related	No
Skin breakdown	Related	Yes
Neurogenic shock	Related	No
Autonomic dysreflexia	Related	Yes

If you determine that the option is related and supporting data are present, it is likely correct. Also, note that this question asks for a specific number of options to choose. As you can see, all options are related in some way, so it is really important to rely on the available data to determine the highest priorities. The only three options with data to support that they are happening are infection, skin breakdown, and autonomic dysreflexia.

Content Area: Medical-Surgical Nursing
Priority Concept: Perfusion
Reference(s): Ignatavicius et al., 2021, pp. 877–881

1040: Based on the highest-risk conditions, the nurse quickly prepares a plan of care for the client and potential interventions.

For each potential intervention, click to specify whether the intervention is indicated or contraindicated in the care of the client.

Potential Intervention	Indicated	Contraindicated
Assist the client in getting back into bed, and position supine.	☐	☒
Check the BP frequently.	☒	☐
Check for bladder distention.	☒	☐
Check for bowel impaction.	☒	☐
Contact the physician.	☒	☐
Place cold packs on the back of the client's neck and in the axilla areas.	☐	☒
Administer sublingual nifedipine.	☐	☒

⚡THINKING SPACE

Rationale: The client is exhibiting symptoms of autonomic dysreflexia including a lower than baseline HR at 60 BPM, BP of 150/90 mm Hg, sweating during the night, nausea, nasal stuffiness, and pounding headaches. The client also reports that the last bowel movement was 4 days ago so the client could be experiencing a bowel impaction, a cause of autonomic dysreflexia. Other risk factors include bladder distention, and the nurse would plan to assess for this occurrence. The nurse would plan to notify the physician and obtain orders for additional interventions if necessary. The nurse would sit the client up because a supine position will exacerbate the hypertension. The nurse would also plan to monitor the BP frequently. If BP elevation does not exceed 150/90 mm Hg, the client should continue to be observed. If the BP exceeds 150/100 mm Hg and a cause is either not found or found but not likely to be eliminated quickly, pharmacologic treatment should be initiated. If BP elevation is between 150/100 and 180/120 mm Hg, the client may be treated with sublingual nifedipine. Because a likely cause is known for this client and because the BP is 150/90 mm Hg, nifedipine is contraindicated at this time. Clients who sustained a spinal cord injury can experience abnormal temperature control as either hypothermia or hyperthermia. Cold packs would cause chills and shaking and could lead to unwanted alterations in temperature.

Test-Taking Strategy

Test-Taking Strategy: Note that this question is asking you to identify potential interventions that are indicated and those that are contraindicated. For each action, think about whether that action could improve/would be necessary or would worsen the autonomic dysreflexia. Remember *GGUV*—GI, gynecologic-urologic, and vascular—and organize your thought process as illustrated in the table.

Potential Intervention	Improve/Necessary or Worsen
Assist the client in getting back into bed, and position supine.	Worsen
Check the BP frequently.	Improve/Necessary
Check for bladder distention.	Improve/Necessary
Check for bowel impaction.	Improve/Necessary
Contact the physician.	Improve/Necessary
Place cold packs on the back of the client's neck and in the axilla areas.	Worsen
Administer sublingual nifedipine.	Worsen

Remember that positioning is important for managing BP abnormalities. Recall that temperature changes can worsen the condition. Note that the BP needs to exceed a certain parameter before antihypertensive medications would be indicated.

Content Area: Medical-Surgical Nursing
Priority Concept: Perfusion
Reference(s): Ignatavicius et al., 2021, pp. 877–881

Sample Question 9.9	Unfolding Case Study: Question 5: Take Action—Multiple Response Select All That Apply
1040: The nurse quickly considers the plan of care and intervenes to manage the complication the client is experiencing.	*Which actions would the nurse perform **immediately?** Select all that apply.* ☒ Catheterize the client. ☒ Loosen the client's clothing. ☒ Remove impacted stool digitally. ☒ Help into bed in an upright position. ☐ Send a urine specimen to the lab for culture and sensitivity. ☐ Teach the client about the measures to prevent autonomic dysreflexia. ☐ Call EMS to transport the client to the hospital.

Rationale: Autonomic dysreflexia is a potentially life-threatening condition in which noxious visceral or cutaneous stimuli cause a sudden massive, uninhibited reflex sympathetic discharge in people with high-level spinal cord injury. The causes of autonomic dysreflexia are typically GI, gynecologic-urologic, and vascular stimulation. Specific risk factors are bladder distention, UTI, epididymitis or scrotal compression, bowel distention or impaction from constipation, or irritation from hemorrhoids. The nurse would immediately take actions to decrease the client's BP and identify and eliminate the noxious stimuli. The client would be helped back into bed in a head-elevated position so as to prevent further increases in the BP. The nurse would loosen clothing because tight clothing causes cutaneous stimulation. The nurse would assess for bladder distention and catheterize the client and digitally remove stool. It is not necessary to call EMS unless immediate measures do not resolve the condition and the condition becomes life-threatening. There are no orders for a culture and sensitivity of the urine, although the physician may prescribe this to rule out UTI. The nurse would obtain the urine specimen and discuss this intervention with the physician; this, however, would not be an immediate intervention. The nurse would teach the client about measures to prevent autonomic dysreflexia, but this is not an immediate intervention; measures to resolve the complication are the priority.

THINKING SPACE

Test-Taking Strategy: Note the strategic word *immediately*. Knowing that the client is experiencing the complication of autonomic dysreflexia, decide whether each listed intervention would address this complication. Remember *GGUV*—GI, gynecologic-urologic, and vascular—and organize your thinking process as noted in the table.

Test-Taking Strategy

Immediate Nursing Action	GGUV
Catheterize the client.	GU
Loosen the client's clothing.	V
Remove impacted stool digitally.	G
Help into bed in an upright position.	V
Send a urine specimen to the lab for culture and sensitivity.	N/A
Teach the client about the measures to prevent autonomic dysreflexia.	N/A
Call EMS to transport the client to the hospital.	N/A

GGUV, GI, gynecologic, urologic, and vascular; *N/A*, not applicable.

Note that catheterizing the client, loosening the client's clothing, removing impacted stool digitally, and assisting to an upright position address GGUV and are the immediate actions. Sending a urine culture, teaching the client about the measures to prevent autonomic dysreflexia, and calling EMS do not directly address the cause and therefore should be eliminated.

Content Area: Medical-Surgical Nursing
Priority Concept: Perfusion
Reference(s): Ignatavicius et al., 2021, pp. 877–881

Sample Question 9.10   Unfolding Case Study: Question 6: Evaluate Outcomes—Matrix Multiple Choice

1050: The nurse has performed the interventions, assesses the client, and makes the following notations in the Nurses' Notes.

Health History	Nurses' Notes	Physician's Orders	Lab Results

VS: T = 99.2°F (37.3°C); HR = 78 BPM; RR = 18 bpm; BP = 132/78 mm Hg.
Client assisted to bed; sitting upright.
Bladder distended, 400 mL urine output via catheterization.
Urine obtained for culture and sensitivity pending physician's order.
Moderate amount of stool removed digitally.
Client teaching initiated about the measures to prevent autonomic dysreflexia.
Reports a mild headache and nasal stuffiness.

1100: The nurse teaches the client about measures to take to prevent episodes of autonomic dysreflexia.

Which client statement indicates that the client understood or requires further teaching? **Place an X in either the Understood or the Requires Further Teaching column.**

Client Statement	Understood	Requires Further Teaching
"I need to follow the bowel regimen every day."	X	☐
"A low-fiber diet will help with the abdominal discomfort and muscle spasms that I get."	☐	X
"It's best to go back to bed during the day and limit the amount of time I spend in the wheelchair to 2 to 3 hours a day."	☐	X
"I should check my bladder to see if it is distended and make sure that I don't allow it to get too full."	X	☐
"I will call 911 immediately to take me to the hospital if I experience any of these symptoms."	☐	X
"I need to have my spouse help me check my skin to be sure there is no redness or skin breakdown."	X	☐

Rationale: The nurse needs to teach the client about the causes of autonomic dysreflexia, measures to take to prevent its occurrence, and actions to take if an episode occurs. The causes of autonomic dysreflexia are typically GI, gynecologic-urologic, and vascular stimulation. Specific risk factors are bladder distention, UTI, epididymitis or scrotal compression, bowel distention or impaction from constipation, or irritation from hemorrhoids. The client needs to be taught about these causes and measures for prevention of this occurrence. Measures to prevent autonomic dysreflexia include emptying the bladder so that it does not become distended, preventing bladder infections, controlling pain with nonpharmacologic or pharmacologic measures as prescribed, eating a high-fiber diet and achieving adequate fluid intake, and performing bowel care including taking stool softeners to avoid stool impaction. It is best that the client be out of bed rather than in bed because of the complications associated with staying in bed, so it is not helpful to limit the time spent in the wheelchair. However, the client should be taught to shift weight to a different position in the wheelchair to prevent scrotal pressure or skin integrity issues. The client needs to be instructed on the signs and symptoms of autonomic dysreflexia so that it can be detected early and immediate interventions to resolve it can be initiated. Finally, the client needs to be instructed on measures to take if autonomic dysreflexia occurs. The client needs to learn how to check the BP and needs to sit up straight if an episode occurs. The client should be taught not to lie down or recline because this can increase the BP even more. The client should monitor the BP during the episode every 5 minutes to check for improvement. The client needs to quickly determine the cause, such as bladder distention, bowel impaction, or skin problems. The client needs to loosen any clothing that is tight, self-catheterize, and quickly do a rectal check for any stool in the rectum. The physician should be notified of the event, even if the symptoms resolve. If the client is unable to resolve the problem, then EMS is called. The client should also carry a medical identification card indicating the risk for autonomic dysreflexia.

Test-Taking Strategy: Note that the question is asking you about evidence to support whether client teaching has been either understood or not understood, therefore necessitating further teaching. For each of the options, decide whether the actions described in the client statement will help to prevent autonomic dysreflexia. Organize your thoughts as illustrated in the table.

Test-Taking Strategy

Client Statement	Helpful/Not Helpful/Not Necessary
"I need to follow the bowel regimen every day."	Helpful
"A low-fiber diet will help with the abdominal discomfort and muscle spasms that I get."	Not Helpful
"It's best to go back to bed during the day and limit the amount of time I spend in the wheelchair to 2 to 3 hours a day."	Not Helpful
"I should check my bladder to see if it is distended and make sure that I don't allow it to get too full."	Helpful
"I will call 911 immediately to take me to the hospital if I experience any of these symptoms."	Not Necessary
"I need to have my spouse help me check my skin to be sure there is no redness or skin breakdown."	Helpful

Recall that a high-fiber diet, rather than a low-fiber diet, is helpful in preventing constipation. Limiting time in the wheelchair is not an option for this client because of complications associated with staying in bed. It is not necessary to call 911 immediately; and this action does not prevent, but rather treats, the problem.

Content Area: Medical-Surgical Nursing
Priority Concept: Perfusion
Reference(s): Ignatavicius et al., 2021, pp. 877–881

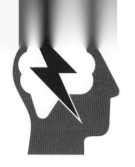

CHAPTER 10

NGN Practice Test: Putting It All Together

As described in Chapter 9, complex clinical scenarios provide the foundation for the NGN test items. Two types of clinical scenarios are part of the NGN starting in 2023: the Unfolding Case Study and the Stand-alone item. Each Unfolding Case Study includes six test items to measure the cognitive skills identified in the NCJMM. Two types of Stand-alone Items will also be included for some candidates taking the NGN—the Trend item and the Bow-tie item. Both item types provide client information that require you to make one or more clinical decisions. Thus these item types can measure more than one CJ cognitive skill.

This chapter allows you the opportunity to practice all of the types of test items you will have on the NGN, starting with Unfolding Cases Studies and ending with Stand-alone Bow-tie and Trend items. The answers, rationales, test-taking strategies, and CJ cognitive skills(s) for each test item are presented at the end of the book. To correctly answer the questions related to these practice clinical scenarios, you'll need to apply one or more CJ cognitive skills from the NCJMM. Chapters 3 through 8 describe these cognitive skills and present test-taking strategies on how to answer test items related to each skill if you need to review them.

 Unfolding Case Studies

Unfolding Case Study 1

Practice Question 10.1	Unfolding Case Study 1

The nurse reviews the medical record of a 56-year-old client who was recently admitted to the ED.

Highlight the client findings in the Nurses' Notes that require **immediate** *follow-up by the nurse.*

Health History	Nurses' Notes	Imaging Studies	Lab Results

2215: Spouse brought client into ED after finding a suicide note and the gun cabinet unlocked. Reports that the client is "not the same person" after being hospitalized 3 months ago with severe COVID-19 and mechanically ventilated for over 2 weeks. Client states that since being discharged from the hospital, has periods of heart palpitations, insomnia, apathy, depressed mood, and anorexia. Reports that drinking alcohol every night helps to relax, but still becomes anxious and depressed at times. Is very worried about getting COVID again because the client's sibling, whom the client recently visited, tested positive yesterday. Has nightmares about the hospital experience because the client nearly died. Lost 35 lb (15.9 kg) during the hospital stay but states still weighs more than 260 lb (117.9 kg). Was considering suicide this evening because the client was afraid of possibly "being reinfected and dying this time." Recently diagnosed with type 2 DM controlled by diet and metformin.

Practice Question 10.2   Unfolding Case Study 1

The nurse reviews the medical record of a 56-year-old client who was recently admitted to the ED.

| Health History | Nurses' Notes | Imaging Studies | Lab Results |

2215: Spouse brought client into ED after finding a suicide note and the gun cabinet unlocked. Reports that the client is "not the same person" after being hospitalized 3 months ago with severe COVID-19 and mechanically ventilated for over 2 weeks. Client states that since being discharged from the hospital, has periods of heart palpitations, insomnia, apathy, depressed mood, and anorexia. Reports that drinking alcohol every night helps to relax, but still becomes anxious and depressed at times. Is very worried about getting COVID again because the client's sibling, whom the client recently visited, tested positive yesterday. Has nightmares about the hospital experience because the client nearly died. Lost 35 lb (15.9 kg) during the hospital stay but states still weighs more than 260 lb (117.9 kg). Was considering suicide this evening because the client was afraid of possibly "being reinfected and dying this time." Recently diagnosed with type 2 DM controlled by diet and metformin.

For each client assessment finding, click or indicate with an X which finding is associated with which client condition. Some findings may be consistent with more than one condition.

Client Finding	Generalized Anxiety Disorder	Clinical Depression	PTSD
Had recent near-death experience	☐	☐	☐
Anorexia	☐	☐	☐
Depressed mood	☐	☐	☐
Apathy	☐	☐	☐
Nightmares	☐	☐	☐
Potential suicide risk	☐	☐	☐
Excessive worry	☐	☐	☐
Insomnia	☐	☐	☐

Practice Question 10.3   Unfolding Case Study 1

The nurse reviews the latest entry (2330) in the Nurses' Notes of a 56-year-old client's medical record.

| Health History | Nurses' Notes | Imaging Studies | Lab Results |

2215: Spouse brought client into ED after finding a suicide note and the gun cabinet unlocked. Reports that the client is "not the same person" after being hospitalized 3 months ago with severe COVID-19 and mechanically ventilated for over 2 weeks. Client states that since being discharged from the hospital, has periods of heart palpitations, insomnia, apathy, depressed mood, and anorexia. Reports that drinking alcohol every night helps to relax, but still becomes anxious and depressed at times. Is very worried about getting COVID again because the client's sibling, whom the client recently visited, tested positive yesterday. Has nightmares about the hospital experience because the client nearly died. Lost 35 lb (15.9 kg) during the hospital stay but states still weighs more than 260 lb (117.9 kg). Was considering suicide this evening because the client was afraid he "might be reinfected and die this time." Recently diagnosed with type 2 DM controlled by diet and metformin.

2330: Social worker (SW) interviewed client and administered several screening assessments for selected mental health conditions. Client admitted to flashbacks about hospitalization and feels guilty about putting family through that experience. States was "lazy" and did not wear a mask or social distance at an important corporate meeting. As a result, the client developed a COVID-19 infection, which worsened and led to the hospital stay and mechanical ventilation. Expressed remorse for upsetting spouse and apologized to her and the SW.

Based on the information in the Nurses' Notes, complete the following sentences from the lists of options provided.

The client *most likely* has _____1 [Select]_____ as the primary potentially life-threatening mental health condition, as evidenced by _____2 [Select]_____ and _____2 [Select]_____. The *priority* for the client's care is to _____3 [Select]_____.

Options for 1	Options for 2	Options for 3
Personality disorder	Anorexia	Begin intensive counseling
Dissociative identity disorder	Nightmares	Ensure personal safety
PTSD	Excessive worry	Start drug therapy
Clinical depression	Flashbacks	Refer to spiritual advisor

Practice Question 10.4   Unfolding Case Study 1

The nurse reviews the latest entry (2330) in the Nurses' Notes of a 56-year-old client's medical record.

Health History	Nurses' Notes	Imaging Studies	Lab Results

2215: Spouse brought client into ED after finding a suicide note and the gun cabinet unlocked. Reports that the client is "not the same person" after being hospitalized 3 months ago with severe COVID-19 and mechanically ventilated for over 2 weeks. Client states that since being discharged from the hospital, has periods of heart palpitations, insomnia, apathy, depressed mood, and anorexia. Reports that drinking alcohol every night helps to relax, but still becomes anxious and depressed at times. Is very worried about getting COVID again because the client's sibling, whom the client recently visited, tested positive yesterday. Has nightmares about the hospital experience because the client nearly died. Lost 35 lb (15.9 kg) during the hospital stay but states still weighs more than 260 lb (117.9 kg). Was considering suicide this evening because the client was afraid he "might be reinfected and die this time." Recently diagnosed with type 2 DM controlled by diet and metformin.

2330: Social worker (SW) interviewed client and administered several screening assessments for selected mental health conditions. Client admitted to flashbacks about hospitalization and feels guilty about putting family through that experience. States was "lazy" and did not wear a mask or social distance at an important corporate meeting. As a result, the client developed a COVID-19 infection, which worsened and led to the hospital stay and mechanical ventilation. Expressed remorse for upsetting spouse and apologized to her and the SW.

The client was diagnosed with PTSD, anxiety, and suicidal risk. Which physician orders would the nurse anticipate for the client at this time? **Select all that apply.**

☐ Begin antidepressant drug therapy.

☐ Admit to acute psychiatric unit.

☐ Refer to case manager.

☐ Refer to spiritual advisor.

☐ Begin intense psychotherapy.

☐ Place on suicide precautions.

☐ Limit visitors to immediate family.

Practice Question 10.5   Unfolding Case Study 1

A 56-year-old client was diagnosed with PTSD after being admitted to the ED because the client's spouse found a suicide note and unlocked gun cabinet. After a thorough evaluation, the client was admitted for one-on-one observation in the acute inpatient psychiatric unit and started on sertraline and psychotherapy. The nurse plans health teaching about the medication for the client and spouse before administering the first dose.

Select five statements that the nurse would include in the health teaching about sertraline.

☐ "This drug is one of the most effective ways to treat PTSD and depression."

☐ "We will be monitoring you for sedation effects while you are here."

☐ "Let me know if you have trouble urinating or having a bowel movement."

☐ "Let me know if you have trouble sleeping or feel nervous while on the drug."

☐ "We will be monitoring you carefully for changes in your vital signs."

☐ "You might experience mild nausea and feel agitated when you start this drug."

☐ "Your liver and kidney function will need to be monitored by lab testing."

Practice Question 10.6 | Unfolding Case Study 1

A 56-year-old client was discharged from the acute psychiatric care unit 2 months ago with a diagnosis of PTSD, anxiety, and clinical depression. The client is following up with the family nurse practitioner (FNP) today. Prior to being examined by the FNP, the office nurse reviews the previous ED admission record and performs an interview regarding the client's current health state.

| Health History | Nurses' Notes | Imaging Studies | Lab Results |

2215: Spouse brought client into ED after finding a suicide note and the gun cabinet unlocked. Reports that the client is "not the same person" after being hospitalized 3 months ago with severe COVID-19 and mechanically ventilated for over 2 weeks. Client states that since being discharged from the hospital, has periods of heart palpitations, insomnia, apathy, depressed mood, and anorexia. Reports that drinking alcohol every night helps to relax, but still becomes anxious and depressed at times. Is very worried about getting COVID again because the client's sibling, whom the client recently visited, tested positive yesterday. Has nightmares about the hospital experience because the client nearly died. Lost 35 lb (15.9 kg) during the hospital stay but states still weighs more than 260 lb (117.9 kg). Was considering suicide this evening because the client was afraid he "might be reinfected and die this time." Recently diagnosed with type 2 DM controlled by diet and metformin.

2330: Social worker (SW) interviewed client and administered several screening assessments for selected mental health conditions. Client admitted to flashbacks about hospitalization and feels guilty about putting family through that experience. States was "lazy" and did not wear a mask or social distance at an important corporate meeting. As a result, the client developed a COVID-19 infection, which worsened and led to the hospital stay and mechanical ventilation. Expressed remorse for upsetting spouse and apologized to her and the SW.

*Based on the ED admission notes and data collected during the nurse's interview with the client, indicate which client findings demonstrate that he is either **Progressing (Improving)** or **Not Progressing (Not Improving)**.*

Client Finding	Progressing (Improving)	Not Progressing (Not Improving)
Has not consumed any alcohol since hospital discharge	☐	☐
States has a more positive outlook without depressed moods, and a better appetite	☐	☐
Has flashbacks and nightmares about once a week	☐	☐
Sleeps most nights for 7–8 hours	☐	☐
States no longer has heart palpitations	☐	☐

Unfolding Case Study 2

Practice Question 10.7   Unfolding Case Study 2

The nurse reviews the preoperative note for a 68-year-old client who is scheduled to have an anterior right THA this morning.

Health History	Nurses' Notes	Imaging Studies	Lab Results

0645: Admitted to the OR for a THA using an anterior surgical approach. History of several surgeries including hysterectomy, appendectomy, and cholecystectomy. 52–pack-year history but quit 2 years ago; BMI of 30.1. History of DVT × 2, hypertension controlled by diet and drug therapy, high cholesterol controlled by statins, and GERD controlled by an antacid PRN. Bilateral hip osteoarthritis with right hip more painful than left. Lives in second-floor apartment in a rural town. Has no transportation and depends on family friends to obtain food and get to medical appointments. Family friends are willing to help with post-operative recovery and transportation. Advance directives on file. Prepped for surgery.

The nurse recognizes that which assessment findings listed below place the client at high risk for postoperative VTE? **Select all that apply.**

☐ History of hypertension
☐ 52–pack-year history
☐ BMI of 30.1
☐ History of high cholesterol
☐ Having a THA
☐ History of cholecystectomy
☐ History of bilateral hip osteoarthritis
☐ History of DVT × 2

Practice Question 10.8   Unfolding Case Study 2

The nurse is assigned to care for a 68-year-old client who had a right THA 2 days ago. The client's pain is being managed with oral opioids and gabapentin. The client is preparing for possible discharge tomorrow. The client has been on apixaban 5 mg orally once a day and has ambulated with assistance 4 times each day in the hall with a walker. The nurse performs a shift assessment and documents the following Nurses' Notes.

Health History	Nurses' Notes	Imaging Studies	Lab Results

1935: Reports was unable to ambulate this evening because of sharp chest pain that hurts worse when taking a deep breath. States has been "belching" since dinner because of eating onions and peppers on a steak. Restless and anxious about pain, but no acute confusion. T = 100°F (37.8°C); HR = 104 BPM; RR = 20 bpm with dyspnea; BP = 114/62 mm Hg; SpO$_2$ = 90% on RA. Right THA incision dry and intact without redness. Right pedal pulse nonpalpable but detected on Doppler; foot warm and not swollen. Posterior tibial and popliteal pulses +2 bilaterally. Able to flex both feet equally; cap refill <3 seconds.

For each client assessment finding, click or indicate with an X which finding is associated with which potential client condition. Some findings may be consistent with more than one condition.

Client Finding	PE	GERD	Respiratory Infection
Chest pain	☐	☐	☐
Belching	☐	☐	☐
Restlessness	☐	☐	☐
Anxiety	☐	☐	☐
T 100°F (37.8°C)	☐	☐	☐
HR 104 BPM	☐	☐	☐
RR 20 bpm with dyspnea	☐	☐	☐
SpO$_2$ 90% on RA	☐	☐	☐

Practice Question 10.9 | Unfolding Case Study 2

The nurse is assigned to care for a 68-year-old client who had a right THA 2 days ago. The client's pain is being managed with oral opioids and gabapentin. The client is preparing for possible discharge tomorrow. The client has been on apixaban 5 mg orally once a day and has ambulated at least 4 times each day in the hall with a walker. The nurse performs a shift assessment and documents the following Nurses' Notes.

Health History	Nurses' Notes	Imaging Studies	Lab Results

1935: Reports was unable to ambulate this evening because of sharp chest pain that hurts worse when taking a deep breath. States has been "belching" since dinner because of eating onions and peppers on a steak. Restless and anxious about pain, but no acute confusion. T = 100°F (37.8°C); HR = 104 BPM; RR = 20 bpm with dyspnea; BP = 114/62 mm Hg; SpO$_2$ = 90% on RA. Right THA incision dry and intact without redness. Right pedal pulse nonpalpable but detected on Doppler; foot warm and not swollen. Posterior tibial and popliteal pulses +2 bilaterally. Able to flex both feet equally; cap refill <3 seconds.

Based on the information in the Nurses' Notes, complete the following sentences from the lists of options provided.

The client **most likely** has ____1 [Select]____ as the *priority* condition as evidenced by ____2 [Select]____ and ____3 [Select]____.

Options for 1	Options for 2	Options for 3
Right leg neurovascular compromise	Chest pain	Tachypnea
	Hypotension	Belching
PE	Bradycardia	Decreased capillary refill
Pneumonia	Nonpalpable right pedal pulse	
GERD		Dyspnea

Practice Question 10.10 | Unfolding Case Study 2

The nurse is assigned to care for a 68-year-old client who had a right THA 2 days ago. The client's pain is being managed with oral opioids and gabapentin. The client is preparing for possible discharge tomorrow. The client has been on apixaban 5 mg orally once a day and has ambulated at least 4 times each day in the hall with a walker. The nurse performs a shift assessment and documents the following Nurses' Notes.

Health History	Nurses' Notes	Imaging Studies	Lab Results

1935: Reports was unable to ambulate this evening because of sharp chest pain that hurts worse when taking a deep breath. States has been "belching" since dinner because of eating onions and peppers on a steak. Restless and anxious about pain, but no acute confusion. T = 100°F (37.8°C); HR = 104 BPM; RR = 20 bpm with dyspnea; BP = 114/62 mm Hg; SpO$_2$ = 90% on RA. Right THA incision dry and intact without redness. Right pedal pulse nonpalpable but detected on Doppler; foot warm and not swollen. Posterior tibial and popliteal pulses +2 bilaterally. Able to flex both feet equally; cap refill <3 seconds.

*The nurse develops a plan of care to manage the client's suspected condition. Select **six actions** that would be appropriate for the nurse to include in the plan of care at this time.*

☐ Obtain venous access.

☐ Place the client in a flat supine position.

☐ Connect the client to a continuous cardiac monitor.

☐ Prepare the client for computed tomography pulmonary angiography (CTPA).

☐ Apply oxygen by NC or mask.

☐ Increase the client's oral apixaban dosage from 5 mg to 10 mg.

☐ Draw blood for laboratory testing, including complete blood count and coagulation studies.

☐ Place the client on continuous oxygen saturation monitoring.

Practice Question 10.11   Unfolding Case Study 2

The nurse is assigned to care for a 68-year-old client who had a right THA 2 days ago. During shift assessment, the nurse documents new onset of symptoms including chest pain and dyspnea. Computed tomography pulmonary angiography (CTPA) confirmed the diagnosis of a submassive PE. The orthopedic surgeon enters the following orders:

Nurses' Notes	Physician Orders	Imaging Studies	Lab Results

1020:
- Fondaparinux 7.5 mg subcutaneously once daily
- Warfarin 5 mg orally once daily
- Supplemental oxygen per NC at 5 L/min
- Continuous pulse oximetry monitoring

The nurse revises the plan of care for the client with confirmed diagnosis of PE. Click or place an X to specify nursing actions that are **Indicated** (appropriate or necessary) and those that are **Contraindicated** (not useful and could be harmful) related to drug therapy for this client.

Potential Nursing Action	Indicated	Contraindicated
Monitor the client's platelet count.	☐	☐
Monitor the client's activated partial thromboplastin time (aPTT).	☐	☐
Assess the client for bleeding or excessive bruising.	☐	☐
Monitor the client's international normalized ratio (INR).	☐	☐
Monitor the client's hematocrit.	☐	☐
Check for availability of protamine sulfate.	☐	☐
Check for availability of phytonadione (vitamin K).	☐	☐

Practice Question 10.12 | Unfolding Case Study 2

A 68-year-old client who had a right THA is returning to the orthopedic surgeon's office for a 6-week follow-up visit. While in the hospital recovering from surgery, the client experienced a PE, which was successfully treated. Today the office nurse conducts a brief assessment before the client is examined by the surgeon and documents the following note.

Health History	Nurses' Notes	Imaging Studies	Lab Results

1015: Walking independently with a cane with full weight bearing; states is able to perform ADLs without assistance. Right hip incision healed with hairline scar and slight distal bruising. Taking warfarin as prescribed and following up on INR testing, but depends mostly on family friends for transportation to the lab. Right arm badly bruised but reports no other bleeding. T = 97.9°F (36.6°C); HR = 86 BPM; RR = 18 bpm; BP = 126/74 mm Hg; SpO$_2$ = 95% on RA. No adventitious breath sounds; no new report of shortness of breath or chest pain. States a loss of 27 lb since hospitalization as part of a new weight loss program. Also reports that left nonsurgical hip is increasingly painful and may soon need to be replaced.

Based on the nurse's brief assessment, which findings indicate that the client is improving or progressing? **Select all that apply.**

☐ No new report of shortness of breath or chest pain

☐ Hip incision healed with hairline scar

☐ SpO$_2$ of 95% on RA

☐ Right arm badly bruised

☐ Recent weight loss of 27 lb

☐ Left hip is becoming more painful

☐ Walking independently with cane

☐ Performing ADLs without assistance

Unfolding Case Study 3

A 64-year-old client presents to the ED and reports a 2-week history of fever and chills, nausea and abdominal pain, sore throat, cough, fatigue and lethargy, and muscle aches. An initial nursing assessment reveals the following:

Health History	Nurses' Notes	Lab Tests	Diagnostic Tests

1000: History of diabetes type 1, hypertension, hyperlipidemia, hypothyroidism. Denies chest pain or shortness of breath. Nonproductive cough, coarse crackles heard in lower lobes bilaterally. Blood glucose levels have been well controlled, but this morning the client reports a level of 375 mg/dL (20.8 mmol/L), prompting the visit to the ED. States recent glycated hemoglobin (A1c) level done 2 months ago was 7.0%. Unable to eat and reports stopping medications 3 days ago because of the nausea and abdominal pain. States has had increased urination despite the inability to tolerate food or fluids. Reports weakness and muscle aches and being confined to bed for the past 3 weeks. Fruity breath odor noted. POC glucose 400 mg/dL (22.2 mmol/L).

VS: T = 100.4°F (38.0°C); HR = 96 BPM; RR = 24 bpm; BP = 142/90 mm Hg; SpO₂ = 91% on RA.

Weight 175 lb (79.37 kg), height 5 feet 9 inches (stated).

Voided: 250 mL.

Medications:

Levothyroxine 125 mcg oral daily
Lisinopril 2.5 mg oral daily
Simvastatin 20 mg oral daily
Insulin glargine 28 units subcutaneous daily
Semaglutide 1 mg subcutaneous weekly

1120: The nurse reviews the recent laboratory and diagnostic test results, which include the following:

Health History	Nurses' Notes	Lab Tests	Diagnostic Tests

Laboratory Test	Results	Normal Reference Range
Glucose	440 mg/dL (24.4 mmol/L) H	74–106 mg/dL (3.9–6.1 mmol/L)
Ketones	86.4 mg/dL (4.8 mmol/L) H	<0 mg/dL (0.0–0.27 mmol/L)
White blood cells (WBCs)	9900/mm³ (6.3 × 10⁹/L)	5000–10,000/mm³ (3.5–12 × 10⁹/L)
Blood urea nitrogen (BUN)	22 mg/dL (9.0 mmol/L) H	10-20 mg/dL (2.9–8.2 mmol/L)
Creatinine (Cr)	1.0 mg/dL (88.3 mcmol/L)	0.6–1.2 mg/dL (53–106 mcmol/L)
Potassium (K)	5.9 mEq/L (5.9 mmol/L) H	3.5-5.0 mEq/L (3.5–5.1 mmol/L)
Sodium (Na)	150 mEq/L (150 mmol/L) H	136-145 mEq/L (136–145 mmol/L)
Thyroid-stimulating hormone (TSH)	4.0 mIU/mL (4.0 mIU/L)	2-10 mIU/mL (0.4–4.8 mIU/L)
D-dimer	15 mcg/mL (112.5 nmol/L) H	<250 ng/mL or <0.4 mcg/mL (<3 nmol/L)
Creatine kinase (CK)	140 U/L (150.5 U/L)	20–200 U/L (20–215 U/L)
C-reactive protein (CRP)	10.2 mg/dL (102 mg/L) H	<1 mg/dL (<10.0 mg/L)
Troponin I	0.01 ng/mL (0.17 mcg/L)	<0.03 ng/mL (<0.35 mcg/L)
Blood culture	Pending	No growth
Urinalysis WBCs	0 (0)	0–4 low-power field
Ketones	Positive H	None
Urine culture	Pending	No growth
Arterial blood gases (ABGs)	pH 7.30 L	pH 7.35–7.45 (7.35–7.45)
	Pco₂ 27 mm Hg L	Pco₂ 35–45 mm Hg (35–45 mm Hg)
	HCO₃ 14 mEq/L L	HCO₃ 21–28 mEq/L (23–29 mEq/L)
	Po₂ 85 mm Hg	Po₂ 80–100 mm Hg (80–100 mm Hg)
SARS-CoV-2 PCR	Positive	Negative

Practice Question 10.13   Unfolding Case Study 3—cont'd

| Health History | Nurses' Notes | Lab Tests | Diagnostic Tests |

Diagnostic Test	Results
Chest x-ray	Bilateral pulmonary infiltrates compatible with COVID-19 pneumonitis
ECG	NSR

*Which four laboratory findings require **immediate** follow-up?*

☐ A1c

☐ BUN

☐ Sodium

☐ Glucose

☐ D-dimer

☐ Potassium

☐ C-reactive protein

☐ Arterial blood gases

Practice Question 10.14   Unfolding Case Study 3

A 64-year-old client presents to the ED and reports a 2-week history of fever and chills, nausea and abdominal pain, sore throat, cough, fatigue and lethargy, and muscle aches. An initial nursing assessment reveals the following:

Health History	Nurses' Notes	Lab Tests	Diagnostic Tests

1000: History of diabetes type 1, hypertension, hyperlipidemia, hypothyroidism. Denies chest pain or shortness of breath. Nonproductive cough, coarse crackles heard in lower lobes bilaterally. Blood glucose levels have been well controlled, but this morning the client reports a level of 375 mg/dL (20.8 mmol/L), prompting the visit to the ED. States recent glycated hemoglobin (A1c) level done 2 months ago was 7.0%. Unable to eat and reports stopping medications 3 days ago because of the nausea and abdominal pain. States has had increased urination despite the inability to tolerate food or fluids. Reports weakness and muscle aches and being confined to bed for the past 3 weeks. Fruity breath odor noted. POC glucose 400 mg/dL (22.2 mmol/L).

VS: T = 100.4°F (38.0°C); HR = 96 BPM; RR = 24 bpm; BP = 142/90 mm Hg; SpO$_2$ = 91% on RA.

Weight 175 lb (79.37 kg), height 5 feet 9 inches (stated).

Voided: 250 mL.

Medications:
Levothyroxine 125 mcg oral daily
Lisinopril 2.5 mg oral daily
Simvastatin 20 mg oral daily
Insulin glargine 28 units subcutaneous daily
Semaglutide 1 mg subcutaneous weekly

1120: The nurse reviews the recent laboratory and diagnostic test results, which include the following:

Health History	Nurses' Notes	Lab Tests	Diagnostic Tests

Laboratory Test	Results	Normal Reference Range
Glucose	440 mg/dL (24.4 mmol/L) H	74–106 mg/dL (3.9–6.1 mmol/L)
Ketones	86.4 mg/dL (4.8 mmol/L) H	<0 mg/dL (0.0–0.27 mmol/L)
White blood cells (WBCs)	9900/mm³ (6.3 × 10⁹/L)	5000–10,000/mm³ (3.5–12 × 10⁹/L)
Blood urea nitrogen (BUN)	22 mg/dL (9.0 mmol/L) H	10–20 mg/dL (2.9–8.2 mmol/L)
Creatinine (Cr)	1.0 mg/dL (88.3 mcmol/L)	0.6–1.2 mg/dL (53–106 mcmol/L)
Potassium (K)	5.9 mEq/L (5.9 mmol/L) H	3.5–5.0 mEq/L (3.5–5.1 mmol/L)
Sodium (Na)	150 mEq/L (150 mmol/L) H	136–145 mEq/L (136–145 mmol/L)
Thyroid-stimulating hormone (TSH)	4.0 mIU/mL (4.0 mIU/L)	2–10 mIU/mL (0.4–4.8 mIU/L)
D-dimer	15 mcg/mL (112.5 nmol/L) H	<250 ng/mL or <0.4 mcg/mL (<3 nmol/L)
Creatine kinase (CK)	140 U/L 150.5 U/L)	20–200 U/L (20–215 U/L)
C-reactive protein (CRP)	10.2 mg/dL (102 mg/L) H	<1 mg/dL (<10.0 mg/L)
Troponin I	0.01 ng/mL (0.17 mcg/L)	<0.03 ng/mL (<0.35 mcg/L)
Blood culture	Pending	No growth
Urinalysis WBCs	0 (0)	0–4 low-power field
Ketones	Positive H	None
Urine culture	Pending	No growth
Arterial blood gases (ABGs)	pH 7.30 L	pH 7.35–7.45 (7.35–7.45)
	Pco$_2$ 27 mm Hg L	Pco$_2$ 35–45 mm Hg (35–45 mm Hg)
	HCO$_3$ 14 mEq/L L	HCO$_3$ 21–28 mEq/L (23–29 mEq/L)
	Po$_2$ 85 mm Hg	Po$_2$ 80–100 mm Hg (80–100 mm Hg)
SARS-CoV-2 PCR	Positive	Negative

Practice Question 10.14 | Unfolding Case Study 3—cont'd

| Health History | Nurses' Notes | Lab Tests | Diagnostic Tests |

Diagnostic Tests

Diagnostic Test	Results
Chest x-ray	Bilateral pulmonary infiltrates compatible with COVID-19 pneumonitis
ECG	NSR

For each client finding below, click or check to specify if the finding is consistent with the disease process of DKA or COVID-19. Each finding may support more than one disease process.

Client Findings	DKA	COVID-19
Fever and chills	☐	☐
Nausea	☐	☐
Abdominal pain	☐	☐
Increased urination	☐	☐
Cough	☐	☐
Lung crackles	☐	☐
High C-reactive protein level	☐	☐
High glucose level	☐	☐
Abnormal ABGs	☐	☐

Practice Question 10.15   Unfolding Case Study 3

A 64-year-old client presents to the ED and reports a 2-week history of fever and chills, nausea and abdominal pain, sore throat, cough, fatigue and lethargy, and muscle aches. An initial nursing assessment reveals the following:

| Health History | Nurses' Notes | Lab Tests | Diagnostic Tests |

1000: History of diabetes type 1, hypertension, hyperlipidemia, hypothyroidism. Denies chest pain or shortness of breath. Nonproductive cough, coarse crackles heard in lower lobes bilaterally. Blood glucose levels have been well controlled, but this morning the client reports a level of 375 mg/dL (20.8 mmol/L), prompting the visit to the ED. States recent glycated hemoglobin (A1c) level done 2 months ago was 7.0%. Unable to eat and reports stopping medications 3 days ago because of the nausea and abdominal pain. States has had increased urination despite the inability to tolerate food or fluids. Reports weakness and muscle aches and being confined to bed for the past 3 weeks. Fruity breath odor noted. POC glucose 400 mg/dL (22.2 mmol/L).

VS: T = 100.4°F (38.0°C); HR = 96 BPM; RR = 24 bpm; BP = 142/90 mm Hg; SpO$_2$ = 91% on RA.

Weight 175 lb (79.37 kg), height 5 feet 9 inches (stated).

Voided: 250 mL.

Medications:

Levothyroxine 125 mcg oral daily
Lisinopril 2.5 mg oral daily
Simvastatin 20 mg oral daily
Insulin glargine 28 units subcutaneous daily
Semaglutide 1 mg subcutaneous weekly

1120: The nurse reviews the recent laboratory and diagnostic test results, which include the following:

| Health History | Nurses' Notes | Lab Tests | Diagnostic Tests |

Laboratory Test	Results	Normal Reference Range
Glucose	440 mg/dL (24.4 mmol/L) **H**	74–106 mg/dL (3.9–6.1 mmol/L)
Ketones	86.4 mg/dL (4.8 mmol/L) **H**	<0 mg/dL (0.0–0.27 mmol/L)
White blood cells (WBCs)	9900/mm³ (6.3 × 10⁹/L)	5000–10,000/mm³ (3.5–12 × 10⁹/L)
Blood urea nitrogen (BUN)	22 mg/dL (9.0 mmol/L) **H**	10-20 mg/dL (2.9–8.2 mmol/L)
Creatinine (Cr)	1.0 mg/dL (88.3 mcmol/L)	0.6–1.2 mg/dL (53–106 mcmol/L)
Potassium (K)	5.9 mEq/L (5.9 mmol/L) **H**	3.5-5.0 mEq/L (3.5–5.1 mmol/L)
Sodium (Na)	150 mEq/L (150 mmol/L) **H**	136-145 mEq/L (136–145 mmol/L)
Thyroid-stimulating hormone (TSH)	4.0 mIU/mL (4.0 mIU/L)	2-10 mIU/mL (0.4–4.8 mIU/L)
D-dimer	15 mcg/mL (112.5 nmol/L) **H**	<250 ng/mL or <0.4 mcg/mL (<3 nmol/L)
Creatine kinase (CK)	140 U/L (150.5 U/L)	20–200 U/L (20–215 U/L)
C-reactive protein (CRP)	10.2 mg/dL (102 mg/L) **H**	<1 mg/dL (<10.0 mg/L)
Troponin I	0.01 ng/mL (0.17 mcg/L)	<0.03 ng/mL (<0.35 mcg/L)
Blood culture	Pending	No growth
Urinalysis		
WBCs	0 (0)	0–4 low-power field
Ketones	Positive **H**	None
Urine culture	Pending	No growth
Arterial blood gases (ABGs)	pH 7.30 **L**	pH 7.35–7.45 (7.35–7.45)
	Pco$_2$ 27 mm Hg **L**	Pco$_2$ 35–45 mm Hg (35–45 mm Hg)
	HCO$_3$ 14 mEq/L **L**	HCO$_3$ 21–28 mEq/L (23–29 mEq/L)
	Po$_2$ 85 mm Hg	Po$_2$ 80–100 mm Hg (80–100 mm Hg)
SARS-CoV-2 PCR	Positive	Negative

Practice Question 10.15   Unfolding Case Study 3—cont'd

| Health History | Nurses' Notes | Lab Tests | Diagnostic Tests |

Diagnostic Test	Results
Chest x-ray	Bilateral pulmonary infiltrates compatible with COVID-19 pneumonitis
ECG	NSR

Complete the following sentence by choosing from the lists of options provided.

The client is at **highest** risk for developing _____ 1 [Select] _____, as evidenced by _____ 2 [Select] _____ and _____ 3 [Select] _____.

Options for 1	Options for 2	Options for 3
Seizures	BUN	Chills
Acute renal injury	Fever	Creatinine levels
Myxedema coma	D-dimer level	Chest x-ray result
Respiratory failure	Lung crackles	TSH level
Thromboembolism	History of hypothyroidism	Immobility

Practice Question 10.16   **Unfolding Case Study 3**

1145: The ED physician documents orders for the client and the nurse is planning care. The nurse rechecks VS and obtains a POC glucose reading. VS: T = 100.4°F (38.0°C); HR = 98 BPM; RR = 24 bpm; BP = 146/92 mm Hg; SpO$_2$ = 89% on RA. POC glucose reading is 500 mg/dL (27.7 mmol/L). The client is alert but lethargic yet arousable. Voiding 200 mL/hr. Dry cough. No shortness of breath. Coarse crackles heard in lower lobes bilaterally. Hospital admission is planned.

Health History	Nurses' Notes	Lab Tests	Diagnostic Tests

1000: History of diabetes type 1, hypertension, hyperlipidemia, hypothyroidism. Denies chest pain or shortness of breath. Nonproductive cough, coarse crackles heard in lower lobes bilaterally. Blood glucose levels have been well controlled, but this morning the client reports a level of 375 mg/dL (20.8 mmol/L), prompting the visit to the ED. States recent glycated hemoglobin (A1c) level done 2 months ago was 7.0%. Unable to eat and reports stopping medications 3 days ago because of the nausea and abdominal pain. States has had increased urination despite the inability to tolerate food or fluids. Reports weakness and muscle aches and being confined to bed for the past 3 weeks. Fruity breath odor noted. POC glucose 400 mg/dL (22.2 mmol/L).
VS: T = 100.4°F (38.0°C); HR = 96 BPM; RR = 24 bpm; BP = 142/90 mm Hg; SpO$_2$ = 91% on RA.
Weight 175 lb (79.37 kg), height 5 feet 9 inches (stated).
Voided: 250 mL.

Medications:
Levothyroxine 125 mcg oral daily
Lisinopril 2.5 mg oral daily
Simvastatin 20 mg oral daily
Insulin glargine 28 units subcutaneous daily
Semaglutide 1 mg subcutaneous weekly

1120: The nurse reviews the recent laboratory and diagnostic test results, which include the following:

Health History	Nurses' Notes	Lab Tests	Diagnostic Tests

Laboratory Test	Results	Normal Reference Range
Glucose	440 mg/dL (24.4 mmol/L) H	74–106 mg/dL (3.9–6.1 mmol/L)
Ketones	86.4 mg/dL (4.8 mmol/L) H	<0 mg/dL (0.0–0.27 mmol/L)
White blood cells (WBCs)	9900/mm^3 (6.3 × 10^9/L)	5000–10,000/mm^3 (3.5–12 × 10^9/L)
Blood urea nitrogen (BUN)	22 mg/dL (9.0 mmol/L) H	10-20 mg/dL (2.9–8.2 mmol/L)
Creatinine (Cr)	1.0 mg/dL (88.3 mcmol/L)	0.6–1.2 mg/dL (53–106 mcmol/L)
Potassium (K)	5.9 mEq/L (5.9 mmol/L) H	3.5-5.0 mEq/L (3.5–5.1 mmol/L)
Sodium (Na)	150 mEq/L (150 mmol/L) H	136-145 mEq/L (136–145 mmol/L)
Thyroid-stimulating hormone (TSH)	4.0 mIU/mL (4.0 mIU/L)	2-10 mIU/mL (0.4–4.8 mIU/L)
D-dimer	15 mcg/mL (112.5 nmol/L) H	<250 ng/mL or <0.4 mcg/mL (<3 nmol/L)
Creatine kinase (CK)	140 U/L (150.5 U/L)	20–200 U/L (20–215 U/L)
C-reactive protein (CRP)	10.2 mg/dL (102 mg/L) H	<1 mg/dL (<10.0 mg/L)
Troponin I	0.01 ng/mL (0.17 mcg/L)	<0.03 ng/mL (<0.35 mcg/L)
Blood culture	Pending	No growth
Urinalysis WBCs	0 (0)	0–4 low-power field
Ketones	Positive H	None
Urine culture	Pending	No growth
Arterial blood gases (ABGs)	pH 7.30 L	pH 7.35-7.45 (7.35–7.45)
	Pco$_2$ 27 mm Hg L	Pco$_2$ 35-45 mm Hg (35–45 mm Hg)
	HCO$_3$ 14 mEq/L L	HCO$_3$ 21–28 mEq/L (23–29 mEq/L)
	Po$_2$ 85 mm Hg	Po$_2$ 80–100 mm Hg (80–100 mm Hg)
SARS-CoV-2 PCR	Positive	Negative

Practice Question 10.16 — Unfolding Case Study 3—cont'd

Health History	Nurses' Notes	Lab Tests	Diagnostic Tests

Diagnostic Tests

Diagnostic Test	Results
Chest x-ray	Bilateral pulmonary infiltrates compatible with COVID-19 pneumonitis
ECG	NSR

*Click or check to indicate whether each potential intervention listed below is either **Anticipated** (appropriate or necessary) or **Contraindicated** (could be harmful)/**Not Helpful** for the client's plan of care at this time.*

Potential Intervention	Anticipated	Contraindicated/ Not Helpful
O_2 per NC	☐	☐
0.45% normal saline infusion	☐	☐
Insulin glargine bolus	☐	☐
Continuous infusion of regular insulin diluted in normal saline	☐	☐
IV potassium	☐	☐
Continuous cardiac monitoring	☐	☐
Enoxaparin subcutaneously daily	☐	☐
Tocilizumab and dexamethasone	☐	☐
Ceftriaxone	☐	☐

Practice Question 10.17   Unfolding Case Study 3

1345: The ED physician orders are initiated and the client with DKA and COVID-19 is transferred to the acute care medical unit for hospital admission. The client is alert and oriented on admission. VS: T = 99.4°F (37.4°C); HR = 88 BPM; RR = 20 bpm; BP = 138/90 mm Hg; SpO$_2$ = 90% on RA. The admitting physician prescribes laboratory studies, and the nurse contacts the laboratory for the tests.

1415: The laboratory results are reported, and the nurse reviews the results and subsequent physician prescriptions.

Health History	Nurses' Notes	Vital Signs	Lab Tests

Laboratory Test	Current Results	Normal Reference Range
Glucose	240 mg/dL (12.6 mmol/L) H	74–106 mg/dL (3.9–6.1 mmol/L)
BUN	18 mg/dL (5.22 mmol/L)	10–20 mg/dL (2.9–8.2 mmol/L)
Cr	1.2 mg/dL (106 mcmol/L)	0.6–1.2 mg/dL (53–106 mcmol/L)
K	4.0 mEq/L (4.0 mmol/L)	3.5–5.0 mEq/L (3.5–5.1 mmol/L)
Na	150 mEq/L (150 mmol/L) H	136–145 mEq/L (136–145 mmol/L)

*Based on the client assessment and laboratory findings, which three actions would be the **priority**?*

☐ Administer IV potassium.

☐ Offer a sports drink for sipping.

☐ Check hourly urine output amounts.

☐ Teach about the ways to prevent dehydration.

☐ Administer 5% dextrose in 0.45% normal saline.

Practice Question 10.18   Unfolding Case Study 3

0700: Hand-off report from the night nurse to the day nurse has been completed. The night nurse reports that the client prescriptions to treat DKA were implemented on the previous evening shift. The client also reports that the client had a comfortable night. Laboratory tests and VS were checked every 4 hours during the night and remained stable. The day nurse assesses the client and reviews the most current laboratory results.

Health History	Nurses' Notes	Vital Signs	Lab Tests

Laboratory Test	Current Results	Normal Reference Range
Glucose	240 mg/dL (12.6 mmol/L) H	74–106 mg/dL (3.9–6.1 mmol/L)
BUN	18 mg/dL (5.22 mmol/L)	10–20 mg/dL (2.9–8.2 mmol/L)
Cr	1.2 mg/dL (106 mcmol/L)	0.6–1.2 mg/dL (53–106 mcmol/L)
K	4.0 mEq/L (4.0 mmol/L)	3.5–5.0 mEq/L (3.5–5.1 mmol/L)
Na	150 mEq/L (150 mmol/L) H	136–145 mEq/L (136–145 mmol/L)

*Which findings indicate that the treatment plan is effective? For each client finding, click or place an X to specify if the finding indicates that the treatment plan is **Effective** or **Ineffective**.*

Previous Client Finding	Current Client Finding	Effective	Ineffective
Glucose 240 mg/dL (12.6 mmol/L)	Glucose 190 mg/dL (10.64 mmol/L)	☐	☐
Potassium 4.0 mEq/L (4.0 mmol/L)	Potassium 4.0 mEq/L (4.0 mmol/L)	☐	☐
Urine output 200 mL/hr	Urine output 45 mL/hr	☐	☐
Na 150 mEq/L (150 mmol/L)	Na 150 mEq/L (150 mmol/L)	☐	☐

Unfolding Case Study 4

A 70-year-old client arrived at the ED for chest heaviness and difficulty breathing. The nurse documents the admission assessment.

*Highlight the client findings in the following medical records that are of **immediate** concern to the nurse.*

Health History	Physical Assessment	Vital Signs	Test Results

1200: 70-year-old client admitted to the ED reporting chest heaviness and difficulty breathing for 2 days. Symptoms are noticed more with activity and subside with rest after a few minutes. Past medical history of type 2 DM, hypertension, hyperlipidemia, hypothyroidism, osteoarthritis. Currently smokes 1 pack cigarettes per day × 20 years. Medications include sliding scale insulin aspart prior to meals and at bedtime, insulin glargine at bedtime, lisinopril, atorvastatin, levothyroxine, and naproxen.

Health History	Physical Assessment	Vital Signs	Test Results

General: Appears nontoxic, well nourished, well hydrated.
Integumentary: Warm, dry, intact.
Respiratory: Lungs clear to auscultation bilaterally, no adventitious sounds. No use of accessory muscles.
Cardiovascular: HR irregularly irregular. S1 and S2 noted, no S3 or S4, no murmurs, rubs, gallops. No peripheral edema.
GI: Abdomen soft, nontender, nondistended. BS present × 4 quads.
Neurologic: Cranial nerves II–XII grossly intact.

Health History	Physical Assessment	Vital Signs	Test Results

1200: VS: T = 36.4°C (97.5°C) oral; HR = 130 BPM; RR = 20 bpm; BP = 108/59 mm Hg; SpO$_2$ = 95% on RA
Height: 165 cm (5 feet 5 inches)
Weight: 81.6 kg (180 lb)
BMI: 30.0
1200: I: 120 mL water (oral)
1230: O: 140 mL clear yellow urine

Health History	Physical Assessment	Vital Signs	Test Results

ECG:
Atrial fibrillation with rapid ventricular response, rate 130 BPM
Acute anterior and lateral MI
Intraventricular conduction delay
No ST elevation

Laboratory Test	Results	Normal Reference Range
Sodium (Na)	136 mEq/L (136 mmol/L)	136–145 mEq/L (136–145 mmol/L)
Potassium (K)	3.8 mEq/L (3.8 mmol/L)	3.5–5.0 mEq/L (3.5–5.1 mmol/L)
Calcium (Ca)	9.2 mg/dL (2.4 mmol/L)	9–10.5 mg/dL (2.25–2.62 mmol/L)
Chloride (Cl)	98 mEq/L (98 mmol/L)	98-106 mEq/L (98–106 mmol/L)
Glucose level	212 mg/dL (11.8 mmol/L) H	74–106 mg/dL (3.9–6.1 mmol/L)
Blood urea nitrogen (BUN)	22 mg/dL (7.8 mmol/L) H	10–20 mg/dL (2.9–8.2 mmol/L)
Creatinine (Cr)	1.0 mg/dL (88.3 mcmol/L)	0.6–1.2 mg/dL (53–106 mcmol/L)
Glomerular filtration rate (eGFR)	70 mL/min/1.73 m^2	>60 mL/min/1.73 m^2
Complete Blood Count (CBC)		
White blood cells (WBCs)	6000/mm^3 (6.0 × 10^9/L)	5000–10,000/mm^3 (3.5–12 × 10^9/L)
Red blood cells (RBCs)	4.6 × 10^{12}/L (4.6 × 10^{12}/L)	4.2–6.1 × 10^{12}/L (4.2–6.2 × 10^{12}/L)
Hemoglobin (Hgb)	Hgb: 13 g/dL (130 g/L)	12–18 g/dL (120–180 g/L)
Hematocrit (Hct)	38% (0.38 volume fraction)	37%–52% (0.37–0.54 volume fraction)
Cardiac Markers		
Troponin T	0.8 ng/mL (0.8 mcg/L) H	<0.1 ng/mL (0.1 mcg/L)

A 70-year-old client arrived at the ED for chest heaviness and difficulty breathing. The nurse is conducting the admission assessment.

| Health History | Physical Assessment | Vital Signs | Test Results |

1200: 70-year-old client admitted to the ED reporting chest heaviness and difficulty breathing for 2 days. Symptoms are noticed more with activity and subside with rest after a few minutes. Past medical history of type 2 DM, hypertension, hyperlipidemia, hypothyroidism, osteoarthritis. Currently smokes 1 pack cigarettes per day × 20 years. Medications include sliding scale insulin aspart prior to meals and at bedtime, insulin glargine at bedtime, lisinopril, atorvastatin, levothyroxine, and naproxen.

| Health History | Physical Assessment | Vital Signs | Test Results |

General: Appears nontoxic, well nourished, well hydrated.
Integumentary: Warm, dry, intact.
Respiratory: Lungs clear to auscultation bilaterally, no adventitious sounds. No use of accessory muscles.
Cardiovascular: HR irregularly irregular. S1 and S2 noted, no S3 or S4, no murmurs, rubs, gallops. No peripheral edema.
GI: Abdomen soft, nontender, nondistended. BS present × 4 quads.
Neurologic: Cranial nerves II–XII grossly intact.

| Health History | Physical Assessment | Vital Signs | Test Results |

1200: VS: T = 36.4°C (97.5°F) oral; HR = 130 BPM; RR = 20 bpm; BP = 108/59 mm Hg; SpO$_2$ = 95% on RA
Height: 165 cm (5 feet 5 inches)
Weight: 81.6 kg (180 lb)
BMI: 30.0
1200: I: 120 mL water (oral)
1230: O: 140 mL clear yellow urine

| Health History | Physical Assessment | Vital Signs | Test Results |

ECG:
Atrial fibrillation with rapid ventricular response, rate 130 BPM
Acute anterior and lateral MI
Intraventricular conduction delay
No ST elevation

Laboratory Test	Results	Normal Reference Range
Sodium (Na)	136 mEq/L (136 mmol/L)	136–145 mEq/L (136–145 mmol/L)
Potassium (K)	3.8 mEq/L (3.8 mmol/L)	3.5–5.0 mEq/L (3.5–5.1 mmol/L)
Calcium (Ca)	9.2 mg/dL (2.4 mmol/L)	9–10.5 mg/dL (2.25–2.62 mmol/L)
Chloride (Cl)	98 mEq/L (98 mmol/L)	98–106 mEq/L (98–106 mmol/L)
Glucose level	212 mg/dL (11.8 mmol/L) H	74–106 mg/dL (3.9–6.1 mmol/L)
Blood urea nitrogen (BUN)	22 mg/dL (7.8 mmol/L) H	10–20 mg/dL (2.9–8.2 mmol/L)
Creatinine (Cr)	1.0 mg/dL (88.3 mcmol/L)	0.6–1.2 mg/dL (53–106 mcmol/L)
Glomerular filtration rate (eGFR)	70 mL/min/1.73 m^2	>60 mL/min/1.73 m^2
Complete Blood Count (CBC)		
White blood cells (WBC)	6000/mm^3 (6.0 × 10^9/L)	5000–10,000/mm^3 (3.5–12 × 10^9/L)
Red blood cells (RBCs)	4.6 × 10^{12}/L (4.6 × 10^{12}/L)	4.2–6.1 × 10^{12}/L (4.2–6.2 × 10^{12}/L)
Hemoglobin (Hgb)	Hgb: 13 g/dL (130 g/L)	12–18 g/dL (120–180 g/L)
Hematocrit (Hct)	38% (0.38 volume fraction)	37%–52% (0.37–0.54 volume fraction)
Cardiac Markers		
Troponin T	0.8 ng/mL (0.8 mcg/L) H	<0.1 ng/mL (0.1 mcg/L)

Based on the assessment findings, the nurse monitors for complications. Complete the following sentence by choosing from the lists of options provided.

The client is at **highest** risk for developing ____ 1 [Select] ____

as evidenced by ____ 2 [Select] ____ .

Options for 1	Options for 2
Fluid volume overload	I&O
Diminished cardiac output	Respiratory assessment
Decreased renal perfusion	Neurologic assessment
VTE	Cardiovascular assessment

A 70-year-old client arrived at the ED for chest heaviness and difficulty breathing. The nurse is conducting the admission assessment.

Health History	Physical Assessment	Vital Signs	Test Results

1200: 70-year-old client admitted to the ED reporting chest heaviness and difficulty breathing for 2 days. Symptoms are noticed more with activity and subside with rest after a few minutes. Past medical history of type 2 DM, hypertension, hyperlipidemia, hypothyroidism, osteoarthritis. Currently smokes 1 pack cigarettes per day × 20 years. Medications include sliding scale insulin aspart prior to meals and at bedtime, insulin glargine at bedtime, lisinopril, atorvastatin, levothyroxine, and naproxen.

Health History	Physical Assessment	Vital Signs	Test Results

General: Appears nontoxic, well nourished, well hydrated.
Integumentary: Warm, dry, intact.
Respiratory: Lungs clear to auscultation bilaterally, no adventitious sounds. No use of accessory muscles.
Cardiovascular: HR irregularly irregular. S1 and S2 noted, no S3 or S4, no murmurs, rubs, gallops. No peripheral edema.
GI: Abdomen soft, nontender, nondistended. BS present × 4 quads.
Neurologic: Cranial nerves II–XII grossly intact.

Health History	Physical Assessment	Vital Signs	Test Results

1200: VS: T = 36.4°C (97.5°F) oral; HR = 130 BPM; RR = 20 bpm; BP = 108/59 mm Hg; SpO_2 = 95% on RA
Height: 165 cm (5 feet 5 inches)
Weight: 81.6 kg (180 lb)
BMI: 30.0
1200: I: 120 mL water (oral)
1230: O: 140 mL clear yellow urine

Health History	Physical Assessment	Vital Signs	Test Results

ECG:
Atrial fibrillation with rapid ventricular response, rate 130 BPM
Acute anterior and lateral MI
Intraventricular conduction delay
No ST elevation

Laboratory Test	Results	Normal Reference Range
Sodium (Na)	136 mEq/L (136 mmol/L)	136–145 mEq/L (136–145 mmol/L)
Potassium (K)	3.8 mEq/L (3.8 mmol/L)	3.5–5.0 mEq/L (3.5–5.1 mmol/L)
Calcium (Ca)	9.2 mg/dL (2.4 mmol/L)	9–10.5 mg/dL (2.25–2.62 mmol/L)
Chloride (Cl)	98 mEq/L (98 mmol/L)	98–106 mEq/L (98–106 mmol/L)
Glucose level	212 mg/dL (11.8 mmol/L) **H**	74–106 mg/dL (3.9–6.1 mmol/L)
Blood urea nitrogen (BUN)	22 mg/dL (7.8 mmol/L) **H**	10–20 mg/dL (2.9–8.2 mmol/L)
Creatinine (Cr)	1.0 mg/dL (88.3 mcmol/L)	0.6–1.2 mg/dL (53–106 mcmol/L)
Glomerular filtration rate (eGFR)	70 mL/min/1.73 m²	>60 mL/min/1.73 m²
Complete Blood Count (CBC)		
White blood cells (WBCs)	6000/mm³ (6.0 × 10⁹/L)	5000–10,000/mm³ (3.5–12 × 10⁹/L)
Red blood cells (RBCs)	4.6 × 10¹²/L (4.6 × 10¹²/L)	4.2–6.1 × 10¹²/L (4.2–6.2 × 10¹²/L)
Hemoglobin (Hgb)	Hgb: 13 g/dL (130 g/L)	12–18 g/dL (120–180 g/L)
Hematocrit (Hct)	38% (0.38 volume fraction)	37%–52% (0.37–0.54 volume fraction)
Cardiac Markers		
Troponin T	0.8 ng/mL (0.8 mcg/L) **H**	<0.1 ng/mL (0.1 mcg/L)

The nurse has completed the admission assessment and is initiating the plan of care. The nurse notes that the cardiologist has been consulted and has ordered further diagnostic testing.

Based on the clinical scenario, complete the following sentence by dragging one answer from each list of options.

The **priority** and **most specific** diagnostic test would be _____1 [Select]_____ to assess for _____2 [Select]_____.

Options for 1	Options for 2
D-dimer level	Blood clots
Chest radiograph	Cardiomegaly
Cardiac catheterization	Hyperthyroidism
Trended electrolyte levels	Hypokalemia or hyperkalemia
Thyroid-stimulating hormone	Blockages and narrowed vessels

Practice Question 10.22   Unfolding Case Study 4

The consulting cardiologist ordered cardiac catheterization for a 70-year-old client suspected of having an MI. Stents were placed, and blood flow was re-established to the affected areas of the heart. The procedure has been completed, and the nurse is monitoring the client on the intermediate care unit. The left femoral vein was used as the insertion site for the procedure.

Choose the interventions the nurse would plan in the care of this client following cardiac catheterization. **Select all that apply.**

☐ Assess for shortness of breath.

☐ Keep both extremities straight.

☐ Encourage activity as tolerated.

☐ Apply a soft knee brace to the left leg.

☐ Position the client in a supine position.

☐ Monitor the client for changes in mental status.

☐ Monitor the VS every 15 minutes initially.

☐ Assess the insertion site for bloody drainage or hematoma.

☐ Apply SCDs to both lower extremities.

☐ Assess circulation, sensation, and motion of the affected extremity.

Practice Question 10.23 — Unfolding Case Study 4

A 70-year-old client was diagnosed with acute MI and post-myocardial heart failure with an ejection fraction of 30%. The nurse is initiating discharge teaching related to medication therapy.

Which information will the nurse teach the client regarding the discharge medications? Choose the **most likely** option for the missing information in the table below by choosing from the lists of options provided.

Medication	Dose, Route, Frequency	Drug Class	Indication
1 [Select]	81 mg orally daily	Antiplatelet	MI prevention
Carvedilol	6.25 mg orally twice daily	Beta blocker	4 [Select]
Atorvastatin	20 mg orally daily	3 [Select]	Atherosclerotic cardiovascular disease
Lisinopril	5 mg orally daily	Angiotensin converting enzyme inhibitor	5 [Select]
Nitroglycerin	2 [Select]	Vasodilator	Acute angina

Options for 1	Options for 2	Options for 3	Options for 4	Options for 5
Aspirin	0.6 mg sublingually every 15 minutes as needed up to 5 times	Fibrate	Acute angina	Hypertension
Ibuprofen		Bile acid sequestrant	Hypertension	Hyperlipidemia
Diclofenac	0.4 mg sublingually every 5 minutes as needed up to 3 times	HMG-CoA reductase inhibitor	Heart failure with reduced ejection fraction	Heart failure with reduced ejection fraction
	0.6 mg sublingually × 1 before strenuous activity			

Practice Question 10.24   Unfolding Case Study 4

The nurse is caring for a 70-year-old client who had a cardiac catheterization yesterday to confirm an MI and has completed discharge teaching using the teach-back method. This morning the nurse is evaluating the client's understanding of the discharge plan of care.

For each of the statements made by the client, click or specify with an X whether the statement indicates an **Understanding** *or* **No Understanding** *of the teaching provided.*

Client Statements	Understanding	No Understanding
"I should walk 1 mile at least once a day in the beginning."	☐	☐
"I will be sure to carry my nitroglycerin with me."	☐	☐
I will check my pulse before, during, and after I do my exercises."	☐	☐
"If I notice my pulse is more than 5 BPM higher than what it usually is, I won't exercise."	☐	☐
"I will exercise indoors as much as possible."	☐	☐
"I will make sure to walk at least 3 times per week."	☐	☐
"I need to avoid straining, so I won't do push-ups or pull-ups."	☐	☐

Stand-alone Items

Stand-alone Item 1: Trend

Practice Question 10.25   **Stand-alone Item 1: Trend**

The nurse is caring for a 56-year-old client admitted 2 days ago from the ED for recurring atrial fibrillation. The client has a history of obesity, heart failure, and hypertension. Today the client reports increasing pitting edema of ankles and is worried about another episode of heart failure. Morning VS are as follows: T = 98°F (36.7°C); HR = 84 BPM; RR = 20 bpm; BP = 158/92. A review of the client's I&O record shows that 24-hour urinary output on hospital day 1 was 750 mL; yesterday urinary output decreased to 535 mL. The nurse reviews the client's lab profile to compare lab results from this morning with those on the day of admission.

*Based on the client's laboratory results, which **six physician's orders** would the nurse anticipate?*

☐ Prepare client for kidney imaging studies.
☐ Administer fluid challenge.
☐ Begin diuretic therapy.
☐ Maintain strict I&O.
☐ Insert indwelling urinary catheter.
☐ Record hourly urinary output.
☐ Weigh client daily before breakfast.
☐ Prepare client for hemodialysis.

Health History	Lab Results	Imaging Studies	Nurses' Notes

Laboratory Test	Laboratory Results on Admission	Laboratory Results Today	Normal Reference Range
Sodium (Na)	141 mEq/L (141 mmol/L)	138 mEq/L (138 mmol/L)	136–145 mEq/L (136–145 mmol/L)
Potassium (K)	5.0 mEq/L (5.0 mmol/L)	5.5 mEq/L (5.5 mmol/L) H	3.5–5.0 mEq/L (3.5–5.0 mmol/L)
Glucose	106 mg/dL (6.0 mmol/L)	100 mg/dL (5.5 mmol/L)	70–110 mg/dL (3.9–6.1 mmol/L)
Calcium (Ca)	9.0 mEq/L (9.0 mmol/L)	8.6 mEq/L (8.6 mmol/L) L	9.0–10.5 mEq/L (9.0–10.5 mmol/L)
Blood urea nitrogen (BUN)	28 mg/dL (10.0 mmol/dL) H	38 mg/dL (13.6 mmol/L) H	8.0–23.0 mg/dL (2.9–8.2 mmol/L)
Creatinine	1.8 mg/dL (157.2 mcmol/L) H	3.1 mg/dL (274.1 mcmol/L) H	0.6–1.2 mg/dL (53–106 mcmol/L)
Hemoglobin (Hgb)	14.2 g/dL (142 g/L)	14.0 g/dL (140 g/L)	14.0–18.0 g/dL (140–180 g/L)
Hematocrit (Hct)	46% (0.46 volume fraction)	44% (0.44 volume fraction)	42%–54% (0.42–0.54 volume fraction)

Stand-alone Item 2: Trend

Practice Question 10.26   Stand-alone Item 2: Trend

The nurse in the surgical unit is caring for a 51-year-old postoperative client with non–small cell lung cancer (NSCLC) of the right lung who had a thoracotomy. The client has a chest tube attached to a stationary closed chest drainage system.

| Health History | Physical Assessment | Vital Signs | Nurses' Notes |

1300: Arrived from the PACU. Alert and oriented × 3. Resting comfortably in bed, no restlessness. Closed chest tube drainage system intact. Upper tube is near the right front lung apex, occlusive dressing dry and intact. Lower tube on the right side near the base of the lung, occlusive dressing dry and intact. Drainage chamber = 70 mL red fluid. Water seal chamber = fluctuation of fluid, no bubbling. Suction control chamber = gentle bubbling. No subcutaneous emphysema. No shortness of breath or difficulty breathing. Lung sounds clear bilaterally. HOB elevated. Trachea midline. O_2 2 L per NC. Having difficulty with coughing and deep breathing and using incentive spirometer. Pain 4/10.
1400: Alert and oriented × 3. Reports nausea. Restless, states pain is 8/10. Closed chest tube drainage system intact. Occlusive dressings dry and intact. Drainage chamber = 170 mL red fluid. Water seal chamber = fluctuation of fluid with intermittent bubbling. Suction control chamber = gentle bubbling. No subcutaneous emphysema. States difficulty breathing due to pain. Lung sounds clear bilaterally. HOB elevated. Trachea midline. O_2 2 L per NC. Refusing to cough and deep breathe or use incentive spirometer due to pain. Able to tolerate respiratory treatment with assistance of respiratory therapist. Nausea and pain medication administered as prescribed.
1500: Sleepy but arousable. Restless, states nausea subsided, pain 7/10. Closed chest tube drainage system intact. Occlusive dressings dry and intact. Drainage chamber = 170 mL red fluid. Water seal chamber = continuous bubbling. Suction control chamber = gentle bubbling. Small amount subcutaneous emphysema around upper tube near the right front lung apex. States difficulty breathing. Lung sounds = crackles in lower lobes bilaterally. Trachea = slight deviation to the left. O_2 2 L per NC. Refusing to cough and deep breathe.

| Health History | Physical Assessment | Vital Signs | Nurses' Notes |

	1300	1400	1500
T	99.6°F (37.5°C)	100.4°F (38.0°C)	101.6 F (38.6°C)
HR	88 BPM	96 BPM	110 BPM
RR	18 bpm	22 bpm	26 bpm
BP	100/62 mm Hg	128/88 mm Hg	140/90 mm Hg
SpO_2	94% on 2 L O_2 per NC	92% on 2 L O_2 per NC	90% on 2 L O_2 per NC

Click (or check with an X) to indicate whether each nursing action listed below is either **Anticipated** (appropriate or necessary) or **Contraindicated** (could be harmful)/**Not Helpful** for the client's plan of care at this time.

Nursing Action	Anticipated	Contraindicated/ Not Helpful
Contact the surgeon.	☐	☐
Clamp the chest tube.	☐	☐
Request an order for a stat chest x-ray.	☐	☐
Monitor the client for continued changes over the next hour.	☐	☐
Request an order for additional pain medication.	☐	☐
Flush the chest drainage tube.	☐	☐
Increase the amount of suction in the suction control.	☐	☐

Stand-alone Item 3: Trend

A 2-year-old child is seen in the ED, where the ED physician diagnoses moderate acute laryngotracheobronchitis.

Health History	Nurses' Notes	Vital Signs	Physical Assessment

Neurologic: Alert and responsive. Resting comfortably in bed, no restlessness. Responsive to verbal and tactile stimuli.

Respiratory: Chest symmetrical. Suprasternal retractions with nasal flaring. Barking cough, labored breathing, use of accessory muscles. Inspiratory wheezes bilaterally.

Cardiovascular: S1 and S2 noted, pulse 110 BPM. No murmurs, rubs, gallops. No cyanosis, edema, clubbing, pulsations. Radial pulses 2+ bilaterally. Pedal pulses 2+ bilaterally.

Health History	Nurses' Notes	Vital Signs	Physical Assessment

	1000	1015	1030
Temperature	99.6°F (37.5°C)	99.4°F (37.4°C)	99.6°F (37.5°C)
Apical pulse	110 BPM	112 BPM	112 BPM
RR	34 bpm	36 bpm	34 bpm
BP	100/62 mm Hg	98/60 mm Hg	98/60 mm Hg
SpO$_2$	94% on RA	92% on RA	90% on RA

The nurse is preparing to collaborate with the ED physician about the child's plan of care. Based on the assessment findings, highlight the interventions the nurse anticipates the ED physician to order. **Select all that apply.**

☐ Oral dexamethasone

☐ Supplemental oxygen

☐ Cool mist via facemask

☐ Intubation with ventilation

☐ Strict NPO status

☐ Nebulized epinephrine every 20 to 30 minutes prn

☐ Limited interaction between the parents and child

Stand-alone Item 4: Bow-tie

Practice Question 10.28   Stand-alone Item 4: Bow-tie

The nurse is assigned to care for a 74-year-old client who was admitted this morning for a spider bite (type unknown) on the left calf that occurred 3 days ago while hiking. Since that time, the leg has become increasingly reddened, hot, swollen, and painful. This morning the bite area started to drain a moderate amount of greenish-yellow exudate, which prompted the client to go to the ED. VS: T = 98.4°F (36.9°C); HR = 85 BPM; RR = 16 bpm; BP = 128/76 mm Hg; SpO$_2$ = 97% on RA. The client's medical history includes type 2 DM, chronic heart failure, and hypertension. The client was admitted for IV drug therapy with ceftriaxone and observation. The nurse is preparing to administer the first dose of ceftriaxone to the client.

Complete the diagram by dragging from the choices below to specify what drug classification ceftriaxone is in, two actions the nurse would take when caring for the client receiving this drug, and two parameters the nurse would monitor to assess the client's progress and the effectiveness of the drug.

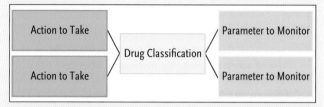

Actions to Take	Drug Classification	Parameters to Monitor
Check for allergy to penicillin before giving drug.	Penicillin	Oxygen saturation
Assess for fluid retention.	Carbapenem	VS
Monitor for seizures.	Cephalosporin	Wound drainage
Avoid giving NSAIDs.	Monobactam	Breath sounds
Assess for dysrhythmias.		Serum potassium

Stand-alone Item 5: Bow-tie

A 72-year-old client is being prepared for hospital discharge following treatment for a new-onset episode of atrial fibrillation. The client's medical history notes that the client has a long-term history of heart failure that has been treated with diet and medications, including furosemide, lisinopril, and carvedilol. Apixaban 5 mg orally twice daily has been added to the home medication regimen. The nurse plans discharge teaching for the client about the new medication.

Complete the diagram by dragging from the choices below to specify the primary adverse effect of apixaban, two points the nurse would teach the client, and two statements that indicate understanding following teaching.

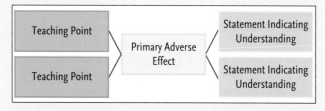

Teaching Points	Primary Adverse Effect	Statements Indicating Understanding
Headaches are a common side effect of the drug and are expected.	Bleeding	"Ibuprofen is best to take if I have a headache."
Right side pain radiating to the shoulder is common.	Hypotension	"I really hope that I don't end up getting gallbladder stones from this drug."
Urinary retention can occur during treatment.	Gallbladder stones	"If I bruise easily or note any blood in my urine I will call my doctor."
Nosebleeds or gum bleeding is a concern.	Renal impairment	"I need to have my blood work checked twice weekly while I am taking this medication."
Persistent tiredness and weakness should be reported to the physician.		"Reactions to the drug are rare but if I get a rash I should have it checked."

Stand-alone Item 6: Bow-tie

Stand-alone Item 6: Bow-tie

The nurse in the birthing suite performs an initial assessment on a newborn and documents the following data in the Nurses' Notes.

Health History	Nurses' Notes	Vital Signs	Lab Results

0800: Newborn of 43 weeks' gestation born via vaginal delivery. Apgar score at 1 minute = 3. Newborn limp, skin color bluish, RR 80 bpm, grunting during breathing with nasal flaring. Lacks cry with minimal response to gentle slap on soles. Nails and umbilical cord stained a yellow-green color. Blood glucose 40 mg/dL (2.2 mmol/L). Profuse scalp hair. Length 23 inches (58.42 cm), weight 5.5 lb (2500 g). SpO_2 = 90% on RA.

Complete the diagram by dragging (or selecting) from the choices below to specify which potential condition the newborn is most likely experiencing, two assessment findings that support that condition, and two potential interventions to treat the condition.

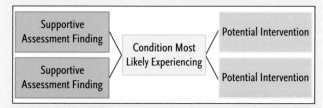

Supportive Assessment Findings	Condition Most Likely Experiencing	Potential Interventions
Skin color bluish	Acrocyanosis	Suctioning
Profuse scalp hair	Meconium aspiration syndrome	Oxygen therapy
Skin dry and cracked without lanugo	Large for gestational age	Early feedings with dextrose
Length 23 inches (58.42 cm), weight 5.5 lb (2500 g)	Transient tachypnea	Phototherapy with a bili-blanket
Nails and umbilical cord stained a yellow-green color		Abdominal decompression with an NG tube

CHAPTER 3

Answers to Practice Questions

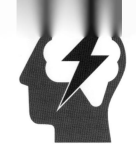

Practice Question 3.1 | **Multiple Response Grouping**

The nurse reviews the assessment findings for a newborn who was born 10 minutes ago via cesarean section at 35 weeks. The newborn's length is 19 in (48.3 cm) and weight is 4.4 lb (2000 g).

*For each body system listed below, click or specify (with an X) the newborn findings that are of **immediate** concern to the nurse. Each body system may support more than one relevant newborn finding.*

Body System	Newborn Finding
Respiratory	☐ Respirations: 40–60 bpm
	☒ Intermittent expiratory grunting
	☐ Fine crackles
	☒ Occasional apneic episodes
Neuromuscular	☒ Arms and legs relaxed
	☐ Crying
	☒ Relaxed body posture
	☒ Diminished reflexes
Cardiovascular	☐ Skin mottled
	☒ Axillary temperature: 96.7°F (35.9°C)
	☐ HR: 132 BPM and regular
	☐ Presence of murmur

Rationale: For the respiratory system, the relevant client findings that would most concern the nurse are the newborn's expiratory grunting and apneic episodes because they indicate respiratory distress and impaired gas exchange. Fine crackles are common and expected, but coarse crackles would be abnormal and concerning to the nurse. The normal/usual newborn RR is 30 to 60 bpm, so the RR is normal and expected. Mottled skin and crying are also typical for newborns. However, the arms and legs of a newborn are usually in a flexed position rather than a relaxed one. The relaxed posture could be the result of hypotonia or muscle atrophy, which could result in respiratory compromise, a significant concern for the nurse. The cardiovascular/metabolic findings, including the presence of a murmur, are typical for a newborn with the exception of the body temperature, which is below normal. A subnormal temperature (hypothermia) may lead to systemic complications such as hypoglycemia and acidosis and would therefore be concerning to the nurse. The normal newborn HR is 100 to 160 BPM.

Test-Taking Strategy: Similar to the approach you would take for the sample questions in this chapter, you would identify normal/usual or abnormal and expected (not relevant), and abnormal and not expected (relevant) client findings for the newborn in this clinical scenario to measure *Recognize Cues.* The newborn's findings can be categorized as shown in the table.

Newborn Assessment Findings	Normal/Usual or Abnormal but Expected (Not Relevant) and Not Requiring Immediate Follow-up	Abnormal and Not Expected (Relevant) and Requiring Immediate Follow-up
Respirations: 40–60 bpm	☒	☐
Intermittent expiratory grunting	☐	☒
Fine crackles	☒	☐
Occasional apneic episodes	☐	☒
Arms and legs relaxed	☐	☒
Crying	☒	☐
Relaxed body posture	☐	☒
Diminished reflexes	☐	☒
Skin mottled	☒	☐
Axillary temperature: 96.7°F (35.9°C)	☐	☒
HR: 132 BPM and regular	☒	☐
Presence of murmur	☒	☐

Recall that a baby born between 34 and 36 weeks is considered to be a late preterm newborn, which may result in abnormal assessment findings. These findings are relevant and require immediate follow-up by the nurse.

Content Area: Maternal-Newborn Nursing
Priority Concept: Gas Exchange
Reference(s): Lowdermilk et al., 2020, pp. 492–503

Practice Question 3.2 | Highlight in Text

The nurse reviews selected data from the medical record of a 54-year-old client who was admitted to the ED with report of diarrhea and weakness.

*Highlight the client findings below in the Nurses' Notes and Laboratory Results that require **immediate** follow-up by the nurse.*

Health History	Nurses' Notes	Imaging Studies	Lab Results

1900: 54-year-old client admitted to the ED with report of severe, watery diarrhea, weakness, and occasional muscle twitching. Has no nausea and vomiting; alert and oriented × 3. Has stage 3 CKD, which has been well managed with diuretics, diet, and fluid restriction. Is not receiving kidney replacement therapy. HR 59 and irregular. Current ECG shows tall peaked T waves, flat P waves, and widened QRS complexes.

Health History	Nurses' Notes	Imaging Studies	Lab Results

1930: Stat lab results.

Laboratory Test Result	Normal Reference Range
Serum sodium 145 mEq/L (145 mmol/L)	136–145 mEq/L (136–145 mmol/L)
Serum potassium 5.9 mEq/L (5.9 mmol/L) **H**	3.5–5.0 mEq/L (3.5–5.0 mmol/L)
Hemoglobin 11.0 g/dL (6.83 mmol/L) **L**	14–18 g/dL (8.7–11.2 mmol/L)
Hematocrit 35% (0.35 volume fraction) **L**	42%–52% (0.42–0.52 volume fraction)
Blood urea nitrogen (BUN) 34 mg/dL (12.14 mmol/L) **H**	10–20 mg/dL (3.6–7.1 mmol/L)
Creatinine 2.8 mg/dL (247.58 mmol/L) **H**	0.6–1.3 mg/dL (53–106 mmol/L)

Rationale: The client has severe watery diarrheal stools that are making him weak and could lead to dehydration, which is of immediate concern to the nurse. The abnormal ECG, dysrhythmia, and muscle twitching suggest that he could have an electrolyte imbalance. Weakness could also be the result of dehydration and/or electrolyte imbalance. The lab results confirm that the client has hyperkalemia, which could be causing cardiac and muscle assessment findings and can be life-threatening if not addressed. The client has an elevated blood urea nitrogen (BUN), which is consistent with both CKD and dehydration, possibly caused by his diarrhea. The nurse would be very concerned about those findings that indicate dehydration because the client could become hypovolemic and progress to shock if not treated. The low hemoglobin and hematocrit are expected for a client who has stage 3 CKD. He has no symptoms of anemia, so these lab results are expected and not relevant. The elevated creatinine is also expected because of his CKD and is not of immediate concern to the nurse at this time because it is not at a life-threatening level. An elevated creatinine is associated only with kidney function and not fluid or dietary status.

Test-Taking Strategy: To determine which client findings are of immediate concern to the nurse, you need to categorize the findings into those that are within normal/usual limits or abnormal but expected (not relevant), or abnormal and not expected (relevant), as shown in the table, to *Recognize Cues.*

Test-Taking
Strategy

Client Findings	Normal/Usual or Abnormal but Expected (Not Relevant) Not Requiring Immediate Follow-up	Abnormal and Not Expected (Relevant) Requiring Immediate Follow-up
Severe, watery diarrhea	☐	☒
Weakness	☐	☒
Occasional muscle twitching	☐	☒
History of stage 3 CKD	☒	☐
Cardiac dysrhythmia	☐	☒
Elevated serum potassium	☐	☒
Low hemoglobin	☒	☐
Low hematocrit	☒	☐
Elevated BUN	☐	☒
Elevated serum creatinine	☒	☐

Once you decide which client findings are either normal or expected and which are abnormal and not expected, you can then highlight the client findings that would be of immediate concern to the nurse at this time and require follow-up. The client's stage 3 CKD likely caused his hyperkalemia, which then resulted in cardiac, muscular, and gastrointestinal manifestations.

Content Area: Medical-Surgical Nursing
Priority Concept: Fluid and Electrolyte Balance
Reference(s): Ignatavicius et al., 2021, pp. 255–256, 1383–1386

Practice Question 3.3   **Drag-and-Drop Cloze**

A 78-year-old client has been hospitalized for the past week for evacuation of a subdural hematoma after a fall. Immediately after surgery, the client was alert and oriented with right-sided hemiparesis. The client's speech was slurred, but client could communicate needs without problem. The client was continent of bowel and bladder most of the time, and began rehabilitative therapies. On the third postoperative day, aspiration pneumonia was confirmed by x-ray and the client was placed on IV antibiotic therapy. Today the nurse reviews the last entry in the Nurses' Notes for an update of the client's condition.

Health History	Nurses' Notes	Imaging Studies	Lab Results

0730: Very drowsy this morning but can be aroused with gentle shaking. Remains oriented × 3. Does not readily respond when spoken to, but eventually answers in 1–2 words. No adventitious or diminished breath sounds. S_1, S_2 present; no additional heart sounds. BS present × 4 and abdomen soft. Had 2 incontinent diarrheal stools during the night. Able to move all extremities but right arm continues to be weak. Skin intact; no reddened areas noted. Plan to send to PT and OT this morning. Temperature this morning has increased from 98°F (36.7°C) last evening to 100.2°F (37.9°C).

Drag (or select) client findings from the choices below to fill in the blanks in the following sentence.

The nurse reviews the notes and recognizes that the client findings that are of *immediate* concern are <u>drowsiness</u>, <u>incontinent diarrheal stools</u>, <u>speech ability</u>, and <u>elevated temperature</u>.

Client Findings

Drowsiness
No adventitious or diminished breath sounds
Right arm weakness
Bowel sounds X 4
Incontinent diarrheal stools
Speech ability
Elevated temperature

Rationale: Immediately after surgery, the client was alert and oriented, communicative, and continent of bowel and bladder. The client began rehabilitative therapies for right hemiparesis and dysarthria (slurred speech), but developed aspiration pneumonia for which treatment was initiated. One week later, the client's LOC changed from alert and oriented to drowsy and oriented. A decrease in LOC suggests that the client is likely clinically deteriorating, and this change would therefore be of immediate concern to the nurse. The client is less communicative and incontinent, which are also significant changes that would concern the nurse. The elevated temperature could be related to cranial surgery or could be caused by an infection. The client's arm weakness was present after surgery, so that finding is expected and not concerning. The client's breath sounds are obviously improved as a result of treatment with antibiotic therapy. Bowel sounds are normal and expected at this time.

Test-Taking Strategy: This clinical scenario is somewhat different from the other test item examples in this chapter because the client's recent health history since hospital admission is presented prior to the current Nurses' Notes entry. To answer this test item correctly, you need to first compare the client's current assessment data with the previous data. Then categorize the client's findings as you would do for the other test items that measure *Recognize Cues*.

Test-Taking
Strategy

Client Findings	Normal/Usual or Abnormal and Expected (Not Relevant) Not Requiring Immediate Follow-up	Abnormal and Not Expected (Relevant) Requiring Immediate Follow-up
Drowsiness	☐	☒
No adventitious or diminished breath sounds	☒	☐
Elevated temperature	☐	☒
Right arm weakness	☒	☐
Bowel sounds X 4	☒	☐
Incontinent diarrheal stools	☐	☒
Speech ability	☐	☒

Content Area: Medical-Surgical Nursing
Priority Concept: Immunity
Reference(s): Ignatavicius et al., 2021, pp. 414–415, 916–918

The nurse reviews part of a Nurses' Notes entry for a 48-year-old client admitted to the inpatient psychiatric unit after a suicide attempt.

Health History	**Nurses' Notes**	Imaging Studies	Lab Results

1100: Admitted to unit for observation and treatment related to a suicide attempt. Attempted to cut both wrists, which are currently bandaged. Client was in a severe motor vehicle accident 5 months ago, resulting in quadriplegia. Has been living in a group home with full-time caregiver for assistance with ADLs since discharge from rehabilitation. Has no family living in the area. Has Stage 3 sacral pressure injury covered with gauze dressing. Recently completed a course of antibiotics for infected sacral wound. Wears an external condom catheter and follows bowel regimen but has frequent problems with urine leakage and bowel incontinence. Is able to transfer with supervision from bed to wheelchair using sliding board. Lost 20 lb (9.1 kg) since the accident and describes appetite as "fair." Does not want to be here because he is "sick of being in hospitals."

Which client findings are of **immediate** concern to the nurse related to risk factors for additional or worsening pressure injuries? **Select all that apply.**

☐ Attempted suicide
☒ Quadriplegic
☒ Current stage 3 sacral wound
☐ ADL dependent
☒ Uses sliding board for transfers
☒ Urinary and bowel incontinence
☐ 48 years of age
☐ Weight loss of 20 lb (9.1 kg)
☐ Fair appetite

Rationale: The nurse recognizes that the client is at high risk for additional or worsening pressure injury due to a number of factors. First, the client already has a stage 3 pressure injury, which resulted in full-thickness skin loss and infection. A local infection can lead to systemic infection and possibly sepsis, a potentially life-threatening health problem. The existence of a pressure injury suggests that the client is vulnerable to skin breakdown. As a result of the client's accident, the client has impaired mobility and is unable to walk. Impaired mobility is a major risk factor for skin breakdown and would be a concern for the nurse. Using a sliding board for transfers can lead to skin friction and shearing, especially due to decreased skin sensation. To add to impaired mobility, the client's skin is frequently soiled by urine and feces. Excessive skin moisture is a major risk factor and would therefore alert the nurse that the client is at high risk for skin and tissue breakdown. The client is not an older adult, meaning that skin should not be thinning to make the client vulnerable for skin integrity issues. Weight loss and fair appetite are likely not of concern at the moment because the client's original weight is not known and quadriplegics have better mobility at a lower weight. The client's ADL dependence is expected and would not cause skin integrity problems.

Test-Taking Strategy

Test-Taking Strategy: To answer this question that measures *Recognize Cues,* you would need to think about what client findings could lead to additional problems with his skin and tissue integrity as categorized in the table.

Client Findings	Normal/Usual, Abnormal or Expected, but Not a Risk Factor for Pressure Injury	Abnormal or Expected, but Is a Risk Factor for Pressure Injury
Attempted suicide	☒	☐
Quadriplegic	☐	☒
Current stage 3 sacral wound	☐	☒
ADL dependent	☒	☐
Uses sliding board for transfers	☐	☒

Client Findings	Normal/Usual, Abnormal or Expected, but Not a Risk Factor for Pressure Injury	Abnormal or Expected, but Is a Risk Factor for Pressure Injury
Urinary and bowel incontinence	☐	☒
48 years of age	☒	☐
Weight loss of 20 lb (9.1 kg)	☒	☐
Fair appetite	☒	☐

As you might expect from the Nurses' Notes, the client has five of the six evidence-based risk factors for predicting pressure injury risk identified by the Braden Scale, as shown in the table.

Braden Scale Risk Factors for Predicting Pressure Injury Risk	Client Risk Factors for Pressure Injury (indicated by an X)
Sensory perception impairment	☒
Moisture excess	☒
Activity impairment	☒
Mobility impairment	☒
Nutrition deficit	☐
Friction and shear problem	☒

The Braden Scale for predicting pressure injury risk is a valid tool frequently used by nurses to assess for risk of skin breakdown. If using the Braden scale, you would determine a score for each of these categories. The scores are totaled and interpreted as:

Score of 15–16	Client is at mild risk for skin breakdown
Score of 12–14	Client is at moderate risk for skin breakdown
Score of less than 11	Client is at severe risk for skin breakdown

The references below include the entire Braden tool if you need to review it.

Content Area: Foundations of Nursing
Priority Concept: Tissue Integrity
Reference(s): Ignatavicius et al., 2021, pp. 440–441; Potter et al., 2021, pp. 1241–1244

Practice Question 3.5   Drop-Down in Table

The nurse reviews the Nurses' Notes documented by the nurse from the last shift who was assigned to care for a 70-year-old client. The client had a right THA 2 days ago and is planning to be discharged tomorrow.

Health History	Nurses' Notes	Imaging Studies	Lab Results

1805: Alert and oriented. Walked in hall tonight with walker independently. Reports increasing pain in right hip and "feeling funny" and anxious for the past hour. Is excited to go home tomorrow and follow up with PT. Husband states that the client has been coughing periodically since stopped walking and returned to the room. No adventitious or abnormal breath sounds. Current VS: T = 99.4°F (37.3°C); HR = 88 BPM; RR = 20 bpm; BP = 102/58 mm Hg; SpO2 = 93% (on RA). Will recheck client and VS in 1 hour.

1922: Reports "a little" difficulty breathing but denies chest pain. VS: T = 99.4°F (37.3°C); HR = 94 BPM; RR = 26 bpm; BP 98/52 = mm Hg; SpO2 88% (on RA). Oxygen initiated at 2/min via NC and HOB in Fowler position. MD notified and awaiting orders.

For each body system listed below, select the client findings that would be of **immediate** concern to the nurse. Each body system may support more than one client finding, but at least one option should be selected for each system.

Body System	Client Findings
Cardiovascular	Hypotension Decreased oxygen saturation
Neurologic	Increased right hip pain Feeling anxious
Respiratory	Difficulty breathing Tachypnea

Options for 1	Options for 2	Options for 3
Tachycardia	Increased right hip pain	Difficulty breathing
Hypotension	Ambulating with walker	Tachypnea
Decreased oxygen saturation	Feeling anxious	Periodic coughing

Rationale: The client is getting ready for discharge the next day but begins to have new onset of symptoms. The cardiovascular findings that are of immediate concern to the nurse are the significant changes in VS. The client became hypotensive with a BP of 98/52 mm Hg. The oxygen saturation also decreased from 93% to 88% on RA. Although the normal oxygen saturation is 95% or greater, it is not unusual for a 70-year-old client to have a 93% level. However, 88% is too low and is of major concern to the nurse. These changes suggest possible clinical decline. Although HR increased, it is not considered tachycardic. The major neurologic change for the client is increased right (surgical) hip pain. The client should be having less hip pain when preparing for discharge to home. The client's anxiety may be due to increased hip pain, impending hospital discharge, or decreased oxygen saturation, and therefore is important to the nurse at this time. New rapid onset of difficulty breathing and tachypnea (RR is 26 bpm) could indicate PE or other cardiopulmonary health problem. Increased respirations are the first sign of a client's clinical deterioration. Many clients who experience a PE also have chest pain and cough, but this client denies chest pain and has only a periodic cough, which could be the result of sinus congestion, dry throat, or allergy.

Test-Taking
Strategy

Test-Taking Strategy: Recall that this client began having new symptoms that worsened within an hour. To answer this test item correctly, you need to categorize the findings into those that are within normal/usual limits or abnormal but expected (not relevant), or abnormal and not expected (relevant), as shown in the table, to *Recognize Cues.*

Client Findings	Normal/Usual or Abnormal and Expected (Not Relevant) Not Requiring Immediate Follow-up	Abnormal and Not Expected (Relevant) Requiring Immediate Follow-up
Increased HR	☒	☐
Hypotension	☐	☒
Decreased oxygen saturation	☐	☒
Right hip pain	☐	☒

Client Findings	Normal/Usual or Abnormal and Expected (Not Relevant) Not Requiring Immediate Follow-up	Abnormal and Not Expected (Relevant) Requiring Immediate Follow-up
Ambulating with walker	☒	☐
Feeling anxious	☐	☒
Difficulty breathing	☐	☒
Tachypnea	☐	☒
Periodic coughing	☒	☐

Content Area: Medical-Surgical Nursing
Priority Concept: Perfusion
Reference(s): Ignatavicius et al., 2021, pp. 588–589

Practice Question 3.6	Multiple Response Select N

The nurse reviews the admission note for a 13-year-old client in the Urgent Care Center.

Health History	Nurses' Notes	Imaging Studies	Lab Results

0850: Parent reports that son started having new GI symptoms 2 days ago, which were "due to something he may have eaten and didn't agree with him." Started with lack of appetite and nausea but has progressed to fever and vomiting with occasional diarrhea. Last night he went to bed earlier than usual and showed no interest in playing video games as he usually does before dinner every night. Parents are divorced; child is with one parent during the school week and the other parent every weekend. Parent is concerned that son does not eat a very healthy diet on the weekends. Both of them prefer "fast food," especially hamburgers. This morning parent noted dark urine in the toilet. Current temperature is 103.2°F (39.6°C). Child states he feels very tired and wants to go home to bed.

Select four client findings that are of **immediate** concern to the nurse.

☒ Anorexia
☐ Occasional diarrhea
☒ Nausea and vomiting
☐ Poor eating habits
☒ Elevated temperature
☐ Fatigue
☐ Wants to sleep
☒ Dark urine

Rationale: The child experienced new GI symptoms 2 days ago that included anorexia, nausea/vomiting, and elevated temperature (fever). These findings are significant and of immediate concern to the nurse because the child could become dehydrated and have electrolyte imbalances. Having dark urine is also of concern because this finding could be due to an increased bilirubin caused by liver inflammation or dysfunction. The child's diarrhea is *not* concerning at this time because it is only occasional and commonly occurs in children with GI distress. Fatigue and desire to sleep are expected because of the client's GI symptoms and would not be of concern for the nurse at this time. A low sodium and/or potassium level can cause fatigue, malaise, and weakness. Hypovolemia caused by fluid loss through vomiting (combined perhaps with occasional diarrhea) can also cause these symptoms. The child's poor eating habits can be addressed later and are not a part of the nurse's current concern for planning care.

Test-Taking Strategy

Test-Taking Strategy: Similar to the other practice questions in this chapter, you need to categorize the client findings as those that are within normal/usual limits or abnormal but expected (not relevant), or abnormal and not expected (relevant), as shown in the table, to *Recognize Cues.* Then you will be able to easily select the correct options.

Client Findings	Normal/Usual or Abnormal and Expected (Not Relevant) Not Requiring Immediate Follow-up	Abnormal and Not Expected (Relevant) Requiring Immediate Follow-up
Anorexia	☐	☒
Occasional diarrhea	☒	☐
Nausea and vomiting	☐	☒
Poor eating habits	☒	☐
Fever	☐	☒
Fatigue	☒	☐
Wants to sleep	☒	☐
Dark urine	☐	☒

Content Area: Pediatric Nursing
Priority Concept: Immunity
Reference(s): Hockenberry et al., 2019, pp. 866–868

CHAPTER 4

Answers to Practice Questions

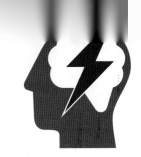

A 45-year-old client diagnosed with CKD requires dialysis. As a candidate for both hemodialysis and peritoneal dialysis, the client decides that peritoneal dialysis is the better option for their lifestyle. The client is hospitalized and undergoes insertion of the peritoneal dialysis catheter, and the first dialysis procedure is ordered. The nurse documents predialysis assessment data and reviews laboratory results.

Health History	Nurses' Notes	Vital Signs	Laboratory Results

1100: T = 98.2°F (36.8°C); apical HR = 90 BPM and regular; BP = 146/98 mm Hg; RR = 16 bpm; breath sounds clear bilaterally. Weight = 160 lb (72.57 kg)

Health History	Nurses' Notes	Vital Signs	Laboratory Results

Test	Result	Normal Reference Range
Blood urea nitrogen (BUN)	30 mg/dL (10.8 mmol/L) **H**	10–20 mg/dL (3.6–7.1 mmol/L)
Creatinine	6.0 mg/dL (528 mcmol/L) **H**	0.5–1.2 mg/dL (44–106 mcmol/L)
Glucose	110 mg/dL (6.1 mmol/L) **H**	70–99 mg/dL (3.9–5.5 mmol/L)
Sodium	150 mEq/L (150 mmol/L) **H**	135–145 mEq/L (135–145 mmol/L)
Potassium	5.5 mEq/L (5.5 mmol/L) **H**	3.5–5.0 mEq/L (3.5–5.0 mmol/L)

During dialysis infusion, the nurse notes a slow inflow of the dialysate and the client complains of pain. On assessment of the catheter, the nurse notes some fibrin clot formation in the dialysis tubing. **Complete the following sentences by choosing from the list of options.**

The nurse recognizes that the slow inflow, presence of fibrin clots, and complaints of pain are **most likely** the result of the <u>initial dialysis treatment</u> due to the <u>surgical procedure.</u>

Options for 1	Options for 2
Peritonitis	Catheter slippage
Initial dialysis treatment	Surgical procedure
Bowel perforation	Lack of aseptic technique
Abdominal pressure	Elevated BP and laboratory results

Rationale: Pain during the inflow of dialysate is common when a client is initially started on peritoneal dialysis therapy following the surgical procedure and catheter placement. Usually, this pain no longer occurs 1 to 2 weeks after receiving these treatments. Warming the dialysate bags before instillation by using a heating pad to wrap the bag or by using the warming chamber of the automated cycling machine will assist in preventing pain. Slow inflow of the dialysate is not uncommon initially but should always be assessed because it could be due to a kink in the tubing or fibrin clots. Fibrin clot formation is not uncommon after catheter placement, although it is also important to know that it can occur with peritonitis. In this client situation fibrin clot formation is most likely an expected finding because the client recently had the catheter placed and because there are no associated findings of peritonitis such as fever. In addition, it is not likely that signs of peritonitis would show just after catheter placement. Milking the tubing may dislodge the fibrin clot and improve flow. Bowel perforation would be exhibited by a brown-colored outflow. Abdominal pressure may occur on inflow and may cause minimal discomfort, but this is an unlikely occurrence in this client situation; also, fibrin clots are not associated with abdominal pressure.

Test-Taking Strategy: The first thing you would do is look at the client data and use knowledge about the peritoneal dialysis procedure and expected and unexpected findings. Think about what the findings presented mean and what could be happening to the client. The elevated BP and laboratory findings are expected in a client with CKD, indicating the need for dialysis. If the catheter slips and is malpositioned, fluid will not drain in or out. Also, note that this scenario presents a client receiving the first dialysis treatment after insertion of the dialysis catheter. Next, look at the options presented and think about what you would expect to note in each of these conditions. Construct a table to help organize your thoughts to answer correctly. In a Drop-Down Rationale item, it is important to select the correct answer for the first option so that you can correctly pair the information with the second option choices.

Condition	Expected Findings
Peritonitis	Fever, not likely to be present initially after insertion, even if there was a lack of aseptic technique
Initial dialysis treatment	Pain, slow inflow, and fibrin clots initially due to a new catheter
Bowel perforation	A complication, but the most likely finding is brown outflow
Abdominal pressure	May be present on inflow, but pain would be minimal and expected; this is unrelated to fibrin clots

Content Area: Medical-Surgical Nursing
Priority Concept: Elimination
Reference(s): Ignatavicius et al., 2021, pp. 1403–1405

Practice Question 4.2 | Drop-Down Rationale

An 80-year-old client who had a cholecystectomy 2 weeks ago was admitted 2 hours ago to the medical-surgical unit from the ED with acute pain located in the left upper abdomen. The client had laboratory testing and contrast-enhanced CT scan of the abdomen. The nurse conducts an admission assessment and reviews the laboratory and diagnostic findings.

| Health History | Nurses' Notes | Vital Signs | Diagnostic Results |

Test	Result	Normal Reference Range
White blood cells (WBCs)	16,000/mm³ (16 × 10⁹/L) **H**	5000–10,000/mm³ (5–10 × 10⁹/L)
Hemoglobin (Hgb)	16 g/dL (160 g/L)	12–18 g/dL (120–180 g/L)
Hematocrit (Hct)	44% (0.44)	37%–52% (0.37–0.52)
Blood urea nitrogen (BUN)	18 mg/dL (6.48 mmol/L)	10–20 mg/dL (3.6–7.1 mmol/L)
Creatinine	0.8 mg/dL (70.6 mcmol/L)	0.5–1.2 mg/dL (44–106 mcmol/L)
Glucose	110 mg/dL (6.1 mmol/L) **H**	70–99 mg/dL (3.9–5.5 mmol/L)
Alanine aminotransferase (ALT)	80 U/L (80 U/L) **H**	4–36 U/L (4–36 U/L)
Aspartate aminotransferase (AST):	88 U/L (88 U/L) **H**	0–35 U/L (0–35 U/L)
Activated partial thromboplastin time (aPTT)	32 sec (32 sec)	30–40 sec (30–40 sec)
Prothrombin time (PT)	11.4 sec (11.4 sec)	11–12.5 sec (11–12.5 sec)
International normalized ratio (INR)	1.0 (1.0)	0.81–1.2 (0.81–1.2)
Amylase	800 U/L (800 U/L) **H**	60–120 U/L (60–120 U/L)
Lipase	320 U/L (320 U/L) **H**	0–160 U/L (0–160 U/L)

CT abdomen with contrast impression: Edema of the uncinate process of the pancreatic head, with peripancreatic fat, consistent with acute interstitial pancreatitis

| Health History | Nurses' Notes | Vital Signs | Diagnostic Results |

1100: T = 99.2°F (36.8°C); HR = 90 BPM; BP = 168/88 mm Hg; RR = 24 bpm; SpO_2 = 89% on RA; lung sounds clear but diminished to auscultation bilaterally and breathing is nonlabored. Bowel sounds are hypoactive in all quadrants. Abdominal pain is 4/10, client receiving prescribed morphine in the ED.

Based on the information in the Nurses' Notes and in the Laboratory and Diagnostic Results, complete the following sentence from the list of options provided,

As a complication of acute pancreatitis, the client is at highest risk for developing **atelectasis** as evidenced by **SpO₂ level**.

Options for 1	Options for 2
Atelectasis	SpO_2 level
Bile duct calculi	PT/INR results
Pulmonary edema	CT abdomen results
Coagulation defects	BUN and creatinine levels

Rationale: Acute pancreatitis is an acute inflammation of the pancreas, and complications associated with acute pancreatitis can sometimes be life-threatening. Atelectasis, bile duct calculi, pulmonary edema, and coagulation defects are all potential complications of acute pancreatitis. Older adults are at risk for developing atelectasis and resultant pneumonia as a complication of acute pancreatitis. The overall clinical presentation, including leukocytosis, hyperglycemia, elevated liver enzymes and pancreatic enzymes, and the CT results, is consistent with acute pancreatitis. The elevation in BP is likely due to pain. Other clinical manifestations include the elevated temperature, RR 24 bpm, SpO_2 89% on RA, and diminished lung sounds bilaterally. These findings point to atelectasis as the most likely complication of this condition. The defining manifestation for atelectasis is the hypoxemia as evidenced by the SpO_2 level.

Test-Taking Strategy

Test-Taking Strategy: Remember to first think about client conditions consistent with the findings or cues. Ask yourself if there are any findings or cues that support or oppose any client conditions. Decide which cues are of concern and which are expected, and establish the significance of the findings within the context of the bigger clinical picture. In a Drop-Down Rationale item type, you have to understand both or all aspects of the concepts being tested in order to receive credit. To answer this question correctly, use the "Supports" or "Opposes" strategy as illustrated in the table below.

Client Finding	Supports Atelectasis	Opposes Atelectasis
SpO_2 89% on RA	☒	☐
Age	☒	☐
Elevated WBC count	☒	☐
Diminished lung sounds bilaterally	☒	☐
RR 24 bpm	☒	☐

Categorizing the findings of each complication listed in the options is a strategy that will help you analyze cues and determine which client findings support or oppose the possible complications. The complication with the most findings in the "Supports" column is most likely the correct answer for the first option. The low SpO_2 level, the elevated RR, and diminished lung sounds bilaterally support atelectasis rather than supporting pulmonary edema. In pulmonary edema, there would be labored breathing, sputum production, and adventitious lung sounds such as rhonchi or crackles. The coagulation study findings would be normal in atelectasis, whereas in coagulation defects these results would be abnormal. The CT results support acute pancreatitis and differentiate bile duct calculi, as this would be noted in the results if this complication were present. The BUN and Cr levels are normal and therefore are not related.

Content Area: Medical-Surgical Nursing
Priority Concept: Elimination
Reference(s): Ignatavicius et al., 2021, pp. 1182–1086

The nurse working at the outpatient pediatric clinic is performing an admission assessment for a 7-year-old child who is accompanied by their parent. The child reports right ear pain for 3 days. The nurse documents the following assessment findings.

Health History	Nurses' Notes	Vital Signs	Diagnostic Results

Reports right ear pain × 3 days described as constant, aching, nonradiating; denies dry mucous membranes, eye drainage, nasal drainage, or throat pain; oropharynx pink, moist, with no redness, swelling, exudate

Reports no sick contacts and has been attending full days of school; reports swimming daily for the past week

Denies neck stiffness; no swelling of the neck, or swollen lymph nodes

Denies cough, wheezing, difficulty breathing; lung sounds clear

Tenderness noted on palpation and manipulation of right auricle with ear canal erythema; no discharge; left auricle nontender

Immunizations up-to-date

Allergies: No known allergies

Health History	Nurses' Notes	Vital Signs	Diagnostic Results

Weight: 55 lb (59th percentile)
Height: 49.25 inches (55th percentile)
BMI: 15.94 (58th percentile)
T: 97.9°F (36.6°C) temporal
HR: 98 BPM
RRs: 18 bpm
BP: 108/70 mm Hg

Complete the following sentence. Drag the words from the options below to fill in each blank.

Clinical findings noted in the assessment that point to otitis externa include **ear pain without fever**, **swimming daily for the past week**, and **tenderness on manipulation of right auricle**.

Options for 1	Options for 2	Options for 3
No sick contacts	Denies neck stiffness	Denies cough
Ear pain without fever	Immunizations up-to-date	No lymphoadenopathy
Attends full school days	Swimming daily for the past week	Tenderness on manipulation of right auricle
Left auricle is nontender to manipulation	Lack of nasal drainage or throat pain	Lung sounds clear to auscultation bilaterally

Rationale: Otitis externa is also known as swimmer's ear and is associated with inflammation and possibly exudate in the external auditory canal. Otitis externa is confirmed when there are no other disorders such as otitis media or mastoiditis. Fever is usually absent, and hearing is unaffected. Often there is tenderness on palpation of the tragus and manipulation of the auricle. The lining of the canal is erythematous and edematous, and discharge may be seen. Another factor that suggests otitis externa is that the child has been swimming daily for the past week. The other findings noted are not risk factors for this problem. Attending full school days heightens the risk for otitis media, which can occur secondary to an upper respiratory infection.

Test-Taking Strategy: Remember to first think about client conditions consistent with the findings or cues. Ask yourself if there are any findings or cues that support or oppose any client conditions. Decide which cues are of concern and establish the significance of the findings within the context of the bigger clinical picture to determine what the findings mean and what is happening to the child. In a Drag-and-Drop Cloze question, partial credit is given if correct and incorrect answers are chosen. Choosing correctly as you begin answering the question will help you choose the greatest number of correct answers. In this question, thinking about the most common conditions that cause ear pain and focusing on the findings will help you answer the question correctly. Otitis externa and otitis media are the most common ear problems in children. Categorize the findings as noted in the table to assist in answering correctly.

Test-Taking Strategy

Client Finding	Otitis Externa	Otitis Media
Ear pain	☒	☒
No fever	☒	☐
No sick contacts	☒	☐
Attends full school days	☐	☒
Swimming daily for the past week	☒	☒
Tenderness noted on palpation and manipulation of the auricle	☒	☐
Erythema in the ear canal	☒	☐

Categorizing the findings of each possible problem using this table is another strategy that will help you analyze cues and determine which condition is most likely occurring. Some findings are related to both common ear problems. The condition with the most findings is most likely the correct answer. You need to rely to some extent on your knowledge base of the differences in clinical manifestations for these two conditions. The absence of fever and the presence of erythema of the external canal leads you to determine that the child is experiencing otitis externa.

Content Area: Pediatric Nursing
Priority Concept: Tissue Integrity
Reference(s): Hockenberry et al., 2019, pp. 898–902

Practice Question 4.4 **Multiple Response Select All That Apply**

Every 30 minutes the nurse is monitoring a 28-year-old client who was admitted 3 hours ago to the labor and delivery unit in the first stage of labor. The nurse suddenly notes late decelerations and frequent episodes of fetal tachycardia in response to FHR decelerations on the monitor.

The nurse determines that these findings indicate which of the following conditions? **Select all that apply.**

- ☐ Breech baby
- ☒ Fetal hypoxemia
- ☒ Metabolic fetal acidemia
- ☐ Strong uterine contractions
- ☒ Uteroplacental insufficiency

Rationale: There are certain FHR patterns associated with physiologic processes for both the birth parent and the fetus. A deceleration can be benign or abnormal. Early decelerations, considered a normal finding, are caused by fundal pressure; breech positions; strong uterine contractions; vaginal examination; and placement of internal monitoring equipment. Late decelerations are caused by fetal hypoxemia due to uteroplacental insufficiency and therefore are considered an abnormal and concerning finding. Metabolic fetal acidemia is characterized by fetal tachycardia in response to FHR decelerations and is a possible condition. In cases of fetal hypoxia, the nurse would observe progressively more frequent episodes of tachycardia after decelerations that are initially transient and later become more consistent. This is because in response to repetitive hypoxic stress from uterine contractions, the fetus initially compensates by increasing its HR, as its ability to increase stroke volume is not very efficient.

Test-Taking Strategy: Remember to first think about client conditions consistent with the findings or cues. Ask yourself if there are any findings or cues that support or oppose any client conditions. Decide which cues are of concern and unexpected and establish the significance of the findings within the context of the bigger clinical picture. For this question, use knowledge about the normal findings during labor and the significance of fetal tachycardia and decelerations. It may be helpful to organize the information by

Test-Taking Strategy

determining causes of early and late decelerations and whether there is the potential to cause fetal harm, or if fetal harm is not likely to result.

Causes	Early Decelerations	Late Decelerations	Potential to Result in Fetal Harm	Not Likely to Result in Fetal Harm
Breech baby	☒	☐	☐	☒
Fetal hypoxemia	☐	☒	☒	☐
Strong uterine contractions	☒	☐	☐	☒
Metabolic fetal acidemia	☐	☒	☒	☐
Uteroplacental insufficiency	☐	☒	☒	☐

Categorizing the cause and whether it is or is not likely to result in fetal harm as illustrated in the table is a strategy that will help you *Analyze Cues*. Then, connecting this analysis with the clinical significance of the FHR patterns will help you select the correct options, recalling that early decelerations are not a cause for concern and that late decelerations are concerning. You may need to rely on your knowledge when presented with questions about FHR patterns. You may want to also create a similar table for variability patterns to assist you with answering questions about this content.

Content Area: Maternal-Newborn Nursing
Priority Concept: Perfusion
Reference(s): Lowdermilk et al., 2020, pp. 363–370

Practice Question 4.5   Multiple Choice Select All That Apply

A 45-year-old client is admitted to the ED because of frequent episodes of chest pain unrelieved by sublingual nitroglycerin. The ECG shows ST segment elevation. Troponin levels are elevated. While awaiting results of diagnostic studies and transfer to the cardiac unit, the nurse monitors the client.
  Vital signs reveal the following:

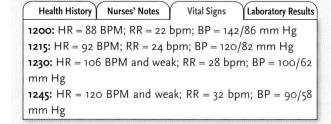

Health History	Nurses' Notes	Vital Signs	Laboratory Results

1200: HR = 88 BPM; RR = 22 bpm; BP = 142/86 mm Hg
1215: HR = 92 BPM; RR = 24 bpm; BP = 120/82 mm Hg
1230: HR = 106 BPM and weak; RR = 28 bpm; BP = 100/62 mm Hg
1245: HR = 120 BPM and weak; RR = 32 bpm; BP = 90/58 mm Hg

*The nurse determines that these vital sign findings **most likely** indicate which complication(s)? **Select all that apply.***

☐ Dysrhythmias
☐ Pulmonary edema
☒ Cardiogenic shock
☐ Cardiac tamponade
☐ Pulmonary embolism
☐ Dissecting aortic aneurysm

Rationale: Cardiogenic shock occurs with severe damage (more than 40%) to the left ventricle. Classic signs include hypotension; a rapid heart rate that becomes weaker; decreased urine output; and cool, clammy skin. RR increases as the body develops metabolic acidosis from shock. Dysrhythmias would be detected by changes in the rate and rhythm of the pulse and would be evidenced on the cardiac monitor and ECG. Although ST segment elevation is noted, there is no evidence of dysrhythmias. Pulmonary edema is evidenced by severe dyspnea and breathlessness and adventitious breath sounds. Cardiac tamponade is accompanied by distant, muffled heart sounds and prominent neck vessels. Pulmonary embolism presents suddenly with severe dyspnea accompanying the chest pain. Dissecting aortic aneurysms usually are accompanied by back pain.

Test-Taking
Strategy

Test-Taking Strategy: Focus on the words *most likely* in the stem of the question. Begin answering this question by analyzing each of the options and thinking about the manifestations of the condition and the most likely effect of each condition on the vital signs. Keeping in mind the pathophysiology associated with each condition will help you determine the most likely effect. As illustrated in the table, cardiogenic shock, cardiac tamponade, and pulmonary embolism are conditions likely to cause the changes with VS noted in this clinical scenario.

Client Condition	Most Common VS Effect: Increase, Decrease, or Both
Dysrhythmias	P: both R: both BP: both (depending on dysrhythmia)
Pulmonary edema	P: increase R: increase BP: increase
Cardiogenic shock	*P: increase R: increase BP: decrease*
Cardiac tamponade	*P: increase R: increase BP: decrease*
Pulmonary embolism	*P: increase R: increase BP: decrease*
Dissecting aortic aneurysm	P: increase R: increase BP: increase

Next, you need to consider the other client data presented including the ECG findings and elevated troponin levels. Next, make the connection between these abnormal findings and the most likely client condition—cardiogenic shock. Although the VS findings in this clinical scenario are also consistent with cardiac tamponade and pulmonary embolism, the other client data are not usually found in these conditions. This will direct you to cardiogenic shock as the correct answer.

Content Area: Medical-Surgical Nursing
Priority Concept: Perfusion
Reference(s): Ignatavicius et al., 2021, pp. 618, 672, 702, 713, 740, 751

Practice Question 4.6   Matrix Multiple Response

At 1300 hours an 86-year-old client with altered mental status who is accompanied by their child is admitted to the medical-surgical unit, and the nurse is performing an assessment. The client has an IV solution of a 1000-mL bag of 0.9% sodium chloride hung at 1200 in the ED that is infusing at 100 mL/hr. One hour after admission the client's child calls the nurse and reports that the client has a pounding headache, is having trouble breathing, and seems scared.

For each assessment finding below, click to specify if the finding is *most likely* consistent with dehydration, circulatory overload, or digoxin toxicity.

Assessment Finding	Dehydration	Circulatory Overload	Digoxin Toxicity
Anorexia	☐	☐	☒
Dry mucous membranes	☒	☐	☐
BUN and creatinine levels	☒	☐	☐
Sodium and potassium levels	☒	☐	☐
Digoxin level	☐	☐	☒
Elevation in BP and RR	☐	☒	☐
Wheezing and congestion bilaterally in lungs	☐	☒	☐
Neck vein distention	☐	☒	☐

Health History	Nurses' Notes	Vital Signs	Laboratory Results

1300: Client is weak and reports has not been able to eat or drink in the past 3 days because of anorexia.
Skin is very dry, dry mucous membranes, sleepy.
The child reports that the client has a H/O heart failure, hypertension, and hyperlipidemia.
Breath sounds clear bilaterally.
Medications include lisinopril, carvedilol, and digoxin.
1400: Client is dyspneic and complaining of chest tightness, coughing and is pale, neck vein distention is seen. Breath sounds wheezing and congestion bilaterally. 500 mL remaining in the IV bag.

Health History	Nurses' Notes	Vital Signs	Laboratory Results

Test	Result	Normal Reference Range
Blood urea nitrogen (BUN)	24 mg/dL (8.64 mmol/L) **H**	10–20 mg/dL (3.6–7.1 mmol/L)
Creatinine	1.8 mg/dL (159.4 mcmol/L) **H**	0.5–1.2 mg/dL (44–106 mcmol/L)
Digoxin level	2.2 ng/mL (2.8 nmol/L) **H**	0.5–2.0 ng/mL (0.64–2.56 nmol/L)
Sodium	148 mEq/L (148 mmol/L) **H**	135–145 mEq/L (135–145 mmol/L)
Potassium	5.2 mEq/L (5.2 mmol/L) **H**	3.5–5.0 mEq/L (3.5–5.0 mmol/L)

Health History	Nurses' Notes	Vital Signs	Laboratory Results

1300: T = 100.2°F (36.8°C); apical HR = 72 BPM and regular; BP = 100/68 mm Hg; RR = 24 bpm; SpO$_2$ = 90% on RA
1400: T = 100.2°F (36.8°C); apical HR = 110 BPM and regular; BP = 152/98 mm Hg; RR = 28 bpm; SpO$_2$ = 89% on RA

Rationale: Dehydration is a condition in which the body has a lower than needed amount of body fluid. At admission this client showed signs of dehydration and reported weakness. The client's skin and mucous membranes were very dry, and the client was sleepy. In addition, the BUN, creatinine, sodium, and potassium are elevated, also noted in dehydration and due to the loss of fluid affecting cellular regulation. The dehydration is likely a result of the client not being able to eat or drink for the last 3 days.

Circulatory overload occurs when the volume of fluid in the body is greater than the body needs and fluid accumulates faster than the circulatory system can compensate for the large volume of fluid. Fluid exists in greater amounts than needed in the extracellular compartments. An elderly client is at risk because of changes in the circulatory system due to the aging process. In addition, those with compromised cardiac function, such as a client with heart failure, are at greatest risk. In this client, 400 mL of fluid is infused into the client during a 1-hour period (inadvertently, because the prescribed rate was 100 mL/hr), and this is the likely cause of the circulatory overload. Some of the signs and symptoms of circulatory overload include headache, dyspnea, orthopnea, wheezing, tightness in the chest, cough, cyanosis, tachypnea, a rapid increase in BP, and distended neck veins.

A client taking digoxin is at risk for digoxin toxicity. The therapeutic digoxin level ranges from 0.5 ng/mL (0.66 nmol/L) to 2.0 ng/mL (2.6 nmol/L). A digoxin level of 2.2 ng/mL (2.8 nmol/L) is above the therapeutic level. Early signs of digoxin toxicity are mental status changes and GI alterations that include anorexia, nausea, vomiting, and diarrhea. Bradycardia or tachycardia can occur and the client develops visual disturbances such as blurred vision and changes in colors.

Test-Taking Strategy

Test-Taking Strategy: Begin answering this question by analyzing the data provided in the Nurses' Notes, Laboratory Results, and Vital Signs tabs of the medical record. For each of the findings, some thought as to whether the finding is consistent with the client condition and why or why not will assist in answering the question correctly. Drawing from your nursing knowledge, try to recall the signs and symptoms of the conditions in the question and then list the findings from the medical record and determine whether they are related or not related. Some findings are the opposite of what you would see; this makes sense because the client is being treated for dehydration with rehydration measures; and so, thinking about the complications of the treatment, it is possible for opposite findings to be noted depending on outcomes of the treatment. Organize your thinking process as illustrated in the table.

Assessment Finding	Dehydration	Circulatory Overload	Digoxin Toxicity
	Dry mucous membranes, mental status changes, weakness, low-grade fever, decreased and concentrated urine, hemoconcentration, elevated BUN and creatinine levels, hypotension	Headache, shortness of breath, cough, elevated BP, puffiness around the eyes, dependent edema, neck vein distention, congestion in the lungs	Anorexia, blurred vision, mental status changes, dysrhythmias, nausea, vomiting, and diarrhea
Anorexia	Not related	Not related	Related
Dry mucous membranes	Related	Not related (opposite)	Not related
BUN and creatinine levels	Related	Not related	Not related
Sodium and potassium levels	Related	Not related	Not related (potassium opposite)
Digoxin level	Not related	Not related	Related
Elevation in BP and RR	Not related (opposite)	Related	Not related
Wheezing and congestion bilaterally in lungs	Not related	Related	Not related
Neck vein distention	Not related (opposite)	Related	Not related

This thinking process demonstrates how to consider the findings in the question and analyze and interpret them, fitting them into the clinical picture. Using visual aids is a very helpful way to ensure you are considering everything you need to and drawing on all available knowledge to direct you to the correct options.

Content Area: Medical-Surgical Nursing
Priority Concept: Fluid and Electrolyte Balance
Reference(s): Ignatavicius et al., 2021, pp. 168–169, 216, 700

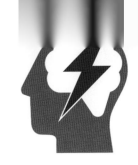

CHAPTER 5

Answers to Practice Questions

Multiple Response Grouping

A 12-year-old client visits the health care clinic for a follow-up visit after laboratory and other testing. The client is accompanied by a parent. The client tells the nurse about an increase in appetite lately and about urinating more frequently than usual. The nurse reviews the client's test results and collects data from the client prior to the client being seen by the physician. The following is documented in the medical record.

Health History	Nurses' Notes	Diagnostic Tests	Lab Results

VS: T = 98.2°F (36.6°C); HR = 78 BPM; BP = 118/70 mm Hg; RR = 16 bpm; SpO$_2$ = 96% on RA; denies pain.
Skin: Warm, dry, intact.
Respiratory: Dry cough. Reports sputum expectoration of white thick mucus following respiratory treatments. Lung sounds clear to auscultation in all lung fields.
GI: Increased appetite. Reports taking pancreatic enzymes with all meals and snacks. Bowel sounds active × 4 quadrants. Regular bowel movements that are brown and fatty.
Weight: 91.5 lb (41.5 kg)
Height: 59.0 inches (149.8 cm)
Parent states that client was diagnosed at 3 years of age with cystic fibrosis (CF).

Health History	Nurses' Notes	Diagnostic Tests	Lab Results

Chest x-ray: Mild lung hyperinflation; no chest infiltrates, atelectasis, or bronchiectasis
Oral glucose tolerance test (OGTT): glucose 240 mg/dL (13.37 mmol/L) 2 hours after administration of the glucose liquid

For each body system, click to select the **priority** client need to prevent a complication of the client's health problem. **Each body system supports one priority client need.**

Body System	Priority Client Need
Respiratory	☒ Oscillatory positive expiratory therapy (PEP)
	☐ Oxygen administration
GI	☒ Pancreatic enzyme therapy
	☐ Low-fat diet
Immune	☐ Prophylactic antibiotic therapy
	☒ Contact precautions with separation from others with CF by at least 6 feet
Endocrine	☒ Insulin administration
	☐ Recombinant human growth hormone administration
Integumentary	☒ High-sodium foods
	☐ Oatmeal baths

Rationale: CF is a condition characterized by exocrine (mucus-producing) gland dysfunction and leads to multisystem involvement. CF is inherited as an autosomal recessive trait. CF leads to decreased pancreatic secretion of bicarbonate and chloride and an increase of sodium and chloride in both sweat and saliva. The primary factor responsible for many manifestations of the health problem is mechanical obstruction caused by the increased viscosity of mucous gland secretions. The mucous glands produce a think, heavy mucoprotein that accumulates and dilates them. Then small passages in organs become obstructed as secretions precipitate or coagulate to form concretions in glands and ducts. Because of the increased viscosity of bronchial mucus, there is a greater resistance to ciliary action, a slower flow rate of mucus, and incomplete expectoration. The retained secretions serve as an excellent medium for bacterial growth. Pulmonary symptoms are produced by the stagnation of mucus with eventual bacterial colonization leading to destruction of lung tissue. The thick mucus also obstructs the bronchi and bronchioles, leading to bronchiectasis, atelectasis, and hyperinflation. Airway clearance therapy (ACT) is a primary need for these clients to assist with the removal of secretions and prevention of pulmonary infection. Chest physiotherapy, percussion and postural drainage, PEP, oscillatory PEP, high-frequency chest compressions, and exercise are among some of the treatments. Oxygen administration may be used for children with acute episodes and exacerbations but must be used cautiously because many children with CF have chronic carbon dioxide retention and oxygen can be harmful. The extent of GI involvement varies. In many clients, the thick secretions block the ducts of the pancreas, leading to cystic dilations then degeneration and progressive diffuse fibrosis. Essential pancreatic enzymes are unable to reach the duodenum, causing impairment in the digestion and absorption of nutrients, particularly fats and proteins. Excessive stool fat (steatorrhea) and foul-smelling stools are characteristic. Biliary obstruction and fibrosis occur in the liver, and extensive liver involvement with fatty infiltration occurs despite adequate nutrition. Pancreatic enzyme therapy is necessary to treat pancreatic insufficiency and is administered with meals and snacks to ensure that digestive enzymes are mixed with food in the duodenum. In addition, because the uptake of fat-soluble vitamins is decreased, water-miscible forms of these vitamins (A, D, E, and K) along with multivitamins are also needed. The client with CF also requires a well-balanced, high-protein, high-calorie diet with unrestricted fat because of the impaired intestinal absorption.

Prevention of infection is critical in the client with CF. Staff, people with CF, and their families need regular and ongoing education to remind them that all persons with CF have some colonization of secretions in the respiratory tract. Therefore clients with CF should separate from others with CF by at least 6 feet to reduce the chance of cross-infection. In addition, contact precautions are needed for all clients regardless of the pathogens present. The client with CF is also advised to wear a mask in common areas of health care facilities. Antibiotics are not administered to the client with CF as a prophylactic measure. If this were done, then a resistance to the antibiotic would develop and it would not be effective when needed to treat an infection. If an infection is confirmed, such as a respiratory infection, then the client is aggressively treated with antibiotics and possible antifungal medications.

The incidence of cystic fibrosis–related diabetes (CFRD) is a concern because the islets of Langerhans decrease in number as the pancreatic fibrosis develops and progresses. CFRD is diagnosed with an OGTT. The result of the OGTT 2 hours after administration of the glucose liquid shows a glucose level of 240 mg/dL (13.37 mmol/L), indicating diabetes. Children with CFRD require close monitoring of blood glucose, administration of insulin injections, diet and exercise management, and glycosylated hemoglobin monitoring. The administration of recombinant human growth hormone is being used to achieve optimum growth in children with CF who have growth delay. There is no indication that this child has a growth delay.

The abnormally high sodium and chloride concentrations in the sweat are a unique characteristic of CF. Parents will often describe their children as tasting "salty" when they kiss the child. Because of the abnormal salt loss, dehydration and hypochloremic and hyponatremic alkalosis during hyperthermic conditions are concerns. Therefore salt replacement therapy is necessary for the person with CF. The recommended dose of salt replacement for people with CF is based on the individual's symptoms, dietary intake, climate conditions, and exercise or activity level. The easiest and best way for people with CF to get extra salt is by adding salt to foods and eating foods that are naturally high in salt. Although salt crystals may deposit on the skin, and oatmeal or other types of baths may be helpful, baths are not the priority need.

Test-Taking
Strategy

Test-Taking Strategy: Note that this question is asking for the *priority client needs,* and the options are organized by body system. You are presented with two possible priority needs within each body system, and you are asked to select one option for each system. Also note that you are asked to choose the priority need to prevent complications associated with CF. Remember that when you are asked to prioritize, some or all of the options presented to you are good choices; however, you need to rank the options in order of priority based on what the question is asking about. In this clinical scenario, certain options prevent complications of CF (what the question is asking you), other options manage complications, and some options are not helpful in preventing or managing complications. Organize your thinking process in this way, as illustrated in the table.

Client Need	Prevents Complications	Manages Complications	Not Helpful in Preventing or Managing Complications
Oscillatory PEP	☒	☐	☐
Oxygen administration	☐	☒	☐
Pancreatic enzyme therapy	☒	☐	☐
Low-fat diet	☐	☐	☒
Prophylactic antibiotic therapy	☐	☐	☒
Contact Precautions with separation from others with CF by at least 6 feet	☒	☐	☐
Insulin administration	☒	☐	☐
Recombinant human growth hormone administration	☐	☒	☐
High-sodium foods	☒	☐	☐
Oatmeal baths	☐	☒	☐

Choose options that prevent complications as the correct answers for each body system, as this most directly relates to the subject of the question, or what the question is asking about. Options that are used to manage complications or are not related to preventing or managing complications of CF are of lesser priority.

Content Area: Pediatric Nursing
Priority Concept: Gas Exchange
Reference(s): Hockenberry et al., 2019, pp. 944–952

Practice Question 5.2   Multiple Response Select N

A 68-year-old client complaining of chest pain is admitted to the medical-surgical nursing unit for acute coronary syndrome. The cardiologist prescribes a continuous IV heparin infusion per protocol. The client weighs 165 lb (74.8 kg), and baseline partial thromboplastin time (PTT) is 32 seconds. A bolus is administered as prescribed and a continuous infusion is initiated based on the protocol noted in the Medication Administration Record.

Health History	Nurses' Notes	Vital Signs	Med Admn Record

Baseline PTT and every 6 or 12 hours after start of continuous infusion based on protocol

Heparin 80 units/kg IV bolus prior to start of continuous infusion

Start heparin 25,000 units in 250 mL D₅W (concentration 100 units/mL) continuous infusion 18 units/kg/hr

Adjust continuous infusion based on the following:
- PTT less than 35 seconds: IV bolus 80 units/kg, increase rate by 4 units/kg/hr, PTT in 6 hours
- PTT 35–45 seconds: IV bolus 40 units/kg, increase rate by 2 units/kg/hr, PTT in 6 hours
- PTT 46–70 seconds (goal): No bolus, no rate change, PTT in 12 hours
- PTT 71–90 seconds: No bolus, decrease rate by 2 units/kg/hr, PTT in 12 hours
- PTT above 90 seconds: No bolus, stop infusion

The next day, the oncoming nurse assigned to monitor the client assesses the client and checks laboratory results. The client states, "I feel OK, I just have a hard time sleeping since I've been in the hospital. My chest pain is better. I had a nosebleed this morning but it stopped. I'm ready for breakfast; it should be here soon." The most recent PTT from 1 hour ago was 92 seconds. The heparin infusion is running at 13.5 mL/hr.

*Select the three priority needs that are of **immediate** concern.*

- ☐ Appetite
- ☐ Chest pain
- ☒ Nosebleed
- ☒ PTT results
- ☒ Heparin infusion
- ☐ Difficulty sleeping

Rationale: The major adverse effects of heparin therapy include heparin-induced thrombocytopenia (HIT) and/or hemorrhage. Other adverse effects include hypersensitivity, local irritation and hematoma, and allergic responses. The priority needs in this scenario that are of immediate concern are the client report of a nosebleed, the PTT results, and the heparin infusion. Nosebleeds can be associated with an adverse effect of HIT or hemorrhage. The PTT results are above the therapeutic range and could also lead to bleeding. The heparin infusion is still running and therefore is of immediate concern. The cardiologist needs to be notified of the nosebleed and supratherapeutic PTT level, and the heparin infusion needs to be stopped. The client is reporting looking forward to having breakfast; this is not a concerning finding related to appetite. The client reports that the chest pain has improved, and therefore this is not an immediate concern. The client's difficulty sleeping since being in the hospital is most likely due to the disruption in routine and is not specifically related to the treatment; therefore this is not of immediate concern.

Test-Taking Strategy

Test-Taking Strategy: Focus on the strategic word *immediate* and note that this question is asking you to prioritize three findings out of a total of six that are of immediate concern to the nurse. Use all the information provided to you in the clinical scenario to help you decide on the three most important findings. In addition, thinking about whether these client needs require immediate follow-up in order to ensure safe client care may help direct you to the correct options. This thinking process is illustrated in the table.

Client Finding	Requires Immediate Follow-up	Does Not Require Immediate Follow-up
Appetite	☐	☒
Chest pain	☐	☒
Nosebleed	☒	☐
PTT results	☒	☐
Heparin infusion	☒	☐
Difficulty sleeping	☐	☒

The client is reporting an appetite, which is normal and does not require follow-up; therefore this option can be eliminated. The client's chest pain is improved and therefore does not require follow-up either, so this option can also be eliminated. Although the client is reporting difficulty sleeping, consider the environment as contributing to this. The nurse would want to take measures to address this to promote sleep, but it is not an immediate client need. This leaves you with the three remaining options of nosebleed, PTT results, and the heparin infusion as the correct answer to this question.

Content Area: Pharmacology
Priority Concept: Perfusion
Reference(s): Burchum & Rosenthal, 2022, pp. 607–610

Practice Question 5.3   Drag-and-Drop Rationale

A 70-year-old client had an exploratory laparotomy with colectomy due to small bowel obstruction. The surgery was completed, and the client has been transferred to the postoperative medical-surgical nursing unit. The client received general anesthesia and has a PCA pump with hydromorphone for pain control. The client has been using the PCA pump every 10 minutes for the last 8 hours. The oncoming nurse receives report and is assessing the client.

Physical Assessment	Nurses' Notes	Vital Signs	Lab Results

T = 98.2°F (36.7°C); HR = 80 BPM; BP = 138/78 mm Hg; RR = 18 bpm; SpO$_2$ = 96% on 2 L/min per NC; pain rated as a 2/10 on a 0 to 10 rating scale

Physical Assessment	Nurses' Notes	Vital Signs	Lab Results

Skin: Warm, dry, intact.
Respiratory: RR 18 bpm, unlabored. SpO$_2$ 96% on 2 L/min per NC. Dry cough, no sputum. Lung sounds clear to auscultation in all lung fields.
Cardiovascular: Apical pulse rate 80 BPM. Heart sounds, regular rate and rhythm.
GI: Bowel sounds active × 4 quadrants. Abdomen rigid to palpation. Dressing over midline abdominal incision intact with scant amount of serosanguineous drainage noted. Dressing changed per surgeon's order, wound cleansed with normal saline, and dressing reapplied. Incision is well approximated; no redness, swelling, tenderness at incision site. Pain 2/10 at the incision site.
Genitourinary: Unable to urinate since arrival to unit 8 hours ago.
Neurologic: Alert and oriented × 3.

Based on the client findings, complete the following sentence by choosing from the lists of options provided.

The client is at **highest** risk for developing <u>urinary retention</u> as evidenced by <u>urine output</u>.

Options for 1	Options for 2
Infection	Urine output
Atelectasis	Temperature
Hemorrhage	BP
Urinary retention	RR
Wound dehiscence	Drainage on dressing

Rationale: The client in the postoperative period is at risk for certain complications related to having surgery. In this scenario, the client is at highest risk for developing urinary retention due to the effects of anesthesia and opioid analgesics, as well as the type of surgery the client had because of manipulation of the tissues surrounding the bladder. Certain positions can also impair voiding reflexes, and a normal voiding position should be assumed whenever possible.

The client's lack of urine output in at least the last 8 hours is evidence that urinary retention may be a complication that is occurring; the client should have a minimum of 30 mL of urine voided per hour on average, and should be able to initiate the urinary stream without difficulty.

In addition, the GI assessment, which revealed a rigid abdomen, is suggestive of urinary retention. Sometimes, straight catheterization following surgery is necessary until the voiding routine is re-established.

Infection can occur after surgery and most often occurs in the wound or incision site. It can be caused by poor aseptic technique or contamination of the site. Signs and symptoms would include warm, red, and tender skin around the wound or incision site; fever; chills; and purulent drainage. Because the client's temperature is normal and the drainage is serosanguineous, which is normal in the early stage of healing, this complication would not be a concern.

Atelectasis can occur because of the effects of anesthesia, analgesia, and immobilization; signs and symptoms include elevated RR, dyspnea, fever, crackles, and productive cough. Because this client's RR is normal, there is no fever, lung sounds are clear, and the cough is dry, atelectasis is most likely not a problem.

Hemorrhage or bleeding can occur after surgery from slipping of a suture or a dislodged clot at an incision site. The client may experience hypotension, weak and rapid pulse, cool and clammy skin, increased RR, restlessness, and, in the later stages, reduced urine output. The client's lack of urine output is a concern; however, in the absence of these other signs and symptoms, hemorrhage is most likely not a complication occurring at this time.

Wound dehiscence occurs when there is separation of wound edges at the suture line. Contributing factors include malnutrition, obesity, radiation to the site, older age, poor circulation, and strain on the suture line. Signs and symptoms include an appearance of underlying tissues at the incision site. The client's incision is well approximated, so this is not a complication that is occurring.

Other complications that can occur after surgery include pneumonia; hypoxemia; PE; hypovolemia; thrombophlebitis; embolus to the brain, heart, or mesentery; deconditioning; paralytic ileus; abdominal distention; nausea and vomiting; UTI; wound evisceration; skin breakdown; intractable pain; and malignant hyperthermia. There are no data that indicate that any of these complications are a concern.

Test-Taking Strategy: Focus on what the question is asking about: postoperative complications. Think about what happens during surgery, including the use of anesthesia, manipulation of tissues, medication administration, and immobility. Because the client had surgery, the client is at risk for all of these complications, so you need to look for the data or evidence that a complication is actually happening. Look at each complication listed in the first column, and use your knowledge of pathophysiology to think about the evidence that is needed to support the presence of this complication. Relate this knowledge back to the data provided in the clinical scenario, as illustrated in the table.

Complication	Supporting Evidence
Infection	None—Temperature is normal; incision site without signs of infection
Atelectasis	None—Lung sounds are clear, SpO$_2$ is normal, RR and work of breathing normal, cough is dry
Hemorrhage	BP normal, pulse normal, RR and work of breathing normal, alert and oriented × 3 Urine output is inadequate; however, without other signs of bleeding, this likely is not related to this complication.
Urinary retention	Inadequate urine output, rigid abdomen
Wound dehiscence	Incision is well approximated Serosanguineous drainage can be a sign of future dehiscence but is also a normal part of the healing process; because incision is not separated, it is not a complication now.

As you can see, some of the findings in the clinical scenario can relate to more than one potential complication; however, the highest risk would be for an actual complication that is confirmed based on the available data. Urinary retention can be confirmed on the basis of inadequate urine output and rigid abdomen, as well as the fact that the client has not urinated for the last 8 hours. Note that there are no data to support infection or atelectasis. The only supporting evidence for hemorrhage is inadequate urine output; recall, however, that this would be a later sign, and in the absence of other signs and symptoms this would not be the priority concern. Although serosanguineous drainage is present, it does not confirm wound dehiscence, and there is evidence to support that this complication is not occurring, as the incision is well approximated; therefore this is not the priority concern at this time. Remember to consider all data presented in the clinical scenario and organize your thinking process in a way that will allow you to make connections; this will make it much easier to decide on the priority client needs.

Content Area: Foundations of Nursing
Priority Concept: Gas Exchange
Reference(s): Potter et al., 2021, p. 1353

Practice Question 5.4   Multiple Response Select All That Apply

A 22-year-old client is brought to the ED by EMS. The client's parent found the client slumped over and unconscious. The client was sitting in the wheelchair eating breakfast when the parent last saw the client, 15 minutes prior. The client was bleeding profusely from both wrists, and the parent reports immediately placing pressure on both wrists, and screaming to the spouse for help and to call EMS. At the scene, EMS reports that the client was unconscious but that the bleeding was controlled and pressure dressings and continuous pressure to both wrists were maintained. EMS reports that the client's BP was 98/60 mm Hg, apical HR was 120 BPM, RR was 16 bpm. Oxygen at 3 L per NC was administered, an IV line was inserted, an infusion of lactated Ringer's was initiated, and the client was transferred to the ED.

On arrival at the ED, the client is arousable but sleepy. Assessment and treatment are immediately initiated, and the client is stabilized and admitted to the hospital. The admission nurse reviews the medical record, performs an assessment, and documents in the Nurses' Notes.

| Health History | Nurses' Notes | Vital Signs | Lab Results |

This 22-year-old client sustained a spinal cord injury in the lower thoracic region 1 year ago from a motor vehicle crash. Client has paraplegia.
No other medical problems.

| Health History | Nurses' Notes | Vital Signs | Lab Results |

T = 101°F (38.3°C); HR = 96 BPM; BP = 116/78 mm Hg; RR = 20 bpm; SpO$_2$ = 94% on RA; wrist pain = 4/10

| Health History | Nurses' Notes | Vital Signs | Lab Results |

Client is alert and oriented. Is sleepy but easily arousable. States is "sick and tired of living this way and is too young to have to be in a wheelchair for the rest of my life." States, "It is my own fault that I am this way, and I am so sorry that they found me this morning. I slashed my wrists using my breakfast knife. I am so useless and do nothing right, even with trying to kill myself."
Has no appetite and is refusing to eat. States wants to sleep and not be bothered by anyone.
Dressings on both wrists are dry and intact. No redness or break in skin integrity noted in other skin areas.
No sensation felt in lower extremities. Unable to move lower extremities.
Last bowel movement 1 day ago. Bowel sounds present in all 4 quadrants.
Abdomen firm. Urinary output 200 mL in the ED via catheterization. States needs to self-catheterize every 6 hours depending on intake.
No respiratory distress. RR = 20 bpm; SpO$_2$ = 94% on RA; wrist pain = 4/10. Pain medication administered in the ED 2 hours ago.
No chest pain; pulse 96 BPM.

Health History	Nurses' Notes	Vital Signs	Lab Results
Test	**Result**	**Normal Reference Range**
Red blood cells (RBCs)	4.7×10^{12} (4.7×10^{12})	$4.2–6.2 \times 10^{12}$/L ($4.2–6.2 \times 10^{12}$/L)
White blood cells (WBCs)	12,000/mm³ (12×10^9/L) **H**	5000–10,000/mm³ ($5–10 \times 10^9$/L)
Platelets	160,000/mm³ (160×10^9/L)	150,000-400,000/ mm³ ($150–400 \times 10^9$/L)
Hemoglobin (Hgb)	14 g/dL (140 g/L)	12–18 g/dL (120–180 g/L)
Hematocrit (Hct)	42% (0.42)	37%–52% (0.37–0.52)

*Which of the following are the priority client needs of **immediate** concern? **Select all that apply.***

☐ Pain

☐ Appetite

☒ Infection

☐ Bleeding

☐ Paraplegia

☒ Suicide risk

☐ Urinary output

Rationale: Suicide or completed suicide is the act of intentionally ending one's own life. A suicide attempt includes all willful, self-inflicted, life-threatening attempts that have not led to death. A risk factor for suicide is a chronic medical condition that affects a person's life ability. A previous attempt at suicide is also a risk factor. A client who has experienced a spinal cord injury with resultant paraplegia may have significant behavioral and emotional reactions as a result of changes in functional ability, body image, role performance, and self-concept. The client needs to be assessed for their reaction to the injury, and it is important that the nurse provide opportunities to listen to the client's concerns. The nurse needs to be realistic about the client's abilities and physical function, but offer hope and encouragement. Aggressive rehabilitation can help most clients live productive and independent lives. This client has two risk factors for suicide: the chronic medical condition and the attempt to commit suicide. The client is also expressing verbal cues of a suicide risk by stating, "It is my own fault that I am this way, and I am so sorry that they found me this morning. I slashed my wrists using my breakfast knife. I am so useless and do nothing right, even with trying to kill myself." Therefore suicide risk is an immediate priority need and concern, and the nurse would implement suicide precautions for this client. Infection is also a priority need for this client. The temperature is elevated at 101°F (38.3°C) and the WBC count is elevated at 12,000/mm^3 (12×10^9 /L), so this needs to be addressed. The client was medicated for pain 2 hours prior in the ED, so although pain is a concern, it is not the priority need at this time and the nurse would continue to monitor pain status. Appetite is not a priority need at this time, although the nurse would closely monitor appetite status and nutritional intake. Bleeding has been controlled and dressings are dry and intact; because this has been stabilized and because the client's VS and RBCs, platelets, and Hgb and Hct levels are in the low-normal range, bleeding is not a priority client need. Paraplegia is a chronic problem and not a priority client need—although the nurse would plan to address this problem at a later time with OT and PT. Urinary output needs to be monitored and the client will need intermittent catheterization, but this is not a priority client need because urinary output in the ED was 200 mL.

Test-Taking Strategy: Begin answering this question by thinking about which client needs noted in the question have immediate safety implications. Then consider whether any data in the clinical scenario provide supporting evidence that this client need is a priority and of immediate concern. Organize your thinking process as illustrated in the table.

Client Need	Immediate Safety Implications	Supporting Evidence
Pain	No	Yes
Appetite	No	Yes
Infection	Yes	Yes
Bleeding	Yes	No
Paraplegia	No	No
Suicide risk	Yes	Yes
Urinary output	No	Yes

If you are able to determine that both immediate safety implications and supporting evidence of this client need are present, then these options are likely correct and would be priority needs of immediate concern. If there is no immediate safety implication, even if there is supporting evidence, then this option would not be of immediate concern and can therefore be eliminated. If an option would be considered an immediate safety concern but there is no supporting evidence, then this option could also be eliminated. Assigning priority to each client need listed in the options will assist in directing you to the correct options: infection and suicide risk.

Content Area: Mental Health Nursing
Priority Concept: Mood and Affect
Reference(s): Ignatavicius et al., 2021, pp. 877–882, 884–887; Varcarolis & Fosbre, 2021, pp. 366–370

Practice Question 5.5   Drop-Down in Table

A 59-year-old postmenopausal client with stage IV bilateral breast cancer had a double mastectomy. The biopsy showed a hormone receptor–positive tumor, and the client was prescribed tamoxifen therapy. One month later the client visits the clinic for a follow-up and tells the nurse completing the intake about experiencing the following over the past month since the last visit:

- Pelvic pain, vaginal discharge, burning on urination
- Hot flashes, dizziness, tenderness and warmth to the left leg
- Weakness, bone pain, joint stiffness
- Constipation, stomach cramps, nausea and vomiting

*For each body system below, click to specify one **priority** concern specific to a complication of tamoxifen therapy.*

Body System	Priority Concerns
Genitourinary	☒ Pelvic pain
	☐ Vaginal discharge
	☐ Burning on urination
Cardiovascular	☐ Hot flashes
	☐ Dizziness
	☒ Tenderness and warmth to left leg
Musculoskeletal	☐ Weakness
	☒ Bone pain
	☐ Joint stiffness
GI	☐ Constipation
	☐ Stomach cramps
	☒ Nausea and vomiting

Rationale: Tamoxifen is an estrogen modulator that blocks the effects of estrogen in breast tissue. It is used to treat breast cancer and for prevention of breast cancer in those who are at high risk for developing it. This medication works by blocking estrogen receptors, which helps to inhibit growth and proliferation of cancer cells. Endometrial cancer is a complication because tamoxifen acts as an estrogen agonist at receptors in the uterus, which can cause proliferation of endometrial tissue, eventually leading to endometrial cancer. In postmenopausal clients, endometrial cancer is often characterized by abnormal menstrual bleeding, so it is an obvious abnormality after menopause. A hysterectomy may be performed as a preventive measure. Another sign of endometrial cancer is pelvic pain. Vaginal discharge may be normal or abnormal and can occur as a side effect of tamoxifen therapy, and should be addressed, but this is not the highest priority. Burning on urination may be a sign of UTI and needs to be followed up on, but it is not specifically related to tamoxifen. Vasomotor symptoms such as hot flashes can occur as a side effect of tamoxifen, but this is not the highest priority and can be addressed routinely. Dizziness may also be associated with tamoxifen therapy but is not the highest priority. Tenderness and warmth in the left leg may be a sign of thromboembolic events, such as DVT, PE, and stroke; therefore this finding is a priority concern. Tamoxifen can cause transient hypercalcemia and subsequent bone pain in clients with bone metastasis, so bone pain is a priority concern and could be an indication of metastasis. In addition, the risk for pathologic fractures with bone metastasis is high. Weakness and joint stiffness are not specifically associated with tamoxifen therapy. Nausea and vomiting commonly occur with tamoxifen therapy; this is a priority concern because of the associated risk of malnutrition, dehydration, and fluid and electrolyte imbalance. Constipation and stomach cramping are not adverse effects that indicate a complication of tamoxifen therapy.

Test-Taking Strategy

Test-Taking Strategy: Note the strategic word *priority*. The first step in answering this question correctly is to determine which of the concerns listed in the question are adverse effects indicating a complication specifically related to tamoxifen therapy. As shown in the table, think about the effects of tamoxifen on the body. First, use your nursing knowledge of this medication, and recall that it blocks the effects of estrogen by blocking estrogen receptors. Recalling the effects of this hormone will help you narrow down which options may be related to complications associated with tamoxifen therapy.

Effects	Specifically Related to Tamoxifen Therapy
Pelvic pain	☒
Vaginal discharge	☒
Burning on urination	☐
Hot flashes	☒
Dizziness	☒
Tenderness and warmth to left leg	☒
Weakness	☐
Bone pain	☒
Joint stiffness	☐
Constipation	☐
Stomach cramps	☐
Nausea and vomiting	☒

From here, you need to prioritize for each body system which of these findings would be of priority concern related to a complication of tamoxifen therapy. Recall that pelvic pain could be a manifestation of endometrial cancer and should be prioritized above vaginal discharge and burning on urination. Tenderness and warmth in the leg are signs of a thrombus and would be the priority over hot flashes and dizziness. Recalling that this medication can cause hypercalcemia in the presence of bone metastasis will assist you in prioritizing bone pain. Remembering that malnutrition, dehydration, and fluid and electrolyte imbalance can occur with nausea and vomiting will assist you in selecting this as the priority.

Content Area: Pharmacology
Priority Concept: Clotting
Reference(s): Burchum & Rosenthal, 2022, p. 1248

Practice Question 5.6	Multiple Response Select N

A 30-year-old pregnant client (G2P1) who is at 35 weeks of gestation presents to the labor and delivery triage unit stating that a sudden gush of fluid occurred 1 hour ago. The nurse collects data and documents the following in the Nurses' Notes.

Health History	Nurses' Notes	Vital Signs	Lab Results

1400:
Client states that they noticed a sudden gush of fluid 1 hour ago at 1300
Has continued to notice fluid leakage sporadically since that time
States that prior to becoming pregnant, smoked cigarettes, 1 pack per day for 13 years; has not smoked during pregnancy
States was diagnosed with chlamydia early in the pregnancy, which was treated with doxycycline

Based on this clinical scenario, select four potential complications that are of **highest priority** to the nurse.

☐ Preeclampsia
☒ Client sepsis
☒ Chorioamnionitis
☐ Client hypertension
☒ Umbilical cord prolapse
☐ Fetal pulmonary hypoplasia
☒ Umbilical cord compression

Rationale: Prelabor rupture of membranes (PROM) is the spontaneous rupture of the amniotic sac with subsequent leakage of amniotic fluid before the onset of labor. This can occur at any gestational age. Preterm prelabor rupture of membranes (pPROM) occurs before week 37 of pregnancy. Risk factors for PROM and pPROM include cigarette smoking; urinary or genital tract infection; previous preterm birth; history of cervical cerclage; short cervical length; contractions during pregnancy; uterine overdistention; bleeding in the second and third trimesters; pulmonary disease; connective tissue disorders; low BMI; and nutritional deficiencies. This client is at risk for pPROM because they are at 35 weeks of gestation and has a history of cigarette smoking and urogenital infection. A number of complications can occur as a result of pPROM. Client complications include chorioamnionitis or bacterial infection of the amniotic cavity, placental abruption, retained placenta and subsequent hemorrhage, sepsis, and death. Fetal complications include intrauterine infection, umbilical cord prolapse and compression, and placental abruption. Pulmonary hypoplasia can occur in the fetus, but this complication occurs before 20 weeks of gestation. Preeclampsia and hypertension in the client are not complications that are specifically related to or caused by pPROM.

Test-Taking Strategy

Test-Taking Strategy: Note the strategic words *highest priority*. Using knowledge and thinking about the pathophysiology and visualizing the possible complications that can occur with ruptured membranes during pregnancy will help direct you to the correct options. Remember that infection and fetal perfusion are the most important considerations with pPROM. Eliminate options that are not complications and are not related to either infection or fetal perfusion. Using a thinking process as illustrated in the table may be helpful to you.

Complication	Yes/No	Infection	Fetal Perfusion
Preeclampsia	No	☐	☐
Client sepsis	Yes	☒	☐
Chorioamnionitis	Yes	☒	☐
Client hypertension	No	☐	☐
Umbilical cord prolapse	Yes	☐	☒
Fetal pulmonary hypoplasia	No	☐	☐
Umbilical cord compression	Yes	☐	☒

Hypertension and preeclampsia are concerning but are not the highest priority in this case because they are not directly related to pPROM. In addition, recall that even though fetal pulmonary hypoplasia is a complication associated with pPROM, lung maturity in the fetus is a concern prior to 20 weeks of gestation; this will assist you in eliminating this option.

Content Area: Maternal-Newborn Nursing
Priority Concept: Perfusion
Reference(s): Lowdermilk et al., 2020, pp. 690-691

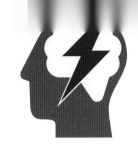

CHAPTER 6

Answers to Practice Questions

Practice Question 6.1 **Multiple Response Grouping**

A 58-year-old client is recovering from an L4–L5 spinal fusion completed 3 hours ago. The client is on the medical-surgical nursing unit, and is prescribed hydromorphone via PCA, 0.2 mg every 10 minutes, with a 4-mg lock-out dose in 4 hours. The nurse is preparing a plan of care for this client.

For each body system below, click to specify the potential intervention that would be appropriate for the initial plan of care to monitor for or prevent adverse effects of hydromorphone. ***Each body system may support more than one potential nursing intervention.***

Body System	Potential Nursing Intervention
Renal	☒ Assess renal function.
	☒ Monitor I&O.
	☐ Maintain fluid restriction.
Respiratory	☒ Assess RR frequently.
	☒ Ensure naloxone is available.
	☐ Place the PCA on hold if RR is less than 18 bpm.
Cardiovascular	☐ Encourage brisk walking.
	☒ Instruct the client to change positions slowly.
	☒ Assess BP and HR frequently.
Gastrointestinal	☐ Administer methylnaltrexone.
	☒ Administer ondansetron as indicated.
	☒ Ensure adequate intake of fluids and fiber.
Urinary	☒ Assess the bladder frequently.
	☒ Prompt the client to void every 4 hours.
	☐ Perform straight catheterization every 4 hours.

Rationale: Hydromorphone is an opioid analgesic used to manage pain. Adverse effects include increased intracranial pressure (ICP), neurotoxicity, respiratory depression, orthostatic hypotension, constipation, emesis, and urinary retention. Other adverse effects include cough suppression, biliary colic, euphoria and dysphoria, sedation, miosis, and birth defects if taken by a pregnant person. Increased ICP can result from hydromorphone owing to retained carbon dioxide from respiratory depression. In addition, opioid-induced neurotoxicity can occur, causing delirium, agitation, myoclonus, and hyperalgesia. Renal impairment, cognitive impairment, and prolonged use are risk factors for increased ICP and neurotoxicity as adverse effects of this medication. Because ICP relates to renal function, assessing renal function, monitoring urinary output, and maintaining hydration and reducing the dose in renal impairment are important measures. Respiratory depression is the most serious adverse effect. The RR needs to be assessed frequently for a client on PCA receiving hydromorphone. The PCA will lock out and would need to be placed on hold if the RR is less than 12 bpm, or as otherwise prescribed. Naloxone, the antidote to opioid analgesics, needs to be available in the event that respiratory depression occurs. Opioid analgesics lower the BP by blunting the baroreceptor reflex and causing dilation to the peripheral vasculature. The nurse needs to teach the client about symptoms of hypotension such as light-headedness and dizziness, and instruct the client to sit or lie down if these symptoms are noticed. Changing positions slowly, while maintaining proper positioning as prescribed by the surgeon, and asking for assistance with activity are important safety measures to prevent hypotension from occurring, or to prevent injury if it does occur. Regularly assessing the BP and HR will alert the nurse to this problem. Constipation is an adverse effect associated with opioid analgesics and occurs as a result of suppression of peristalsis. Fecal impaction, tearing, hemorrhoids, and bowel perforation can result. Initially the nurse would promote motility by ensuring adequate fluid and fiber intake, encouraging activity, and administering prophylactic stimulants such as senna and stool softeners such as docusate. Lactulose or sodium phosphate, stronger osmotic laxatives, may be needed if these measures do not work. Methylnaltrexone, a medication that blocks mu receptors in the intestine, may be given as a last resort for opioid-induced constipation but is not an appropriate intervention initially. Emesis can occur through stimulation of the chemoreceptor trigger zone in the brain. Remaining still and taking an antiemetic, such as ondansetron, help with this effect if it occurs. Hydromorphone can cause urinary retention by increasing tone in the bladder sphincter, increasing tone in the detrusor muscle, and interfering with voiding by suppressing awareness of bladder stimuli. Clients need to be prompted to void every 4 hours. The nurse needs to assess for urinary retention by monitoring I&O and palpating for bladder distention every 4 to 6 hours. Intermittent straight catheterization may be needed if this complication occurs but is not performed unless clients cannot void on their own.

Test-Taking Strategy: Note that this question is asking for the *appropriate potential nursing interventions* and that the options are organized by body system. You are presented with three possible interventions within each body system, and you are asked to select one or more option for each system. When answering questions about medications, you should think about how safety is addressed with each of the options presented and whether the option monitors for or prevents an adverse effect of the medication. Organize your thinking process in this way, as illustrated in the table.

Potential Intervention	Addresses Potential Adverse Effect	Does Not Address Potential Adverse Effect
Assess renal function.	☒	☐
Monitor I&O.	☒	☐
Maintain fluid restriction.	☐	☒
Assess RR frequently.	☒	☐
Ensure naloxone is available.	☒	☐
Place the PCA on hold if RR is less than 18 bpm.	☐	☒
Encourage brisk walking.	☐	☒
Instruct the client to change positions slowly.	☒	☐
Assess BP and HR frequently.	☒	☐
Administer methylnaltrexone.	☐	☒
Administer ondansetron as indicated.	☒	☐
Ensure adequate intake of fluids and fiber.	☒	☐
Assess the bladder frequently.	☒	☐
Prompt the client to void every 4 hours.	☒	☐
Perform straight catheterization every 4 hours.	☐	☒

Choose options that address adverse effects as the correct answers for each body system, because this most directly relates to the subject of the question, or what the question is asking about. Options that are unrelated to monitoring for or managing adverse effects can be eliminated.

Content Area: Pharmacology
Priority Concept: Gas Exchange
Reference(s): Burchum & Rosenthal, 2022, p. 277

Practice Question 6.2   Multiple Response Select N

A 72-year-old client with a history of peripheral vascular disease has an arterial leg ulcer that is open and draining copious amounts of drainage. The client is admitted to the medical-surgical nursing unit for wound care management. The initial plan is to pack the wound with sterile saline–moistened gauze and then cover with a dry sterile dressing, with daily dressing changes and as needed. The nurse noted that the client was requiring multiple dressing changes each day owing to the excessive drainage, and initiates a wound care team consultation. The client is seen by the wound care team, and the physician prescribes negative-pressure wound therapy (NPWT).

Which five interventions would the nurse include in the plan of care for the client to maintain and ensure a good seal during NPWT?

- ☒ Identify air leaks using a stethoscope.
- ☐ Shave the hair on the skin around the wound.
- ☒ Make sure the periwound skin surface area is dry.
- ☒ Avoid wrinkles when applying the transparent film.
- ☒ Fill uneven skin surfaces with a skin barrier product.
- ☒ Frame the periwound area with a hydrocolloid dressing.
- ☐ Cut the transparent film to extend ½ inch beyond the wound perimeter.
- ☐ Use as many additional dressing layers as needed for identified air leaks.

Rationale: NPWT treats acute and chronic wounds and is a helpful treatment for clients with wounds with copious amounts of drainage. Maintaining an airtight seal is important for NPWT to be effective. To avoid loss of suction, or negative pressure, the wound and dressing must stay sealed. Interventions to assist in maintaining an airtight seal include identifying air leaks using a stethoscope and repairing them with transparent dressing; filling uneven skin surfaces with a skin barrier product; making sure the periwound skin surface is dry; avoiding wrinkles when applying the transparent film; and framing the periwound area with a hydrocolloid dressing. Rather than shaving, the hair on the skin around the wound needs to be clipped per agency policy. Only one or two additional dressing layers should be used for air leaks because multiple layers reduce moisture vapor transmission and cause maceration of the wound. The transparent film should be cut to extend 1 to 2 inches beyond the wound perimeter.

Test-Taking Strategy

Test-Taking Strategy: Note that this question is asking you to identify five interventions out of a total of eight listed interventions that the nurse would plan in the care of a client receiving NPWT. Use knowledge about this treatment and the information provided to you in the clinical scenario to help you decide on the five appropriate interventions. Note that the question focuses on maintaining a good seal for NPWT. Thinking about the interventions that would help with this, and then the interventions that either do not help or pose a safety risk, will assist you in answering the question correctly. This thinking process is illustrated in the table.

Intervention	Helps Maintain/ Ensure Seal	Does Not Help Maintain/Ensure Seal or Poses Safety Risk
Identify air leaks using a stethoscope.	☒	☐
Shave the hair on the skin around the wound.	☐	☒
Make sure the periwound skin surface area is dry.	☒	☐
Avoid wrinkles when applying the transparent film.	☒	☐
Fill uneven skin surfaces with a skin barrier product.	☒	☐
Frame the periwound area with a hydrocolloid dressing.	☒	☐
Cut the transparent film to extend ½ inch beyond the wound perimeter.	☐	☒
Use as many additional dressing layers as needed for identified air leaks.	☐	☒

Shaving hair poses a safety risk because of the possibility of injury and therefore can be eliminated. From here, use your nursing knowledge to eliminate the option stating to cut the transparent film ½ inch beyond the wound perimeter and the option that states to use as many additional dressing layers as needed for air leaks, noting that these interventions would not help to maintain or ensure a good seal.

Content Area: Foundations of Nursing
Priority Concept: Tissue Integrity
Reference(s): Potter et al., 2021, pp. 999, 1263–1264

Practice Question 6.3   Drag-and-Drop Rationale

A 44-year-old postoperative client returned to the nursing unit from the PACU following bilateral mastectomy. The client has four Jackson-Pratt drains from the incisional areas on the chest. The nurse assesses VS and performs the physical assessment.

Based on the client findings, complete the following sentence by choosing from the lists of options provided.

To ensure client safety, the nurse plans to **first administer enoxaparin** to address **thrombus risk**.

Health History	Physical Assessment	Vital Signs	Orders

Alert and oriented. Incisional pain rated 2/10.
Bilateral incisions on the chest covered with a dry sterile dressing, clean, dry, and intact.
Lung sounds clear to auscultation bilaterally. S1S2, no S3S4. +2 peripheral pulses, no edema.
4 Jackson Pratt drains from the incisional areas: #1 with 5 mL of sanguineous drainage, #2 with 10 mL of sanguineous drainage, #3 with 5 mL of sanguineous drainage, #4 with 10 mL of sanguineous drainage, compressed for suction.

Options for 1	Options for 2
Administer enoxaparin	Pain
Administer pain medication	Infection
Increase supplemental oxygen	Hypoxemia
Empty and compress surgical drains	Thrombus risk

Health History	Physical Assessment	Vital Signs	Orders

BP = 146/72 mm Hg; HR = 70 BPM; RR = 20 bpm; T = 98.2°F (36.8°C); SpO_2 = 97% at 3 L per NC

Health History	Physical Assessment	Vital Signs	Orders

Monitor VS per unit protocol
Titrate oxygen to maintain SpO_2 greater than 92%
Monitor incision site for signs of bleeding
Monitor and maintain surgical drains
Enoxaparin 40 mg subcutaneously daily
Apply sequential compression devices (SCDs) below the knee bilaterally for venous thrombosis prevention
Pan management via PCA pump
Clear liquids advance to regular as tolerated
Incentive spirometry per unit protocol
Ondansetron 4 mg IV every 4 hours as needed for nausea

Rationale: Taking into consideration all of the client data in this clinical scenario, the major concern would be the potential complication for thrombus formation as a postoperative complication. Enoxaparin, classified as an anticoagulant or low–molecular-weight heparin, is given to postoperative clients as a preventive measure for thrombus formation. To ensure client safety, the nurse would plan to first administer the enoxaparin to address thrombus risk. The other options may be needed but are not the priority at this time. Pain is expected after surgery and needs to be well managed to promote healing. The client's pain is currently rated 2/10, and because the client has a PCA pump as noted in the Orders, it would not be a priority for the nurse to administer pain medication. Hypoxemia can occur after surgery, related to the effects of anesthesia and immobility in the postoperative period. The client's SpO$_2$ is 97% on 3 L per NC, and there is no evidence of hypoxemia; therefore the nurse would not need to increase the oxygen flow rate. Maintaining the surgical drains is an important measure so that body fluids are adequately drained and do not build up in the affected area, leading to infection. Because there is only 5 to 10 mL of drainage in each drain, it is not the priority to empty and compress the surgical drains at this time. In addition, the Physical Assessment notes indicate that the drains were already compressed for suction.

Test-Taking Strategy: Focus on what the question is asking about: nursing interventions to ensure client safety and the rationale behind them. Note the strategic word *first.* This word may indicate that some or all of the options are correct, and you need to decide which intervention should be planned first. Once you have determined the intervention, then consider the rationale for that intervention. Think about the potential complications of surgery. Because the client had surgery, the client is at risk for pain, infection, hypoxemia, and thrombus, and so you need to decide which intervention needs to be planned *first* for client safety considerations. Using this knowledge and the data provided in the clinical scenario, organize your thought process as illustrated in the table. There needs to be supporting evidence for options in order for the option to be correct.

Intervention	Supporting Evidence Indicating Priority Intervention
Administer enoxaparin	Recent surgery—prevents thrombus
Administer pain medication	Not needed—pain 2/10, using PCA
Increase supplemental oxygen	Not needed—97% 3 L per NC
Empty and compress surgical drains	Not needed—not full yet; already compressed

The client's pain assessment, SpO$_2$, and surgical drain assessments do not indicate the need for intervention at this time and therefore do not need to be addressed first. Because administering enoxaparin is a preventive measure to reduce the risk of thrombus following surgery, this intervention should be done first. Note that the second part of the question requires you to demonstrate that you know the reason for choosing the first option. Use your nursing knowledge to recall that enoxaparin is an anticoagulant commonly used after surgery to prevent the formation of a thrombus as a result of the surgery.

Content Area: Medical-Surgical Nursing
Priority Concept: Clotting
Reference(s): Burchum & Rosenthal, 2022, p. 596; Potter et al., 2021, p. 1349

Practice Question 6.4   **Multiple Response Select All That Apply**

A 22-year-old client presents to the outpatient clinic reporting feeling "down" and stating having difficulty maintaining responsibilities with school. States experiencing a hard time finding friends, that peers in class don't think the client is smart, and that they make fun of the client behind the client's back. When asked about family dynamics, the client states is not speaking to parents and that the only support system is the client's partner. States "putting myself through school." Describes not being able to meet assignment deadlines and thinks about considering quitting school. The client is referred to the counseling and psychological center and is beginning group therapy.

Based on this scenario, which of the following interventions would the psychiatric nurse plan for the client? **Select all that apply.**

☒ Set realistic goals for behavior modification.

☒ Reward the client for practicing new behaviors.

☐ Provide positive regard for adaptive behaviors only.

☒ Encourage the client to practice behavior modifications.

☐ Help the client identify negative qualities and experiences.

☒ Help the client identify their own behaviors needing change.

☒ Reinforce self-worth with time and attention by giving one-to-one time.

Rationale: This client is experiencing decreased self-esteem, which could be related to perceived lack of belonging, perceived lack of respect from others, lack of success in role functioning, a disturbed relationship with parents or caregivers, and feeling targeted by peers. Although not reported, a psychiatric disorder could also be a factor for this client. The nurse would help the client to describe self in positive ways, fulfill personally significant roles, and engage in meaningful interaction with others. Interventions that should be planned for this client include setting realistic goals for behavior modification; rewarding the client for practicing new behaviors; encouraging the client to practice behavior modifications; helping the client to identify own behaviors needing change; and reinforcing self-worth with time and attention by giving one-on-one time. Rather than providing positive regard for adaptive behaviors only, the nurse needs to give unconditional positive regard and avoid acknowledgement or reinforcement of negative behaviors. Instead of helping the client identify negative qualities and experiences, the nurse would help the client identify positive qualities and accomplishments.

Test-Taking Strategy: Note that this question is asking you choose interventions that the nurse would plan for this client based on the information described in the clinical scenario. To decide on the appropriate interventions for the plan of care, first you need to determine based on the information in the scenario that the client is experiencing problems with self-esteem. Next, for each intervention listed, determine whether that intervention would improve or not improve self-esteem. Organize your thinking process as illustrated in the table.

Intervention	Improves Self-Esteem	Does Not Improve Self-Esteem
Set realistic goals for behavior modification.	☒	☐
Reward the client for practicing new behaviors.	☒	☐
Provide positive regard for adaptive behaviors only.	☐	☒
Encourage the client to practice behavior modifications.	☒	☐
Help the client identify negative qualities and experiences.	☐	☒
Help the client identify their own behaviors needing change.	☒	☐
Reinforce self-worth with time and attention by giving one-on-one time.	☒	☐

If you focus on the outcome of improving self-esteem, then you will be able to determine which interventions are appropriate in the plan of care for this client. Options that describe new behaviors, realistic goals, self-worth, and changing behaviors are aligned with actions that would improve self-esteem. Options that are limited in scope or that focus on negative adaptations are the actions that would not improve self-esteem and therefore should be eliminated.

Content Area: Mental Health Nursing
Priority Concept: Stress and Coping
Reference(s): Varcarolis & Fosbre, 2021, p. 66

Practice Question 6.5   Matrix Multiple Choice

A 32-year-old client is in the neurologic unit after sustaining a head injury after falling from a ladder while working in the garage. The client is unable to eat or drink because of unconsciousness. The intensivist prescribes central line insertion and total parenteral nutrition (TPN) to be administered for nutritional support.

*Place an X to indicate whether each potential intervention listed below is either **Anticipated** (appropriate or necessary) or **Contraindicated** (is unnecessary or is harmful) for the client's plan of care at this time.*

Potential Intervention	Anticipated	Contraindicated
Administer insulin.	X	☐
Assess for diaphoresis.	X	☐
Monitor IV site.	X	☐
Follow Droplet Precautions.	☐	X
Monitor blood glucose level every 6 hours.	X	☐
Shut the infusion off if the bag is empty while waiting for the next TPN bag to become available.	☐	X

Rationale: TPN, also called parenteral nutrition (PN), involves IV administration of complex and highly concentrated solution that contains nutrients and electrolytes. It is formulated to meet the client's nutritional needs. This nutritional support is provided for clients who are unable to digest or absorb nutrition orally or enterally. Clients who are in highly stressed physiologic states such as sepsis, head injury, or burns are candidates for TPN. TPN needs to be administered through a central venous catheter (CVC). Safe administration of TPN requires management of the CVC and insertion site to prevent infection, and ongoing and careful monitoring to prevent metabolic complications. Hypoglycemia and hyperglycemia are potential complications of TPN therapy. The nurse needs to monitor for diaphoresis and needs to assess the blood glucose level every 6 hours to monitor for these complications. For clients receiving TPN who are conscious, other signs and symptoms of these potential complications include shakiness, confusion, loss of consciousness, thirst, headache, lethargy, and increased urination. In addition, to prevent hypoglycemia the TPN should not be abruptly discontinued, but rather tapered down. If an infusion bag of TPN completes, and it is necessary to wait for the next TPN infusion bag, the nurse would infuse a solution of 10% glucose until the TPN infusion bag is available. IV 50% dextrose or glucagon needs to be available to treat hypoglycemia if it occurs. TPN also should not be suddenly increased but instead should be tapered up to prevent hyperglycemia. Insulin may be required during therapy, especially if the client has DM. The client is at risk for infection because of the CVC and because the client is receiving TPN. The nurse needs to monitor the IV site for signs of infection and intervene accordingly to prevent infection and to address it if it is suspected. On the basis of TPN therapy, the nurse does not need to follow Droplet Precautions but instead should follow Standard Precautions, unless the client is on Transmission-Based Precautions for another transmissible disease.

Test-Taking Strategy: Note that the question is asking you about actions or interventions that are either anticipated or contraindicated. An anticipated action is one that would be appropriate or necessary, whereas, as noted in this question, a contraindicated action is one that is unnecessary or could be harmful. The first step in answering this question correctly is to determine which of the potential interventions listed in the options are helpful or not helpful or unnecessary or potentially harmful as they relate to the care necessary for a client receiving TPN. As shown in the table, think about the effects of TPN on the body. Use your nursing knowledge of the indications and effects of TPN.

Test-Taking Strategy

Potential Intervention	Helpful or Not Helpful/ Unnecessary or Harmful
Administer insulin.	Helpful
Assess for diaphoresis.	Helpful
Monitor IV site.	Helpful
Follow Droplet Precautions.	Unnecessary
Monitor blood glucose level every 6 hours.	Helpful
Shut the infusion off if the bag is empty while waiting for the next TPN bag to become available.	Harmful

From here, you can determine that any helpful intervention is a correct option, but any intervention that is not necessary or is harmful is an incorrect option. Recall that blood glucose changes can occur with TPN; therefore any option related to monitoring for complications or managing blood glucose levels would be helpful. Droplet Precautions are not needed for TPN therapy and therefore are unnecessary. Shutting off the infusion before the next bag is available could be harmful because of a drop in blood glucose levels and therefore is incorrect.

Content Area: Pharmacology
Priority Concept: Fluid and Electrolyte Balance
Reference(s): Burchum & Rosenthal, 2022, pp. 999, 1124

Practice Question 6.6   Multiple Response Select N

A 46-year-old client was admitted to the hospital after reporting increased thirst, increased hunger, and increased urination for the last 7 days. On admission, the client's blood glucose level was significantly elevated, and the client was treated for DKA. After being stabilized, the client was discharged to home with a diagnosis of new-onset DM. The home care nurse is visiting the client and is providing teaching on self-management and measures to prevent hospitalization. The client tells the home care nurse about often feeling hungry, irritable, shaky, and weak and having a headache.

Based on the client's reported symptoms, which five measures would the home care nurse plan to teach this client to implement when these symptoms occur?

- ☒ Eat 6 saltine crackers.
- ☒ Eat 3 graham crackers.
- ☒ Drink 120 mL of fruit juice.
- ☒ Drink 240 mL of skim milk.
- ☒ Consume 6 to 10 hard candies.
- ☐ Consume 4 tablespoons of honey.
- ☐ Drink 120 mL of a diet soft drink.
- ☐ Decrease intake of carbohydrates.
- ☐ Administer insulin based on sliding scale.

Rationale: Clients with DM need to be taught how to manage hypoglycemia at home. The client's symptoms (feeling hungry, irritable, shaky, weak, headache) are indicative of possible hypoglycemia. To manage or treat hypoglycemia at home if the client is conscious, they should be taught to do one of the following: eat 6 saltine crackers, eat 3 graham crackers, or drink 120 mL of fruit juice, 240 mL of skim milk, or 120 mL of nondiet or regular soft drink. The client can also consume 6 to 10 hard candies or 1 tablespoon of honey or syrup. The client would not be instructed to administer insulin based on the sliding scale or to decrease the intake of carbohydrates, as this would worsen the hypoglycemia; these measures would be used to manage hyperglycemia.

Test-Taking Strategy

Test-Taking Strategy: Note that this clinical scenario describes symptoms consistent with hypoglycemia. Thinking about the pathophysiology and recalling the measures that are necessary to manage hypoglycemia will help direct you to the correct options. Remember that the food item given needs to be the correct item and in the correct amount in order to adequately raise the blood glucose, while also not causing the blood glucose to go too high. Using a thinking process as illustrated in the table may be helpful to you.

Food Item	Correct Item	Correct Amount
6 saltine crackers	Yes	Yes
3 graham crackers	Yes	Yes
120 mL of fruit juice	Yes	Yes
240 mL of skim milk	Yes	Yes
6 to 10 hard candies	Yes	Yes
4 tablespoons of honey	Yes	No
120 mL of diet soft drink	No	No

Food items that are correct items and are also correct in the amount should be chosen as interventions for this scenario. Note that only 1 tablespoon of honey should be given to avoid raising the blood glucose too high. Also note that 120 mL of nondiet (rather than diet) soft drink can be given in the event of hypoglycemia. The last two options should be eliminated, noting that decreasing the intake of carbohydrates and administering insulin based on the sliding scale would further worsen the hypoglycemia. This leaves you with the five correct options: the saltine crackers, graham crackers, fruit juice, skim milk, and hard candies.

Content Area: Medical-Surgical Nursing
Priority Concept: Glucose Regulation
Reference(s): Ignatavicius et al., 2021, p. 191

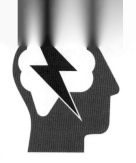

Answers to Practice Questions

Practice Question 7.1 **Multiple Response Select All That Apply**

An occupational nurse is called for emergency assistance to a 42-year-old victim of an accident in which the victim's index and middle finger were completely severed by a machine saw. The victim is sitting on the floor leaning against a wall and the fingers are seen on the floor 2 feet away from the client.

Health History	Nurses' Notes	Vital Signs	Laboratory Results

0800:
VS: T = 98.2°F (36.7°C); HR = 120 BPM; RR = 22 bpm;
BP = 132/84 mm Hg

What actions would the nurse take? **Select all that apply.**

- ☒ Call 911 (EMS).
- ☒ Elevate the affected hand above heart level.
- ☒ Place the fingers in a waterproof sealed plastic bag.
- ☒ Check the victim for airway or breathing problems.
- ☐ Place the waterproof sealed bag containing the fingers on ice.
- ☒ Apply direct pressure to the amputation sites with layers of dry gauze.
- ☐ Remove the dry gauze after 10 minutes to check the status of the bleeding.
- ☒ Ensure that the amputated fingers are transported to the hospital with the victim.

Rationale: The nurse needs to call 911 in the event of a traumatic amputation. Emergency care is necessary while waiting for transport of the victim to the hospital. The nurse assesses the victim for airway or breathing problems, examines the amputation sites, and applies direct pressure with layers of dry gauze. The hand is elevated above the victim's heart level to decrease the bleeding. Once the dressing has been applied it is not removed, in order to prevent dislodging of the clot that may form. The nurse would wrap the completely severed fingers in dry sterile gauze and place them in a waterproof sealed plastic bag. The bag is placed in ice water, never directly on ice, as 1 part ice and 3 parts water. The nurse ensures that the amputated parts are transported to the hospital with the victim. While waiting for EMS to arrive, the nurse stays with the client and monitors the client's status including VS.

Test-Taking Strategy

Test-Taking Strategy: Think about the goals of care for a victim of a traumatic amputation. Bleeding needs to be stopped and adequate peripheral perfusion to the residual part needs to be maintained. The goal for the amputated part is to preserve perfusion for possible reattachment. With these goals in mind, read each option and think about how the action will achieve the goal. This will assist in answering correctly. A simple "Yes/No/Why or Why Not" approach with some thought as to the rationale for each option will help you organize the information in a way that will help to answer correctly, as noted in the table.

Nursing Actions	Yes	No	Why or Why Not
Call 911 (EMS).	☒	☐	Emergency care needed for traumatic event
Elevate the affected hand above heart level.	☒	☐	To decrease bleeding and swelling

Nursing Actions	Yes	No	Why or Why Not
Place the fingers in a waterproof sealed plastic bag.	☒	☐	To preserve the fingers for reattachment
Check the victim for airway or breathing problems.	☒	☐	To ensure cardiopulmonary stability
Place the waterproof sealed bag containing the fingers on ice.	☐	☒	Not directly on ice—rather, in ice water; direct ice could damage tissue
Apply direct pressure to the amputation site with layers of dry gauze.	☒	☐	To decrease bleeding
Remove the dry gauze after 10 minutes to check the status of the bleeding.	☐	☒	May dislodge any formed clots
Ensure that the amputated fingers are transported to the hospital with the victim.	☒	☐	For possible reattachment

Remember that test-taking strategies are useful ways to organize information in order to answer a test question. With multiple response questions, the "Yes/No/Why or Why Not" approach is a helpful way to think through each option.

Content Area: Medical-Surgical Nursing
Priority Concept: Perfusion
Reference(s): Ignatavicius et al., 2021, p. 1048

Practice Question 7.2   **Drag-and-Drop Cloze**

The nurse is preparing to administer medications to a hospitalized 82-year-old client recovering from an acute exacerbation of heart failure. The client was taking eight different routine medications at home and is started on three additional medications to be taken while in the hospital. Recognizing the safety risks of polypharmacy and the importance of safe medication administration, the nurse takes steps to prevent medication errors.

Complete the following sentence. Drag or select words from the options below to fill in each blank.

To promote medication administration safety and to prevent medication errors, the nurse checks at least <u>two</u> client identifier(s), reads medication labels at least <u>three</u> time(s), and documents medication administration <u>as soon as medications are given</u>.

Options for 1	Options for 2	Options for 3
One	One	As soon as medications are given
Two	Two	Immediately before medications are given
Three	Three	After medications are given and after leaving the room
Four	Four	Before removing the medications from the dispensing system

Rationale: Medication administration is an integral aspect of the nurse's role. Safe medication administration and preventing medication errors requires careful attention and nursing actions. To safely administer medications, the nurse needs to follow the rights of medication administration, prepare medications for only one client at a time, use at least *two* client identifiers each time medications are administered, read labels at least *three* times and compare the medication administration record with medication labels, not allow any interruptions, verify all high-risk medications with another licensed nurse, question unusually large or small doses, and document all medications *as soon as they are given.*

Test-Taking Strategy: Visualizing the nursing actions in this question is the first step in answering correctly. Thinking about how each action promotes safety and focusing on certain strategic words, such as *at least* in this question, will be a helpful strategy. In a Drag-and-Drop Cloze question, partial credit is given if correct and incorrect answers are chosen. Choosing correctly as you begin answering each part of the question will help you in choosing the greatest number of correct answers. For the first two response columns, you will have to rely on your knowledge of how many identifiers need to be checked and how many times labels need to be checked based on best practice guidelines in order to answer correctly. Remember that safety is a central concept for medication administration. For the third response column, looking at each option and thinking through whether that nursing action would promote safety or would not promote safety during medication administration, in terms of accurate medication administration documentation, will help you narrow down your options and answer correctly. Organizing your thought process using a table format, or just thinking about it in this way, will help you use the process of elimination and narrow down your answers.

Nursing Action	Safety	Possible Outcomes
Documenting medication administration as soon as medications are given	Promotes	Accurate documentation
Documenting medication administration immediately before medications are given	Does not promote	Inaccurate documentation
Documenting medication administration after medications are given and after leaving the room	Does not promote	Inaccurate documentation
Documenting medication administration before removing the medications from the dispensing system	Does not promote	Inaccurate documentation

Documenting medication administration as soon as medications are given promotes safety. Looking at the other options, documenting medication administration immediately before medications are given or before removing medications from the dispensing system does not promote safety. There are many things that could occur before the medication is given, such as interruptions or client refusal, resulting in inaccurate documentation. Although you may be drawn to choose documenting after medication administration and after leaving the room, remember that interruptions could occur and could result in inaccurate documentation; therefore documenting as soon as they are given is the safest action.

Content Area: Foundations of Nursing
Priority Concept: Perfusion
Reference(s): Potter et al., 2021, p. 606

Practice Question 7.3   Matrix Multiple Response

A 65-year-old client was hospitalized and treated for symptoms of heart palpitations and extreme shortness of breath. On admission, diagnostic studies showed the following:

Health History	Nurses' Notes	Vital Signs	Diagnostic Studies

- ECG: atrial fibrillation
- CT of the lungs: negative for embolism
- Chest x-ray: enlarged left ventricle

The nurse is preparing the client for discharge and provides teaching about prescribed medications.

For each medication listed, click in the box to specify the teaching point the nurse would provide to the client. Each teaching point may support more than one medication.

Teaching Point	Amiodarone	Metoprolol	Warfarin
Routine laboratory monitoring	☐	☐	☒
Monitor and report signs of bleeding	☐	☐	☒
Monitor and report shortness of breath	☒	☒	☐
Monitor BP and HR	☒	☒	☐
Consume consistent amounts of green leafy vegetables	☐	☐	☒

Rationale: Amiodarone is an antidysrhythmic used to treat atrial fibrillation. It causes blood vessels to dilate and can lead to dizziness and hypotension. The client is taught how to check the HR and BP. An adverse effect of amiodarone is pulmonary toxicity, and if the client experiences shortness of breath, it could be an indication that this effect is occurring, warranting prescriber notification. Metoprolol is a beta-adrenergic blocker and causes the HR and BP to decrease, so the client needs to make sure the HR and BP are within prescribed parameters before taking this medication, so that they do not drop too low. Metoprolol can also cause shortness of breath, coughing, and wheezing; if these occur, the prescriber is notified. The client taking amiodarone or metoprolol is taught safety measures such as moving slowly from a sitting or lying to a standing position and to immediately sit or lie down if dizziness or light-headedness occurs. The client is also instructed to contact the prescriber if these symptoms persist. Warfarin is an anticoagulant that requires routine laboratory monitoring for coagulation studies, specifically the international normalized ratio (INR), and dose adjustments are made based on the INR. Because warfarin slows clotting, an adverse effect is bleeding, and the client needs to monitor and report signs of bleeding. Green leafy vegetables contain vitamin K, which is the antidote for warfarin. The client needs to consume consistent amounts of green leafy vegetables so that the vitamin K from these foods remains at a consistent level in the body and does not inhibit the effects of the warfarin.

Test-Taking Strategy: An important nursing action is to provide teaching to a client. Begin to answer this question by thinking about the medication classifications. Sometimes you will be easily able to recognize medication names and their classifications, and other times you need to rely on knowledge. For example, metoprolol has a common suffix *(-lol)*, which helps you determine that this medication belongs to the beta-adrenergic blocker classification. From here, you may need to use your knowledge and determine the other medication classifications. Rather than trying to learn every medication and everything about it, learn medications by associating them with a specific classification. Indications, side and adverse effects, and primary nursing considerations and teaching points for a classification will be similar, so if you can associate a medication with a classification, this will really help you in answering pharmacology questions. Organizing information in the format shown in the table when answering pharmacology questions will be a helpful strategy in answering these questions correctly. In this question, recalling the medication classifications and associated side and adverse effects and primary nursing considerations will help you determine the teaching points specific to each medication.

Medication Classification	Indications	Side/Adverse Effects	Primary Nursing Considerations/Teaching Points
Warfarin (anticoagulant)	Long-term prophylaxis of thrombosis	Bleeding	Multiple drug-drug and drug-food interactions. Review medications and diet to identify any interactions. Monitor for bleeding: bruising, urine, stool. Safety measures
Amiodarone (antidysrhythmic)	Management of atrial and ventricular dysrhythmias	Pulmonary, cardiac, liver, and thyroid toxicity. Ophthalmic effects. Photosensitivity	Monitor for signs and symptoms of toxicity. Measure HR and BP. Report episodes of light-headedness or dizziness
Metoprolol (beta-adrenergic blocker)	Treatment of hypertension, angina, heart failure, myocardial infarction	Bradycardia, reduced cardiac output, heart block, rebound cardiac excitation	Measure HR and BP. Monitor for and report adverse effects such as light-headedness or dizziness, cough, wheezing

Content Area: Pharmacology
Priority Concept: Perfusion
Reference(s): Burchum & Rosenthal, 2022, pp. 168–170, 559–560, 612–616; Ignatavicius et al., 2021, pp. 653–654

Practice Question 7.4   Matrix Multiple Choice

The nurse is caring for an 80-year-old client on the medical-surgical unit admitted with complicated UTI. The client takes lisinopril and metformin at home and is started on antibiotics for infection and antipyretics as needed. The physician ordered the Modified Early Warning Score (MEWS) to be calculated every 4 hours to monitor for signs of septic shock. Assessment findings include RR, 12 bpm; HR, 110 BPM; systolic BP, 92 mm Hg; temperature, 100.5°F (38.1°C); and the client is currently alert and responsive. The client's MEWS is currently a 2 and is documented as follows:

	+3	+2	+1	0	+1	+2	+3
RR				X			
HR					X		
Systolic BP			X				
T				X			
Mental status				X			

MEWS Scoring Key

RR (bpm)		Systolic BP (mm Hg)	
<9	+2	≤70	+3
9–14	0	71–80	+2
15–20	+1	81–100	+1
21–29	+2	101–199	0
≥30	+3	≥200	+2
HR (BPM)		**T**	
<40	+2	<35°C / 95°F	+2
41–50	+1	35-38.4°C / 95–101.1°F	0
51–100	0	≥38.5°C / 101.3°F	+2
101–110	+1	**Mental Status**	
111–129	+2	Alert	0
≥130	+3	Reacts to voice	+1
		Reacts to pain	+2
		Unresponsive	+3

*Based on this assessment, click in the box to specify nursing actions that are **Indicated** (appropriate or necessary) and those that are **Contraindicated** (could be harmful).*

Nursing Action	Indicated	Contraindicated
Perform hourly VS, urine output, neurologic, and cardiopulmonary measurements	☒	☐
Administer prescribed daily BP medication	☐	☒
Administer ibuprofen for fever	☐	☒
Administer prescribed antibiotics	☒	☐
Notify the physician of an increase in the MEWS	☒	☐

Rationale: Sepsis and septic shock are complications and potential bodily responses to infection. Sepsis and septic shock can cause tissue damage, organ failure, and death if left untreated. Older adults are at risk for developing sepsis, and UTI can lead to this complication. Because the progression of sepsis occurs over time, there are subtle changes in the clinical manifestations as the condition develops. The MEWS system is a tool that is helpful in detecting these subtle changes related to a declining condition. The higher the score, the higher likelihood of the need for intensive care. With a MEWS of 2, the nurse would perform hourly observations, administer prescribed antibiotics, and contact the physician if the MEWS increases. Additional actions may be taken, such as checking the lactate level, checking blood cultures followed by administering antibiotics, administering IV fluids, and administering vasopressors depending on how the client presents and how the condition evolves. Administering the client's prescribed BP medication is contraindicated and could be harmful because the BP is low. Use of aspirin-containing products and or NSAIDs is a risk factor for shock and would be contraindicated in managing the fever; alternative antipyretics such as acetaminophen would be used.

Test-Taking Strategy: You need to use knowledge about the effects of sepsis and septic shock on the body to assist in answering this question. Consider the strategic words *indicated* and *contraindicated* and visualize the possible outcomes from each of the nursing actions. Using the strategy of looking at each option and thinking through whether that nursing action would promote safety or would not promote safety, as well as the possible outcomes, will assist in answering the question correctly.

Test-Taking Strategy

Nursing Action	Safety	Possible Outcomes
Perform hourly VS, urine output, neurologic, and cardiopulmonary measurements	Promotes	Assists in detecting clinical deterioration
Administer prescribed daily BP medication	Does not promote	Dangerous reduction in BP causing further clinical deterioration
Administer ibuprofen for fever	Does not promote	Increased likelihood that shock will occur
Administer prescribed antibiotics	Promotes	Treat infection and reduce risk for sepsis and septic shock
Notify the physician of an increase in the MEWS	Promotes	Detect clinical deterioration suggestive of sepsis and septic shock and determine the need for additional treatment

Performing hourly VS, urine output, neurologic, and cardiopulmonary measurements; administering prescribed antibiotics; and notifying the physician of an increase in the MEWS are all actions that promote safety by allowing the nurse to detect subtle changes of clinical deterioration that may be associated with the complications of sepsis and septic shock, and the need for additional treatment. Administering ibuprofen and BP medication would not promote safety and could harm the client, and therefore these actions are contraindicated.

Content Area: Medical-Surgical Nursing
Priority Concept: Perfusion
Reference(s): Ignatavicius et al., 2021, pp. 743–745; https://www.mdcalc.com/modified-early-warning-score-mews-clinical-deterioration

---

| **Practice Question 7.5** | **Multiple Response Select All That Apply** |

A 48-year-old client underwent laparoscopic cholecystectomy and is transferred to the surgical outpatient unit. The nurse performs a postoperative assessment and documents in the Nurses' Notes.

| Health History | Nurses' Notes | Diagnostic Studies | Laboratory Results |

1100:
VS: T = 99.2°F (37.3°C); HR = 92 BPM; RR = 16 bpm; BP = 118/72 mm Hg; SpO$_2$ = 97% on RA
Alert and oriented. Dressing dry and intact. IV 5% dextrose/lactated Ringer's infusing at 100 mL/hr. Has not voided. Pain 4/10.

The nurse would take which actions in managing this client's care in the immediate postoperative period? **Select all that apply.**

☐ Keep the head of the bed flat.
☒ Assist to the bathroom to void.
☒ Assess incision sites frequently.
☒ Administer antiemetics as needed.
☐ Maintain strict NPO status.
☒ Administer pain medication.
☒ Encourage use of the incentive spirometer.

Rationale: Care of the client in the immediate postoperative period following laparoscopic cholecystectomy includes keeping the head of the bed elevated to avoid aspiration and promote comfort, assisting the client to the bathroom to void, assessing incision sites frequently, administering antiemetics as needed, offering food and water when fully awake, administering pain medication as needed, and encouraging the use of the incentive spirometer while awake. Keeping the head of the bed flat would be contraindicated and could result in aspiration, particularly if the client is experiencing nausea and vomiting. In addition, this position causes stress on the abdominal incision sites. It is not necessary to maintain NPO status; but food and water need to be offered after the client is alert to prevent aspiration.

Test-Taking
Strategy

Test-Taking Strategy: Note the strategic word *immediate,* and think about the nursing actions necessary in caring for a client immediately after laparoscopic cholecystectomy, as well as general nursing actions for clients undergoing surgery. Using the "Yes/No/Why or Why Not" approach with some thinking processes as to the rationale for each option will help you organize the information in a way that will help you answer correctly, as noted in the table.

Nursing Actions	Yes	No	Why or Why Not
Keep the head of the bed flat.	☐	☒	Could result in aspiration; postoperative clients often have nausea and vomiting; may cause stress on the incision sites.
Assist to the bathroom to void.	☒	☐	Ensuring adequate voiding after surgery is important because urinary retention can occur from anesthesia. Ambulation is also important to prevent respiratory and circulatory complications.
Assess incision sites frequently.	☒	☐	Monitor for bleeding, drainage, opening of incisions, infection.
Administer antiemetics as needed.	☒	☐	Nausea and vomiting are common effects of anesthesia.
Maintain strict NPO status.	☐	☒	Would be used prior to surgery but is not needed following surgery; need to ensure adequate oral intake after surgery, maintain nutrition and hydration once safe to do so.
Administer pain medication.	☒	☐	Pain management in the immediate postoperative period is important in promoting comfort, mobility, and recovery.
Encourage use of the incentive spirometer.	☒	☐	Important in preventing atelectasis and resultant pneumonia.

Remember that test-taking strategies are useful ways to organize information in order to answer a test question. With multiple response questions, the "Yes/No/Why or Why Not" approach is a helpful way to think through each option and will assist you in choosing the correct answers.

Content Area: Medical-Surgical Nursing
Priority Concept: Tissue Integrity
Reference(s): Ignatavicius et al., 2021, p. 1181

Practice Question 7.6   Drop-Down Rationale

The nurse is caring for a 70-year-old client with cellulitis on both lower extremities caused by methicillin-resistant *Staphylococcus aureus (MRSA)* and who is being treated with IV vancomycin. The next dose of vancomycin is due now, and the nurse checks the laboratory results.

Health History	Nurses' Notes	Vital Signs	Laboratory Results

Test	Result	Normal Reference Range
Vancomycin trough level	16 mcg/mL (11.3981 mcmol/L)	10–20 mcg/mL (10.3498–13.7998 mcmol/L)
White blood cells (WBCs)	10,000/mm³ (10×10^9 /L)	5000–10,000/mm³ (5–10×10^9 /L)
Blood urea nitrogen (BUN)	20 mg/dL (7.1 mmol/L)	10–20 mg/dL (3.6–7.1 mmol/L)
Creatinine	0.6 mg/dL (53 mcmol/L)	0.5–1.2 mg/dL (44–106 mcmol/L)

Based on this information, which action would the nurse take? Complete the following sentence by choosing from the list of options.

The nurse would **administer the next dose as prescribed** because **the trough level is normal**.

Options for 1	Options for 2
Hold the next dose	The WBC count is high
Administer a lower dose	The trough level is normal
Administer the next dose orally	The creatinine level indicates toxicity
Administer the next dose as prescribed	The BUN level is high but not toxic

Rationale: Vancomycin is classified as an antimicrobial and works by inhibiting bacterial cell wall synthesis. It is indicated for treatment of serious infections, including infections caused by MRSA. Vancomycin can be administered orally, intravenously, and rectally. IV administration is indicated for systemic infections. Dosages need to be reduced in renal impairment, and trough levels need to be monitored for IV vancomycin. The trough level is the lowest concentration of the medication in the client's bloodstream; therefore the specimen should be collected just prior to administration of the vancomycin. The peak level is the highest concentration of the medication in the client's bloodstream. A peak level is drawn 1 hour to several hours after the medication is administered, depending on the medication. Vancomycin trough levels of 10 to 20 mcg/mL (10.3498 to 13.7998 mcmol/L) are recommended for best outcomes. A trough level of 16 mcg/mL (11.3981 mcmol/L) is normal and in the expected range and indicates that the kidneys are adequately excreting the medication as expected; therefore the nurse can administer the next dose as prescribed based on this information. The reference range for vancomycin peak levels is 20 to 40 mcg/mL (13.7998 to 27.5995 mcmol/L). The normal WBC count is 5000 to 10,000/mm³ (5 to 10×10^9/L). The normal BUN level is 10 to 20 mg/dL (3.6 to 7.1 mmol/L). The normal creatinine level is 0.5 to 1.2 mg/dL (44 to 106 mcmol/L).

Test-Taking Strategy: First, it is necessary to know the normal or therapeutic trough level for vancomycin and the normal reference ranges for the WBC count, BUN, and creatinine. From there, it may be helpful to look at the options for the second response column first and determine the appropriate action in terms of dosage adjustment for these findings. This may help you choose the correct answer for the first response column. Refer to the table for an illustration applying this strategy.

Test-Taking Strategy

Laboratory Result	Action and Rationale
The WBC count is normal, not high.	No specific action is indicated, as the value is normal.
The trough level is normal and in expected range.	Same dosage can be administered; level is in the expected range and indicates that the kidneys are adequately excreting the medication as expected.
The creatinine level is normal, not toxic.	No specific action is indicated, as the value is normal.
The BUN is normal, not high or toxic.	No specific action is indicated, as the value is normal.

Using knowledge to determine that the WBC count, BUN, and creatinine level are normal will assist in answering. Next, if you can determine that the trough level is normal, you can then decide that the same dosage would be indicated. This will assist in directing you to administer the next dose as prescribed as a safe and appropriate nursing action based on this clinical scenario.

Content Area: Pharmacology
Priority Concept: Elimination
Reference(s): Burchum & Rosenthal, 2022, p. 1045

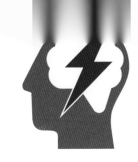
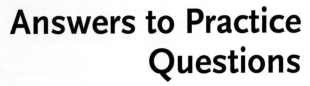

| Practice Question 8.1 | Matrix Multiple Choice |

The nurse is preparing a 68-year-old client in a rehabilitation center for discharge to home. The client was transferred from the hospital 2 weeks ago following treatment for a right cerebral stroke. On admission to the rehabilitation center, the following findings were documented.

| Health History | Nurses' Notes | Vital Signs | Physician's Orders |

T = 98.6°F (36.0°C); HR = 92 BPM; BP = 132/78 mm Hg; RR = 20 bpm; SpO$_2$ = 95% on RA

| Health History | Nurses' Notes | Vital Signs | Physician's Orders |

Client is accompanied by spouse, who will be the primary caregiver when the client returns home.

Alert and oriented and understands about receiving rehabilitative therapy before returning to home. States doesn't really have "much to rehab" and is fine but will do what the doctor says to get home.

Has left-side weakness and seems impulsive with movements. Able to move right arm and leg with adequate strength noted.

Has difficulty focusing and attention span is short; spouse is assisting in answering questions.

Spouse notes that the client's judgment is impaired and is concerned about the client's safety because of the client's impulsivity.

Client also exhibits left-sided neglect; lacks proprioception. Has homonymous hemianopsia.

| Health History | Nurses' Notes | Vital Signs | Physician's Orders |

PT and OT evaluation and initiate a treatment plan as needed

Low-fat diet

Out of bed as much as tolerated

Begin to prepare client and spouse for discharge to home

Referral to case manager to plan discharge

Clopidogrel 75 mg oral daily

Carvedilol 3.125 mg oral twice daily

Docusate 100 mg oral daily

Simvastatin 20 mg oral daily

The nurse consults with the case manager about the plan for home care. Collaboration with the client and spouse and the case manager reveals that the spouse will need assistance with the client's personal needs and ADLs and with ambulation and PT. A home care aide is scheduled to visit the client daily for 3 hours a day. In addition, PT is planned for home visits 3 times weekly. The nurse implements a teaching plan for the client and spouse and monitors the client's readiness for discharge.

Which client or spouse statement/observation indicates that the home care instruction is either understood or requires further teaching? **Place an X in either the <u>Understood</u> column or the <u>Requires Further Teaching</u> column.**

Client or Spouse Statement/Observation	Understood	Requires Further Teaching
Client places the right arm into the shirt sleeve first when putting the shirt on.	☐	☒
Spouse states: "It will help vision if I approach my spouse from the right side."	☒	☐
Spouse states: "I will talk to the home care aides when they come, to be sure they get all of the care done during the first hour after they arrive."	☐	☒
Client turns the head to the right and then to the left before taking on an activity.	☒	☐
Client states: "I know that I need to call for help if I need to use the bathroom."	☒	☐
Client states: "I can skip the stool softener medication if I have a bowel movement."	☐	☒
Client picks up a washcloth with the left hand to wash the face.	☒	☐

Rationale: A right cerebral stroke occurs in the right side of the brain. The effects of a right cerebral stroke may include left-sided weakness or paralysis and sensory impairment. The client tends to deny deficits, such as the weakness or paralysis. Visual problems include an inability to see the left visual field of each eye. Unilateral neglect, also known as unilateral inattention, occurs most commonly in clients who have had a right cerebral stroke. This problem places the client at risk for injury, especially falls, because of the inability to recognize the physical impairment on one side of the body or a lack of proprioception (body position sense). The client needs to be taught to touch and use both sides of the body. When dressing, the client needs to be reminded to dress the affected side first, which would be the client's left side. In addition, the client should be encouraged to use the affected side so that attention is paid to the deficit. The client can use the unaffected side to assist with using the affected (neglected) side. For example, the client can use the unaffected hand to hold the affected hand to perform the activity, such as washing the face. In homonymous hemianopsia, vision is lost on the same side of the visual field in both eyes. The client should be approached from the unaffected visual side so that the client can sense someone approaching. In addition, the client is taught to turn the head from side to side to scan the environment and expand the visual field. Because of the client's short attention span, activities should be divided into short steps rather than being done all at one time. Trying to complete all care and activities in 1 hour can also be very frustrating to the client. Because of the left side weakness, the client is at risk for injury, so the client needs to be encouraged to call for assistance when getting out of bed or for other activities that can cause injury. Stool softeners need to be taken on a daily basis as prescribed to assist in promoting bowel elimination because of the risk of constipation caused by decreased mobility. In addition, stool softeners prevent the Valsalva maneuver during defecation to prevent increased ICP.

Test-Taking Strategy

Test-Taking Strategy: Begin answering this question by thinking about the physical manifestations following a stroke, and remember that if the stroke affects the right side of the brain, then deficits will be noted on the left side, whereas if the stroke affects the left side of the brain, then deficits will be noted on the right side. Focusing on the fact that this client experienced a right-sided stroke, evaluate each of the statements or observations and consider whether the action will be helpful or not helpful for a client experiencing left-sided physical deficits. Organize your thinking process as illustrated in the table.

Client or Spouse Statement/Observation	Helpful	Not Helpful
Client places the right arm into the shirt sleeve first when putting the shirt on.	☐	☒
Spouse states: "It will help vision if I approach my spouse from the right side."	☒	☐
Spouse states: "I will talk to the home care aides when they come, to be sure they get all of the care done during the first hour after they arrive."	☐	☒
Client turns the head to the right and then to the left before taking on an activity.	☒	☐
Client states: "I know that I need to call for help if I need to use the bathroom."	☒	☐
Client states: "I can skip the stool softener medication if I have a bowel movement."	☐	☒
Client picks up a washcloth with the left hand to wash the face.	☒	☐

Caregiving for this client will be helpful by ensuring that others approach the client from the right side, encouraging the client to turn the head to the right and then the left when scanning the environment, and reminding the client to call for help to go to the bathroom. Also recall that both sides need to be used and the affected side should not be neglected so that strength can be regained over time on that side. Looking at the other options, note that it will not be helpful for the client to place the right arm into the right sleeve of the shirt first because of the physical limitations on the left side. Clustering care in the first hour will cause exhaustion and depletion and will also delay recovery. Lastly, recall the pharmacologic concepts surrounding use of stool softeners, remembering that they work best as a preventive measure, and so even with bowel movements occurring, they should still be taken.

Content Area: Medical-Surgical Nursing
Priority Concept: Perfusion
Reference(s): Ignatavicius et al., 2021, pp. 908–912

A 16-year-old client was admitted to the mental health residential treatment center. The nurse performs an admission assessment and documents the following findings.

Health History	Nurses' Notes	Vital Signs	Lab Results

T = 96.4°F (35.7°C); HR = 40 BPM; BP = 88/48 mm Hg; RR = 16 bpm; SpO$_2$ = 92% on RA
Height: 5 ft 6 inches
Weight: 88 lb (40 kg)
BMI: 15.99 kg/m²

Health History	Nurses' Notes	Vital Signs	Lab Results

Client is accompanied by a parent. The parent consistently interrupts the client during the interview.

Parent states that the client is compulsive and always has to have everything in perfect order otherwise becomes anxious.

Parent states, "I was just like my child when I was that age and always had to look perfect and be perfect with everything that I did. I know my child is very skinny, but that is how I was when I was a teenager and I had to starve myself like my child does in order to keep my hourglass figure."

Client reports not socializing much because of being too busy exercising and reports constant exercising all day long, at least 10 times a day for an hour each session. Reports the need to burn off calories and stay in control of weight.

States hardly eats because of feeling fat and feeling appearance is fat. Is very fearful of gaining weight; describes restrictive eating patterns.

Loves to collect food recipes and cookbooks and prepare huge meals for other people but doesn't eat with them.

Denies alcohol or drug misuse.

Denies suicidal thoughts.

Denies food binging and purging, or use of laxatives or enemas.

Reports amenorrhea for the past 3 months.

Face is hollowed with sunken eyes.

Skin is pale, hair dry and thin.

Growth of lanugo on skin, skin is yellow tinged.

Complains of dizziness and skipped heart beats.

An interdisciplinary treatment approach was instituted to treat the client's eating disorder and included nutritional consultation, weight restoration therapy, and intensive psychotherapy and counseling. In addition, family therapy was planned. After 70 days of treatment, the interdisciplinary team meets to discuss the client's readiness for discharge to home and use of outpatient support services.

*The nurse evaluates the client for acceptable outcome criteria indicating readiness for discharge. For each factor below, click to specify if the finding indicates readiness for discharge. **Each factor may support more than one finding.***

Factor	Finding
Physiological	☒ Weight: 102 lb (46.3 kg)
	☒ Eating 80% of each of the 3 meals delivered by the dietary department and 2 snacks
	☐ Electrolyte results indicate:
	• **Potassium**: 3.2 mEq/L (3.2 mmol/L) L (normal reference range: 3.5–5.0 mEq/L [3.5–5.0 mmol/L])
	• **Sodium**: 130 mEq/L (130 mmol/L) L (normal reference range: 135–145 mEq/L [135–145 mmol/L])
	• **Chloride**: 95 mEq/L (95 mmol/L) L (normal reference range: 98–106 mEq/L [98–106 mmol/L])
Psychological	Client states:
	☐ "I really need to walk around the nursing unit 10 times a day and do 45 laps each time. I was doing 50 laps each time but cut down to 45."
	☐ "I counted my calories that I ate for the day and it came to 950. I think that's more than enough but I need to keep counting the calories to be sure."
	☒ "I am clear about what triggers my disruptive eating patterns and I know what alternative behaviors I need to take to help this."
Social	Client states:
	☐ "My best friend asked if I would go to lunch with some of our friends but I'm not going to go because I have nothing to wear that makes me look good. All my clothes are too tight."
	☒ "My parent is taking me and my siblings to that new movie that just came out; it'll be fun. I'm really looking forward to sharing a big box of popcorn and drinking a cola!"
	☐ "I have no interest in going to my prom this year. I've gained this weight and people in my class are definitely going to notice that."
Family Support	☐ Parent states will be sure that the child eats at least 3 full meals a day and 2 snacks and will remove and throw away any "teen magazines" or other distracting books or magazines that are in the child's bedroom.
	☒ Parent states that all of the children are going to take a 15-minute walk every evening after dinner.
	☒ Parent states, "My child seems to want to stay close to home, but I'm encouraging my child to spend some time with friends from school. I think these peer relationships are important."
Follow-up	☐ Parent states that family therapy sessions are not necessary since the problem is with the one child "and not the family."
	Client states:
	☐ "I have an appointment with the nutrition person in 2 weeks, but I'm thinking that if I maintain my weight and eat like I'm supposed to, then I can cancel it."
	☒ "The nurse at my school says there is a support group for students with eating problems and that they meet weekly. Do you think that this will help me?"

Rationale: Individuals with anorexia nervosa, an eating disorder, have intense irrational beliefs about their shape and weight. They engage in self-starvation behaviors and express intense fear of gaining weight. Physiologic outcome criteria for a client with anorexia nervosa include that the client consume a healthy diet and adequate daily calories per kilogram of body weight, demonstrate and maintain ideal body weight, maintain normal fluid and electrolyte levels, and demonstrate skin turgor and muscle tone that indicate that the nutritional state is proportionate with physiologic and metabolic needs. The client is 102 lb (46.3 kg), which reflects a 14-lb weight gain since admission. A weight less than 90 lb (40.9 kg) can be life-threatening. Although 102 lb (46.3 kg) may not be the ideal weight, it does indicate a gain of 14 lb. Eating 80% of each meal and 2 snacks is a positive outcome for the client. If the client's electrolyte levels are abnormal, this is not a positive outcome and needs to be addressed because of the adverse and in some situations life-threatening effects on the body; this does not meet acceptable criteria for discharge. This client's electrolyte levels are low: normal levels are potassium is 3.5 to 5.0 mEq/L (3.5–5.0 mmol/L); sodium 135 to 145 mEq/L (135–145 mmol/L); and chloride 98 to 106 mEq/L (98–106 mmol/L). An extreme regimen of physical exercise in an effort to burn unwanted calories and a focus on counting calories indicate compulsive behavior. In addition, cutting laps from 50 to 45 and thinking that 950 calories a day is sufficient is unhealthy thinking. However, the ability to identify triggers for disruptive eating patterns and strategies that will manage impaired behaviors is positive criterion. These clients express a disturbance in the way their body weight, size, or shape is experienced or viewed and see themselves as fat, although they are grossly underweight. Thinking that clothes are too tight or that classmates will notice a weight gain is a negative outcome. However, viewing a social activity such as a movie as fun and looking forward to sharing popcorn and drinking a cola is a positive outcome. The family's ability to relate to one another and to the client in a meaningful way is important. Clients with anorexia nervosa should not be forced to eat or be punished for not eating because these methods only make them fight more for control. The client should not be forced to eat or controlled in any way because this can disrupt the positive progression. Removing items from the client's room, such as magazines, is controlling and punitive and will not help in the healing process. Rather, giving the client control and responsibility provides the client with the opportunity to grow, develop, and take charge of one's own life. Peer relationships are important and should be encouraged. Taking a 15-minute walk every evening after dinner is a positive activity; the parent shows that exercise in some form is important and acceptable and healthy. Exercise within limits is important to maintain physical and emotional wellness. Family therapy is helpful to identify strategies to deal with behaviors effectively. Follow-up appointments with a nutritional therapist are important to ensure that adequate progression is made and that weight reaches normal and is maintained because starvation is life-threatening. Any faltering from the plan of care can be identified and addressed early. Support groups provide a safe, supportive setting that gives clients the opportunity to share problems and discuss strategies for management of symptoms.

Test-Taking Strategy: A simple "positive/negative" thinking process can be applied to help you answer this question correctly. Using the table, consider each finding and whether it would be an adaptive or maladaptive outcome for a client with anorexia nervosa.

Test-Taking
Strategy

Finding	Positive (Adaptive)	Negative (Maladaptive)
Weight: 102 lb (46.3 kg)	☒	☐
Eating 80% of each of the 3 meals delivered by the dietary department and 2 snacks	☒	☐
Electrolyte results indicate: Potassium 3.2 mEq/L (3.2 mmol/L); sodium 130 mEq/L (130 mmol/L); chloride 95 mEq/L (95 mmol/L)	☐	☒
"I really need to walk around the nursing unit 10 times a day and do 45 laps each time. I was doing 50 laps each time but cut down to 45."	☐	☒
"I counted my calories that I ate for the day and it came to 950. I think that's more than enough but I need to keep counting the calories to be sure."	☐	☒
"I am clear about what triggers my disruptive eating patterns and I know what alternative behaviors I need to take to help this."	☒	☐
"My best friend asked if I would go to lunch with some of our friends but I'm not going to go because I have nothing to wear that makes me look good. All my clothes are too tight."	☐	☒
"My parent is taking me and my siblings to that new movie that just came out; it'll be fun. I'm really looking forward to sharing a big box of popcorn and drinking a cola!"	☒	☐
"I have no interest in going to my prom this year. I've gained this weight and people in my class are definitely going to notice that."	☐	☒
Parent states will be sure that the child eats at least 3 full meals a day and 2 snacks and will remove and throw away any "teen magazines" or other distracting books or magazines that are in the child's bedroom.	☐	☒
Parent states that all of the children are going to take a 15-minute walk every evening after dinner.	☒	☐
Parent states, "My child seems to want to stay close to home, but I'm encouraging my child to spend some time with friends from school. I think these peer relationships are important."	☒	☐
Parent states that family therapy sessions are not necessary since the problem is with the one child "and not the family."	☐	☒
"I have an appointment with the nutrition person in 2 weeks, but I'm thinking that if I maintain my weight and eat like I'm supposed to, then I can cancel it."	☐	☒
"The nurse at my school says there is a support group for students with eating problems and that they meet weekly. Do you think that this will help me?"	☒	☐

In evaluating each of these findings, look for words or indicators that indicate progression toward a successful outcome. Consider negative words, such as "I have no interest," and associate these with a negative or maladaptive outcome. On the other hand, evaluate positive words, such as "support groups," as being aligned with a positive or adaptive outcome. Using this thinking process will help you organize your evaluation and answer this question correctly.

Content Area: Mental Health Nursing
Priority Concept: Stress and Coping
Reference(s): Varcarolis & Fosbre, 2021, pp. 186–188, 190–192

Practice Question 8.3   **Multiple Response Select N**

A 68-year-old client is admitted to the ED with a diagnosis of atrial fibrillation and rapid ventricular response. The ED physician completes the history and physical, and prescribes IV amiodarone to treat the dysrhythmia.

Health History	Nurses' Notes	Vital Signs	Lab Results

A 68-year-old client presents to the ED at 1215 with complaints of "heart fluttering" and shortness of breath that started 2 hours ago. Associated with fatigue and dizziness, worsened by activity. No alleviating factors, symptoms are constant. Denies chest pain, losing consciousness, and difficulty breathing while lying down. Reports past medical history of hypertension, hyperlipidemia, and type 2 DM. Family history is negative for cardiac events.

Speaks in short sentences, appears short of breath while talking. Skin is warm, dry, and intact throughout. Rapid, irregular HR, 120–140 BPM on auscultation. Lung sounds clear to auscultation in all fields. No peripheral edema.

Health History	Nurses' Notes	Vital Signs	Lab Results

12:15: T = 98.8°F (37.1°C); apical HR = 120–140 BPM and irregular; RR = 22 bpm; BP = 128/76 mm Hg; SpO$_2$ = 95% on RA

Health History	Nurses' Notes	Vital Signs	Lab Results

1215: Client admitted to ED. Received orders for IV amiodarone.

1230: Admission assessment completed. Amiodarone started. Continuous VS monitoring and cardiac monitor in place. Cardiac monitor shows shortened PR interval, narrowed QRS complex, atrial fibrillation with an irregular rate of 120–140 BPM.

1300: Follow-up VS and assessment completed. Client reports tremors, light sensitivity, lack of appetite with nausea, vomiting × 1 undigested food, no hematemesis. BP 90/56 mm Hg, HR 102 BPM. Cardiac monitor shows prolongation of previously shortened PR interval, widening of previously narrowed QRS complex, atrial fibrillation converted to sinus rhythm. HR regular at 102 BPM. 2+ pitting peripheral edema.

Select the four findings that indicate a therapeutic outcome of medication therapy.

☐ Reports of tremors
☐ Reports of photosensitivity
☐ BP 90/56 mm Hg
☒ HR regular at 102 BPM
☒ Prolongation of the PR interval
☒ Widening of the QRS complex
☐ Peripheral edema 2+ pitting bilaterally
☐ Reports of anorexia, nausea, and vomiting
☒ Atrial fibrillation converted to sinus rhythm

Rationale: Amiodarone is an antidysrhythmic used for treatment and prevention of atrial fibrillation and other cardiac dysrhythmias. For this client experiencing atrial fibrillation with rapid ventricular response, IV therapy is a lifesaving measure. The client comes to the ED with elevated HR, shortened PR interval, narrowed QRS complex, and atrial fibrillation, as noted on the cardiac monitor. Amiodarone primarily affects the atrioventricular node and slows conduction; therefore on follow-up assessment after starting the medication, client findings that indicate a therapeutic outcome include HR regular at 102 BPM (previously irregular at 120 to 140 BPM), prolongation of the PR interval (previously shortened), widening of the QRS complex (previously narrowed), and conversion of the rhythm from atrial fibrillation to sinus rhythm. Reports of tremors; photosensitivity; and anorexia, nausea, and vomiting are adverse (as opposed to therapeutic) outcomes associated with amiodarone use. BP of 90/56 mm Hg (previously 128/76 mm Hg) indicates hypotension, which can occur as an adverse outcome (not therapeutic) in some clients receiving this medication. Peripheral edema is an abnormal finding and may be associated with cardiotoxicity and heart failure, which is another possible adverse outcome (not therapeutic) of this medication.

Test-Taking Strategy: Evaluate each of the options in this question, thinking about whether the finding is consistent with a therapeutic outcome or an adverse outcome, recalling that amiodarone is used for its antidysrhythmic properties. Also think about the normal and abnormal findings. Using the table, consider each finding and whether it would be a therapeutic or normal and expected outcome or an adverse or abnormal and unexpected outcome.

Finding	Therapeutic Outcome	Adverse Outcome
Reports of tremors	☐	☒
Reports of photosensitivity	☐	☒
BP 90/56 mm Hg	☐	☒
HR regular at 102 BPM	☒	☐
Prolongation of the PR interval	☒	☐
Widening of the QRS complex	☒	☐
Peripheral edema 2+ pitting bilaterally	☐	☒
Reports of anorexia, nausea, and vomiting	☐	☒
Atrial fibrillation converted to sinus rhythm	☒	☐

Think about cardiac monitoring findings when a client is experiencing atrial fibrillation with rapid ventricular response. The HR will be elevated, the PR interval shortened, the QRS complex narrowed, and morphology reflective of fibrillation in the atria. Knowing that amiodarone is used to address the problems with cardiac conduction, consider these options as the answers, and then further evaluate them to determine whether they indicate a therapeutic outcome. Also recall that, although amiodarone can be very beneficial and in some cases lifesaving, there are adverse outcomes; therefore monitoring the client and evaluating for therapeutic as well as adverse outcomes is integral to promoting safe client care. The incorrect options are not specifically related to cardiac conduction and would be good options to consider as possible adverse outcomes of amiodarone.

Content Area: Pharmacology
Priority Concept: Perfusion
Reference(s): Burchum & Rosenthal, 2022, pp. 559–560

Practice Question 8.4   **Matrix Multiple Choice**

A 39-year-old client is being seen in the outpatient pain management clinic. The client was in a motor vehicle accident 1 year ago and sustained an injury to the cervical and lumbar spine and has been experiencing neck and back pain since the injury. The client has tried conservative measures, including ice and heat, massage, and PT. The client has also tried acetaminophen, NSAIDs, muscle relaxants, and opioid analgesics, and the pain has become intolerable again even with these measures. The pain management specialist has added amitriptyline to the treatment plan, and the nurse provides teaching to the client about the plan. The client returns to the clinic 1 month later for follow-up evaluation.

Which observations indicate that the treatment plan is effective? **For each client statement/observation, click to specify if the statement indicates that the treatment plan is Effective or Ineffective.**

Statement/Observation	Effective	Ineffective
Client states: "My back and neck are sore after PT."	☒	☐
Client states: "I have been walking a mile each day before going to work."	☒	☐
Client states: "I need to wear my neck collar all the time because I need it for added support."	☐	☒
Client ambulates to the examination room and is limping and leaning the hand on the wall while walking.	☐	☒
Client states: "I know that new medication is used for depression but it has helped my pain too."	☒	☐

Rationale: Amitriptyline is a tricyclic antidepressant that can reduce pain of neuropathic origin. It can be used either on its own or in conjunction with opioid analgesics for chronic pain. This medication works by inhibiting norepinephrine uptake, thereby reducing pain. This medication is particularly helpful in the management of chronic back pain and neuropathic pain. PT is often used in conjunction with medication therapy for chronic pain management. It is normal and expected for there to be some pain or discomfort after PT because of exercising muscles associated with the injury and would be an indicator of effectiveness of the treatment plan. The client's ability to walk a mile before going to work and the ability to continue working are both indicators of effectiveness as well. The client statement that the medication has helped the pain also provides evidence of an effective treatment plan. The need to wear a neck collar all the time for support and limping and leaning on the wall during ambulation are signs that the treatment plan may not be adequate or may be ineffective and would need to be addressed further.

Test-Taking Strategy: Note that this question is asking about evidence of an effective treatment plan for a client with chronic pain. You need to look for signs that pain management interventions are indicating either an improvement and expected outcome or a declining and unexpected outcome. Organize your thought process using an approach as outlined in the table.

Test-Taking
Strategy

Observation	Improving/ Expected	Declining/ Unexpected
Client states: "My back and neck are sore after PT."	☒	☐
Client states: "I have been walking a mile each day before going to work."	☒	☐
Client states: "I need to wear my neck collar all the time because I need it for added support."	☐	☒
Client ambulates to the examination room and is limping and leaning the hand on the wall while walking.	☐	☒
Client states: "I know that new medication is used for depression but it has helped my pain too."	☒	☐

You may think that soreness in the neck and back after PT is not an improvement; however, continued adherence to the treatment plan is important, and some soreness is expected after these activities because the affected muscles are targeted during therapy. Increased activity and functionality, such as walking and going to work, are signs of improvement as well. Any client statement regarding relief of pain is also an indication of improvement. The report of using the neck collar all the time is an indication that the pain is not adequately controlled with other measures; a neck collar should not be needed all the time or on a long-term basis. Objective signs such as limping are indicators of a lack of improvement or a decline in the client's progress and therefore may indicate that the treatment plan is inadequate or ineffective.

Content Area: Pharmacology
Priority Concept: Tissue Integrity
Reference(s): Burchum & Rosenthal, 2022, p. 310

Practice Question 8.5   Drop-Down Cloze

A 58-year-old client is admitted to the medical-surgical unit at 0600 from the ED with abdominal pain, fatigue, dizziness, and bright red blood in the stool, and is diagnosed with GI hemorrhage. The nurse reviews the medical record on admission.

| Health History | Nurses' Notes | Physician's Orders | Lab Results |

Past medical history: DM, osteoarthritis, depression
Social history: Smokes cigarettes 1 pack per day for 10 years, drinks 3 glasses of wine nightly, denies other recreational drug use
Medications: Metformin 500 mg twice daily, ibuprofen 800 mg three times daily for joint pain, citalopram 10 mg daily

| Health History | Nurses' Notes | Physician's Orders | Lab Results |

Complete blood count (CBC)
Prothrombin time (PT)
Partial thromboplastin time (aPTT)
International normalized ratio (INR)
Type and crossmatch
1 unit PRBCs if hemoglobin is less than 8.0 g/dL (80 g/L), repeat hemoglobin and hematocrit level 2 hours after transfusion is complete
Bowel preparation (polyethylene glycol as directed) for colonoscopy
Obtain consent for colonoscopy
Pantoprazole 40 mg intravenously every 8 hours
Bowel rest, NPO
Normal saline IV maintenance fluids at 125 mL/hr
Hydromorphone 1 mg IV push every 3 hr as needed for pain
GI specialist consultation

| Health History | Nurses' Notes | Physician's Orders | Lab Results |

0800: Received and reviewed laboratory results. Started blood transfusion per protocol. Administering 1 unit PRBCs. Client reports continued abdominal pain, fatigue, dizziness. VS stable.
1200: 1 unit PRBCs completed. VS stable throughout transfusion. Client reports abdominal pain is unchanged. States no longer feels dizzy and feels less fatigued.
1400: Hemoglobin and hematocrit result updated. T = 98.8°F (37.1°C); apical HR = 82 BPM and regular; RR = 18 bpm; BP = 122/74 mm Hg; SpO_2 = 95% on RA.

| Health History | Nurses' Notes | Physician's Orders | Lab Results |

0800:

Test	Result	Normal Reference Range
Complete Blood Count		
Red blood cells (RBCs)	4.5 (4.5 × 10^{12})	4.2–6.2 × 10^{12}/L (4.2–6.2 × 10^{12}/L)
White blood cells (WBCs)	8000/mm³ (8 × 10^9/L)	5000–10,000/mm³ (5–10 × 10^9/L)
Platelets	180,000/mm³ (180 × 10^9/L)	150,000–400,000/mm³ (150–400 × 10^9/L)
Hemoglobin (Hgb)	7.6 g/dL (76 g/L) L	12–18 g/dL (120–180 g/L)
Hematocrit (Hct)	32% (0.32) L	37%–52% (0.37–0.52)
Coagulation Studies		
aPTT	32 seconds	30–40 sec
PT	12.5 seconds	11–12.5 sec
INR	1.0	0.81–1.2
Fecal Occult Blood Test		
Occult blood	Detected	Negative
Type and Crossmatch		
Type and crossmatch	O positive No antibodies detected	

1400:

Test	Result	Normal Reference Range
Hemoglobin (Hgb)	9.0 g/dL (90 g/L) L	12-18 g/dL (120–180 g/L)
Hematocrit (Hct)	39% (0.39)	37%–52% (0.37–0.52)

Based on the client findings, complete the following sentence by choosing from the lists of options provided.

The nurse determines that the **blood transfusion** was effective, as evidenced by the **hemoglobin level** and the **report about fatigue and dizziness** .

Options for 1	Options for 2	Options for 3
Pantoprazole	Hemoglobin level	VS
Hydromorphone	Coagulation studies result	Abdominal pain
Blood transfusion	Fecal occult blood test result	Report about fatigue and dizziness

Rationale: GI bleeding can occur in the upper or lower GI tract. In this clinical scenario, the location of bleeding would be determined once the client undergoes the colonoscopy. Certain risk factors increase the likelihood of this health problem, such as smoking, use of NSAIDs and selective serotonin reuptake inhibitors, alcohol consumption, and a history of DM. The client's subjective complaints of abdominal pain, dizziness, and fatigue are supportive of GI bleeding. The client's laboratory results, specifically the hemoglobin and hematocrit levels, are below normal range and are consistent with anemia, likely secondary to the bleeding. The physician ordered PRBCs to be administered, and the client's hemoglobin level necessitates this order. In addition, the physician ordered pantoprazole, which is a proton pump inhibitor. This is an important part of the treatment plan for a client with GI bleeding. Pain management is also often necessary for the client with this problem, and hydromorphone is the treatment for this, as well as bowel rest (NPO status). Based on this clinical scenario, the nurse determines that interventions were effective, specifically the blood transfusion, as evidenced by the hemoglobin and hematocrit levels and the reports of dizziness and fatigue being improved. Although pantoprazole and hydromorphone have been administered, the evidence does not exist to support these interventions as being effective at this time. The client's abdominal pain is still present; this does not provide information to confirm these interventions as being effective. The coagulation studies results were normal and unrelated to these interventions, and the fecal occult blood test result does not provide additional evaluative information for these interventions.

Test-Taking Strategy: Note that this question is asking you to evaluate whether certain interventions (blood transfusion, medications) were effective, and to decide based on the evidence of that evaluation. Recall that blood transfusions are used to treat acute blood loss and anemia. Also remember that pantoprazole and hydromorphone are components of the treatment plan for GI bleeding. Look at the options for all three columns in the question. Then connect the evidence (columns 2 and 3 in the question) with the interventions (column 1), as illustrated in the table.

Evidence	Intervention
Hemoglobin level improved	**Blood transfusion**
Coagulation studies results—normal	Not specific to a listed intervention
Fecal occult blood test result—positive	Not specific to a listed intervention
VS—normal	Hydromorphone (nonspecific)
Abdominal pain unchanged	Hydromorphone and pantoprazole
Reports about dizziness—no longer feels dizzy and is less fatigued	**Blood transfusion**

Note that the question is asking for an intervention that is supported by two different sources of evidence. Consider the evidence first: The improved hemoglobin level and report about dizziness and that the client no longer feels dizzy provide specific information about the client's anemia and the effectiveness of the blood transfusion. The results of the coagulation studies and the fecal occult blood test do not provide information specific to the blood transfusion, the hydromorphone, or the pantoprazole. The VS (noted as stable and are normal) may provide information about the effectiveness of the hydromorphone, but this information is nonspecific. The abdominal pain would provide evidence for the effectiveness of hydromorphone and pantoprazole, but the client's pain is unchanged. Note that the only intervention that is supported by two sources of evidence is the blood transfusion, which may be another strategy to assist you in choosing the correct options.

Content Area: Medical-Surgical Nursing
Priority Concept: Perfusion
Reference(s): Ignatavicius et al., 2021, pp. 1108–1109

Practice Question 8.6 — Highlight in Text

A 3-day-old newborn is seen in the outpatient pediatric clinic for a post-hospital follow-up appointment. The nurse reviews the health history and notes the following.

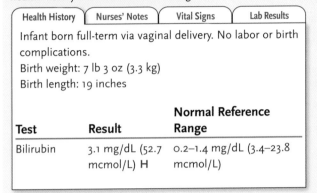

| Health History | Nurses' Notes | Vital Signs | Lab Results |

Infant born full-term via vaginal delivery. No labor or birth complications.
Birth weight: 7 lb 3 oz (3.3 kg)
Birth length: 19 inches

Test	Result	Normal Reference Range
Bilirubin	3.1 mg/dL (52.7 mcmol/L) H	0.2–1.4 mg/dL (3.4–23.8 mcmol/L)

The nurse performs an assessment on the newborn and obtains a blood specimen for evaluation of the bilirubin level. The following notes are documented.

Click to highlight the findings that indicate the need for follow-up in the 3-day-old newborn.

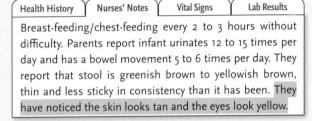

| Health History | Nurses' Notes | Vital Signs | Lab Results |

Breast-feeding/chest-feeding every 2 to 3 hours without difficulty. Parents report infant urinates 12 to 15 times per day and has a bowel movement 5 to 6 times per day. They report that stool is greenish brown to yellowish brown, thin and less sticky in consistency than it has been. They have noticed the skin looks tan and the eyes look yellow.

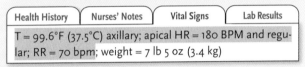

| Health History | Nurses' Notes | Vital Signs | Lab Results |

T = 99.6°F (37.5°C) axillary; apical HR = 180 BPM and regular; RR = 70 bpm; weight = 7 lb 5 oz (3.4 kg)

| Health History | Nurses' Notes | Vital Signs | Lab Results |

Test	Result	Normal Reference Range
Bilirubin	4.8 mg/dL (81.6 mcmol/L) H	0.2 –1.4 mg/dL (3.4–23.8 mcmol/L)

Rationale: Hyperbilirubinemia occurs when an excessive amount of bilirubin accumulates in the blood. The most common evidence of hyperbilirubinemia is the relatively mild and self-limited physiologic jaundice, or icterus neonatorum. Physiologic jaundice is not associated with any pathologic process. Although almost all newborns experience elevated bilirubin levels, only about half demonstrate observable signs of jaundice. Normal values of unconjugated bilirubin are 0.2 to 1.4 mg/dL (3.4–23.8 mcmol/L). In all newborns, levels must exceed 5 mg/dL (85 mcmol/L) before jaundice is observable. Because this 3-day-old has a serum bilirubin level of 4.8 mg/dL (81.6 mcmol/L), signs of jaundice such as tan-colored skin and yellow eyes are not expected and are a concern requiring follow-up for evaluation of pathologic jaundice associated with a disease process. Newborns will urinate up to 20 times a day because the bladder involuntary empties when stretched by a volume of 15 mL. Transitional stools appear by the third day after initiation of feeding and are greenish brown to yellowish brown, thin, and less sticky than meconium. A bowel movement 5 to 6 times a day is expected depending on the frequency of feeding. Normal VS are temperature 97.7°F to 98°F (36.5°C to 37°C) axillary, apical HR 120 to 140 BPM, and RR 30 to 60 bpm. The temperature, apical HR, and RR are elevated, warranting follow-up. The serum bilirubin level of 4.8 mg/dL (81.6 mcmol/L) requires follow-up because of observable signs of jaundice in this newborn. The bilirubin level will rise and peak before it returns to a normal level in physiologic jaundice. Depending on age, it could peak as high as 12 mg/dL (204 mcmol/L) before dropping down to a normal range.

Test-Taking Strategy: This question is asking you to evaluate the findings that indicate the need for follow-up in the 3-day-old newborn. You need to use knowledge and recall normal findings in a newborn infant and expected progression of the jaundice that occurs, differentiating physiologic from pathologic jaundice. Create a table and organize your thinking process by considering findings that are consistent with expected outcomes or outcomes that are abnormal and/or indicate the need for follow-up.

Test-Taking Strategy

Finding	Expected/ Normal Outcome	Unexpected Outcome/Requires Follow-up
Breast-feeding/chest-feeding every 2 to 3 hours without difficulty	☒	☐
Urinates 12 to 15 times per day	☒	☐
Has a bowel movement 5 to 6 times per day	☒	☐
Stool is greenish brown to yellowish brown, thin and less sticky in consistency than it has been	☒	☐
Skin looks tan and eyes look yellow	☐	☒
Temperature 99.6°F (37.5°C) axillary	☐	☒
Apical HR 180 BPM	☐	☒
RR 70 bpm	☐	☒
Weight 7 lb 5 oz (3.4 kg)	☒	☐
Serum bilirubin level 4.8 mg/dL (81.6 mcmol/L)	☐	☒

Content Area: Maternal-Newborn Nursing
Priority Concept: Elimination
Reference(s): Hockenberry et al., 2019, pp. 198, 205, 257–259

CHAPTER 10

Answers to Practice Questions

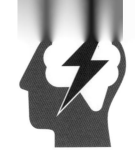

Unfolding Case Study 1

Content Area: Mental Health Nursing
Priority Concept: Stress and Coping
Reference(s): Halter et al., 2022, pp. 252–255; 277–281; 299–302; 475–483

Practice Question 10.1   Unfolding Case Study 1

The nurse reviews the medical record of a 56-year-old client who was recently admitted to the ED.

*Highlight the client findings in the Nurses' Notes that require **immediate** follow-up by the nurse.*

Health History	Nurses' Notes	Imaging Studies	Lab Results

2215: Spouse brought client into ED after finding a suicide note and the gun cabinet unlocked. Reports that the client is "not the same person" after being hospitalized 3 months ago with severe COVID-19 and mechanically ventilated for over 2 weeks. Client states that since being discharged from the hospital, has periods of heart palpitations, insomnia, apathy, depressed mood, and anorexia. Reports that drinking alcohol every night helps to relax, but still becomes anxious at times. Is very worried about getting COVID again because the client's sibling, whom the client recently visited, tested positive yesterday. Has frequent nightmares about the hospital experience because the client nearly died. Lost 35 lb (15.9 kg) during the hospital stay but states still weighs more than 260 lb (117.9 kg). Was considering suicide this evening because the client was afraid of possibly "being reinfected and dying this time." Recently diagnosed with type 2 DM controlled by diet and metformin.

Rationale: The client was brought to the hospital because the client was planning suicide, a life-threatening problem which is an immediate concern for the nurse. Because of the client's near-death experience with COVID-19, the client is having physical, psychological, and emotional manifestations that are likely contributing to suicide risk, including palpitations, depressed mood, insomnia, anorexia, apathy, anxiety, and frequent nightmares. Therefore these symptoms and behaviors are also concerning to the nurse. Although alcohol is an ineffective coping strategy for the client, the nurse is not concerned about this behavior at this time because it is not immediately life-threatening. The client's weight and diabetes are important for overall health but are not necessarily related to suicide risk. Therefore these client findings are not of immediate concern to the nurse at this time.

Test-Taking Strategy: Remember to first identify normal/usual or abnormal and expected (not relevant) client findings versus abnormal and not expected (relevant)

Test-Taking
Strategy

findings to determine which findings require immediate follow-up by the nurse. The client's findings in the Nurses' Notes can be categorized as shown in the table to help *Recognize Cues* in this case study.

Client Finding	Normal/Usual or Abnormal but Expected (Not Relevant) and Not Requiring Immediate Follow-up	Abnormal and Not Expected (Relevant) and Requiring Immediate Follow-up
Insomnia	☐	☒
Heart palpitations	☐	☒
Anxiety	☐	☒
Anorexia	☐	☒
Depressed mood	☐	☒
Apathy	☐	☒
Drinks alcohol every night	☒	☐
Nightmares	☐	☒
Overweight	☒	☐
Type 2 DM	☒	☐
Planned suicide earlier today	☐	☒

Review the factors that contribute to the client's risk for suicide. The client's reported physical, psychological, and emotional behaviors are indicative of clinical depression and anxiety, which make the client at current risk for suicide and are therefore of immediate concern to the nurse.

CJ Cognitive Skill: Recognize Cues

Practice Question 10.2   Unfolding Case Study 1

The nurse reviews the medical record of a 56-year-old client who was recently admitted to the ED.

| Health History | Nurses' Notes | Imaging Studies | Lab Results |

2215: Spouse brought client into ED after finding a suicide note and the gun cabinet unlocked. Reports that the client is "not the same person" after being hospitalized 3 months ago with severe COVID-19 and mechanically ventilated for over 2 weeks. Client states that since being discharged from the hospital, has periods of heart palpitations, insomnia, apathy, depressed mood, and anorexia. Reports that drinking alcohol every night helps to relax, but still becomes anxious and depressed at times. Is very worried about getting COVID again because the client's sibling, whom the client recently visited, tested positive yesterday. Has nightmares about the hospital experience because the client nearly died. Lost 35 lb (15.9 kg) during the hospital stay but states still weighs more than 260 lb (117.9 kg). Was considering suicide this evening because the client was afraid of possibly "being reinfected and dying this time." Recently diagnosed with type 2 DM controlled by diet and metformin.

For each client assessment finding, click or indicate with an X which finding is associated with which client condition. Some findings may be consistent with more than one condition.

Client Finding	Generalized Anxiety Disorder	Clinical Depression	PTSD
Had recent near-death experience	☒	☒	☒
Anorexia	☒	☒	☐
Depressed mood	☐	☒	☒
Apathy	☐	☒	☒
Nightmares	☐	☐	☒
Potential suicide risk	☐	☒	☒
Excessive worry	☒	☐	☐
Insomnia	☒	☒	☒

Rationale: The nurse analyzes the client's findings to determine which mental health conditions the client is likely experiencing. PTSD can occur after any traumatic event that is not part of one's usual life experience. Clients who experience a highly traumatic event that has the potential for actual or threatened death often respond with fear similar to what this client expressed. Adults who have PTSD often have comorbidities including anxiety disorders, clinical depression, and/or dissociative disorders. In this client's case, the near-death experience as a result of a severe COVID-19 infection most likely led to PTSD, depression, and anxiety.

Clients who have generalized anxiety disorder display excessive worry, which can affect their sleep patterns and appetite. Some clients have anorexia, whereas others respond to excessive stress by eating more than usual. Clients who have major clinical depression can also be anorexic or overeat. They tend to lack energy, are apathetic, and experience a negative or depressed mood, often every day. These negative and depressed thoughts place them at risk for suicide. Clients who have PTSD have many of the same physical and emotional behaviors that are common in clients with anxiety and depression. Two additional common behaviors seen in clients with PTSD are nightmares and flashbacks. Flashbacks are intense, repeated episodes of reliving the traumatic experience while a client is fully awake. Nightmares and flashbacks are very scary for the client and can lead to thoughts of suicide as an escape.

Test-Taking Strategy: Many of the client's findings are common behaviors associated with more than one mental health condition. To add to that challenge in answering this test item, many clients who have PTSD also have other mental health conditions, including anxiety and clinical depression. Use the table to help decide which client findings represent supporting data for each mental health condition in this item measuring *Analyze Cues.*

Test-Taking
Strategy

Client Finding (Assessment Data)	Supporting Data for Generalized Anxiety Disorder? Yes or No	Supporting Data for Clinical Depression? Yes or No	Supporting Data for PTSD? Yes or No
Had recent near-death experience	Yes	Yes	Yes
Anorexia	Yes	Yes	No
Depressed mood	No	Yes	Yes
Apathy	No	Yes	Yes
Nightmares	No	No	Yes
Potential suicide risk	No	Yes	Yes
Excessive worry	Yes	No	No
Insomnia	Yes	Yes	Yes

Apply nursing knowledge and retrieve information about the characteristics and assessment findings for each condition. Once you review these data in the table, you can more easily determine which mental health conditions the client *may be* experiencing to answer the test item.

CJ Cognitive Skill: Analyze Cues

Practice Question 10.3   Unfolding Case Study 1

The nurse reviews the latest entry (2330) in the Nurses' Notes of a 56-year-old client's medical record.

| Health History | Nurses' Notes | Imaging Studies | Lab Results |

2215: Spouse brought client into ED after finding a suicide note and the gun cabinet unlocked. Reports that the client is "not the same person" after being hospitalized 3 months ago with severe COVID-19 and mechanically ventilated for over 2 weeks. Client states that since being discharged from the hospital, has periods of heart palpitations, insomnia, apathy, depressed mood, and anorexia. Reports that drinking alcohol every night helps to relax, but still becomes anxious and depressed at times. Is very worried about getting COVID again because the client's sibling, whom the client recently visited, tested positive yesterday. Has nightmares about the hospital experience because the client nearly died. Lost 35 lb (15.9 kg) during the hospital stay but states still weighs more than 260 lb (117.9 kg). Was considering suicide this evening because the client was afraid of possibly "being reinfected and dying this time." Recently diagnosed with type 2 DM controlled by diet and metformin.

2330: Social worker (SW) interviewed client and administered several screening assessments for selected mental health conditions. Client admitted to flashbacks about hospitalization and feels guilty about putting family through that experience. States was "lazy" and did not wear a mask or social distance at an important corporate meeting. As a result, the client developed a COVID-19 infection, which worsened and led to the hospital stay and mechanical ventilation. Expressed remorse for upsetting spouse and apologized to her and the SW.

Based on the information in the Nurses' Notes, complete the following sentences from the lists of options provided.

The client **most likely** has <u>PTSD</u> as the primary mental health condition, as evidenced by <u>nightmares</u> and <u>flashbacks</u>. The **priority** for the client's care is to <u>ensure personal safety</u>.

Options for 1	Options for 2	Options for 3
Personality disorder	Anorexia	Begin intensive
Dissociative identity	Nightmares	counseling
disorder	Excessive worry	Ensure personal safety
PTSD	Flashbacks	Start drug therapy
Clinical depression		Refer to spiritual
		advisor

Rationale: The client likely has several mental health conditions, including PTSD and clinical depression. However, the primary life-threatening mental health condition is PTSD due to his history of a near-death experience as a result of having severe COVID-19 infection. The client expresses being afraid of getting the infection again and perhaps not survive a second event. Since surviving that experience, the client developed new emotional and physical behaviors. Two of the classic differentiating behaviors associated with PTSD and not with other mental health conditions are nightmares and flashbacks. Excessive worry and anorexia are associated more with anxiety than with PTSD. The client is at suicide risk because the client was planning how to end his life; therefore the priority for the client's care is safety. Safety is always the priority for any client. Once safety is ensured, the client may start drug therapy, begin counseling, and/or need a spiritual advisor.

Test-Taking Strategy

Test-Taking Strategy: To answer this test item measuring the CJ cognitive skill *Prioritize Hypotheses,* first determine which of the potential client conditions are life-threatening to narrow down the choices. Clients who experience PTSD and clinical depression have the potential for suicide, which is obviously life-threatening. Next, review the supporting client findings for each of these two disorders by using the table.

Client Finding (Assessment Data)	Supporting Evidence for PTSD? Yes or No	Supporting Evidence for Clinical Depression? Yes or No
Anorexia	No	Yes
Nightmares	Yes	No
Excessive worry	No	No
Flashbacks	Yes	No

As displayed in the table, there is only one client finding that supports clinical depression, but *two* findings that support the presence of PTSD. The test item required you to identify *two* client findings for the condition, and only PTSD has evidence of two supporting findings. Therefore you would conclude that the client's primary condition is PTSD.

For the second sentence of the test item, you need to decide what the client's priority need is based on the diagnosis of PTSD. The client was planning suicide, but the suicide note and unlocked gun cabinet were found before the client could actually commit this action. The priority for the client, then, is to keep the client safe at all times. Safety is the priority for all clients and is ensured by using a variety of nursing and collaborative interventions.

CJ Cognitive Skill: Prioritize Hypotheses

Practice Question 10.4   **Unfolding Case Study 1**

The nurse reviews the latest entry (2330) in the Nurses' Notes of a 56-year-old client's medical record.

Health History	Nurses' Notes	Imaging Studies	Lab Results

2215: Spouse brought client into ED after finding a suicide note and the gun cabinet unlocked. Reports that the client is "not the same person" after being hospitalized 3 months ago with severe COVID-19 and mechanically ventilated for over 2 weeks. Client states that since being discharged from the hospital, has periods of heart palpitations, insomnia, apathy, depressed mood, and anorexia. Reports that drinking alcohol every night helps to relax, but still becomes anxious and depressed at times. Is very worried about getting COVID again because the client's sibling, whom the client recently visited, tested positive yesterday. Has nightmares about the hospital experience because the client nearly died. Lost 35 lb (15.9 kg) during the hospital stay but states still weighs more than 260 lb (117.9 kg). Was considering suicide this evening because the client was afraid of possibly "being reinfected and dying this time." Recently diagnosed with type 2 DM controlled by diet and metformin.

2330: Social worker (SW) interviewed client and administered several screening assessments for selected mental health conditions. Client admitted to flashbacks about hospitalization and feels guilty about putting family through that experience. States was "lazy" and did not wear a mask or social distance at an important corporate meeting. As a result, the client developed a COVID-19 infection, which worsened and led to the hospital stay and mechanical ventilation. Expressed remorse for upsetting spouse and apologized to her and the SW.

The client was diagnosed with PTSD, anxiety, and suicidal risk. Which physician orders would the nurse anticipate for the client at this time? **Select all that apply.**

- ☒ Begin antidepressant drug therapy.
- ☒ Admit to acute psychiatric unit.
- ☐ Refer to case manager.
- ☐ Refer to spiritual advisor.
- ☒ Begin intense psychotherapy.
- ☒ Place on suicide precautions.
- ☒ Limit visitors to immediate family.

Rationale: The desired outcome for this client's care is to ensure safety because of potential suicide. The orders would be focused on ways to keep the client safe, including admission to the acute psychiatric unit for one-on-one observation and treatment with medication and psychotherapy. The client would also be placed on suicide precautions, which usually include:

- Observing the client swallow each dose of medication
- Removing glass and knives from meal trays to prevent self-injury
- One-on-one observation of the client at all times
- Documentation of client's behaviors and verbal statements every 15 to 30 minutes

Visitors would likely be limited to a small number of immediate family members to prevent the client from obtaining devices from others that could cause self-harm. Immediate family members could provide support and encouragement for the client during the hospital stay. A case manager can help plan for the client's discharge to ensure continuity of care to keep the client safe at home or in another setting but would not help ensure immediate safety. A spiritual advisor may be requested by the client but is not usually ordered.

Test-Taking
Strategy

Test-Taking Strategy: To answer this question measuring *Generate Solutions,* remember that the *priority* desired outcome is to ensure the client's safety. Therefore review each choice in the test item to determine if the intervention or order would promote the client's immediate safety. Use the table to help with this determination.

Potential Physician's Order	Promotes Client's Immediate Safety? Yes or No
Begin antidepressant drug therapy.	Yes
Admit to acute psychiatric unit.	Yes
Refer to case manager.	No
Refer to spiritual advisor.	No
Begin intense psychotherapy.	Yes
Place on suicide precautions.	Yes
Limit visitors to immediate family.	Yes

Note that this question asks you to identify the physician orders that you would anticipate for the client at this time. Think about the client's conditions and immediate needs. The potential orders that promote the client's immediate safety and are marked by a "Yes" are the correct responses to the test item.

CJ Cognitive Skill: Generate Solutions

Practice Question 10.5   **Unfolding Case Study 1**

A 56-year-old client was diagnosed with PTSD after being ad-mitted to the ED because the client's spouse found a suicide note and unlocked gun cabinet. After a thorough evaluation, the client was admitted for one-on-one observation in the acute inpatient psychiatric unit and started on sertraline and psycho-therapy. The nurse plans health teaching about the medication for the client and spouse before administering the first dose.

Select five statements that the nurse would include in the health teaching about sertraline.

- ☒ "This drug is one of the most effective ways to treat PTSD and depression."
- ☐ "We will be monitoring you for sedation effects while you are here."
- ☐ "Let me know if you have trouble urinating or having a bowel movement."
- ☒ "Let me know if you have trouble sleeping or feel nervous while on the drug."
- ☒ "We will be monitoring you carefully for changes in your vital signs."
- ☒ "You might experience mild nausea and feel agitated when you start this drug."
- ☒ "Your liver and kidney function will need to be monitored by lab testing."

Rationale: Sertraline is a selective serotonin reuptake inhibitor (SSRI) that can be very effective in managing clinical depression and/or PTSD. Side effects of the drug include insomnia, nervousness, anxiety, agitation, and mild nausea. Although not common, this drug, like most antidepressants, can affect liver and kidney function, which should be monitored through frequent lab testing. The nurse would monitor VS to help assess for a rare adverse drug reaction called serotonin syndrome. This syndrome is likely due to overaction of central nervous system receptors and is usually dose related or the result of drug interactions. Symptoms include elevated temperature, HR, and BP; delirium; muscle spasms; abdominal pain; diarrhea; and possible seizures. Severe manifestations can lead to shock or possibly death. Urinary retention, constipation, and sedation more commonly occur in clients who take other classes of antidepressants, especially tricyclic antidepressants.

Test-Taking Strategy: Remember that health teaching about side and adverse effects is particularly important for clients starting new drug therapy. If the client responds to and tolerates the medication, the client will likely continue taking it after being discharged. Also recall that sertraline is classified as an SSRI. Apply knowledge of antidepressant drug therapy as shown in the table to help delineate which side or adverse effects can occur when clients are prescribed SSRIs.

Test-Taking Strategy

Potential Drug Side or Adverse Effect	Occurs Commonly in Clients Taking SSRIs? Yes or No
Sedation effects	No
Urinary retention and constipation	No
Insomnia and nervousness	Yes
Increased VS	Yes
Mild nausea	Yes
Agitation	Yes
Liver and/or kidney impairment	Yes

Based on the side or adverse effects for which you responded with a "Yes" for SSRIs such as sertraline, you can then select the appropriate options in the test item that would be included in health teaching to measure *Take Action.*

CJ Cognitive Skill: Take Action

Practice Question 10.6   Unfolding Case Study 1

A 56-year-old client was discharged from the acute psychiatric care unit 2 months ago with a diagnosis of PTSD, anxiety, and clinical depression. The client is following up with the family nurse practitioner (FNP) today. Prior to being examined by the FNP, the office nurse reviews the previous ED admission record and performs an interview regarding the client's current health state.

| Health History | Nurses' Notes | Imaging Studies | Lab Results |

2215: Spouse brought client into ED after finding a suicide note and the gun cabinet unlocked. Reports that the client is "not the same person" after being hospitalized 3 months ago with severe COVID-19 and mechanically ventilated for over 2 weeks. Client states that since being discharged from the hospital, has periods of heart palpitations, insomnia, apathy, depressed mood, and anorexia. Reports that drinking alcohol every night helps to relax, but still becomes anxious and depressed at times. Is very worried about getting COVID again because the client's sibling, whom the client recently visited, tested positive yesterday. Has nightmares about the hospital experience because the client nearly died. Lost 35 lb (15.9 kg) during the hospital stay but states still weighs more than 260 lb (117.9 kg). Was considering suicide this evening because the client was afraid of possibly "being reinfected and dying this time." Recently diagnosed with type 2 DM controlled by diet and metformin.

2330: Social worker (SW) interviewed client and administered several screening assessments for selected mental health conditions. Client admitted to flashbacks about hospitalization and feels guilty about putting family through that experience. States was "lazy" and did not wear a mask or social distance at an important corporate meeting. As a result, the client developed a COVID-19 infection, which worsened and led to the hospital stay and mechanical ventilation. Expressed remorse for upsetting spouse and apologized to her and the SW.

Based on the ED admission notes and data collected during the nurse's interview with the client, indicate which client findings demonstrate that he is either **Progressing (Improving)** or **Not Progressing (Not Improving)**

Client Finding	Progressing (Improving)	Not Progressing (Not Improving)
Has not consumed any alcohol since hospital discharge	☒	☐
States has a more positive outlook without depressed moods, and a better appetite	☒	☐
Has flashbacks and nightmares about once a week	☐	☒
Sleeps most nights for 7–8 hours	☒	☐
States no longer has heart palpitations	☒	☐

Rationale: Prior to the psychiatric hospital stay, the client consumed alcohol every night to help relax. However, since discharge, the client says he has not consumed alcohol to help cope with the situation. Today the client does not have insomnia, anorexia, or palpitations, and states not experiencing the depressed moods experienced prior to hospitalization. All of these client findings show that the client has improved and is progressing. The client still reports flashbacks and nightmares, which does not indicate improvement, but is sleeping better.

Test-Taking Strategy

Test-Taking Strategy: This test item requires you to compare the client's initial findings before the inpatient psychiatric unit stay with current findings during this follow-up visit. Use the table to help you determine if the client has improved, and is therefore progressing, to answer this test item measuring *Evaluate Outcomes.*

Client Finding Before Psychiatric Unit Stay	Client Finding During Current Provider Visit	Current Finding Demonstrates Client Is Progressing or Improving? Yes or No
Reports that drinking alcohol every night helps to relax	Has not consumed any alcohol since hospital discharge	Yes
Has anorexia and is depressed at times	States has a more positive outlook without depressed moods, and a better appetite	Yes
Has flashbacks and nightmares	Has flashbacks and nightmares at least once a week	No
Has insomnia	Sleeps most nights for 7–8 hours	Yes
Has heart palpitations	States no longer has heart palpitations	Yes

Creating a table as illustrated will help you organize your thoughts to help answer the question. Use the findings that are answered with a "Yes" as the correct responses for the test item.

CJ Cognitive Skill: Evaluate Outcomes

Unfolding Case Study 2

Content Area: Medical-Surgical Nursing
Priority Concept: Clotting
Reference(s): Burchum & Rosenthal, 2019, pp. 612–616; Ignatavicius et al., 2021, pp. 587–592, 1009–1010

> **Practice Question 10.7**   **Unfolding Case Study 2**

The nurse reviews the preoperative note for a 68-year-old client who is scheduled to have an anterior right THA this morning.

Health History	Nurses' Notes	Imaging Studies	Lab Results

0645: Admitted to the OR for a THA using an anterior surgical approach. History of several surgeries including hysterectomy, appendectomy, and cholecystectomy. 52–pack-year history but quit 2 years ago; BMI of 30.1. History of DVT × 2, hypertension controlled by diet and drug therapy, high cholesterol controlled by statins, and GERD controlled by an antacid PRN. Bilateral hip osteoarthritis with right hip more painful than left. Lives in second-floor apartment in a rural town. Has no transportation and depends on family friends to obtain food and get to medical appointments. Family friends are willing to help with postoperative recovery and transportation. Advance directives on file. Prepped for surgery.

The nurse recognizes that which assessment findings listed below place the client at high risk for postoperative VTE? **Select all that apply.**

☐ History of hypertension
☒ 52–pack-year history
☒ BMI of 30.1
☐ History of high cholesterol
☒ Having a THA
☐ History of cholecystectomy
☐ History of bilateral hip osteoarthritis
☒ History of DVT × 2

Rationale: VTE is the development of one or more blood clots and includes DVT and PE. The nurse needs to recognize that the client has multiple risk factors for developing VTE, which can be potentially life-threatening. The client has a 52–pack-year smoking history but quit 2 years ago. However, long-term smoking exposure causes vasoconstriction and vessel damage, which predispose the client to clot development. A BMI of over 30 indicates that the client is obese; clients who are obese are at higher risk of VTE and other postoperative complications than clients who are within a normal weight range. For unknown reasons, orthopedic injuries and surgery increase VTE risk. Clients who have a history of VTE are at higher risk for recurrence than are clients who do not have that history.

Hypertension is an arterial health problem affecting peripheral vessels and would not likely contribute to developing a peripheral venous or pulmonary clot. High cholesterol can contribute to hypertension and atherosclerosis development in small arterial vessels. A surgical history of cholecystectomy, GERD, and current bilateral osteoarthritis are unrelated to one's risk for VTE.

Test-Taking Strategy: Recall that all clients having major orthopedic surgery are at risk for VTE. However, this client has additional findings making the client especially prone to this postoperative complication. Use the table to help you decide which assessment findings to select to *Recognize Cues* that should concern the nurse.

Client Assessment Finding	Can Contribute to Developing VTE	Does Not Typically Contribute to Developing VTE
History of hypertension	☐	☒
52–pack-year history	☒	☐
BMI of 30.1	☒	☐
History of high cholesterol	☐	☒
Having a THA	☒	☐
History of cholecystectomy	☐	☒
History of bilateral hip osteoarthritis	☐	☒
History of DVT × 2	☒	☐

Apply your knowledge of VTE pathophysiology to help you determine the correct responses. Based on this table, select all of the client findings that are marked with an X under "Can Contribute to Developing VTE" to correctly answer the test item.

CJ Cognitive Skill: Recognize Cues

Practice Question 10.8   Unfolding Case Study 2

The nurse is assigned to care for a 68-year-old client who had a right THA 2 days ago. The client's pain is being managed with oral opioids and gabapentin. The client is preparing for possible discharge tomorrow. The client has been on apixaban 5 mg orally once a day and has ambulated with assistance 4 times each day in the hall with a walker. The nurse performs a shift assessment and documents the following Nurses' Notes.

Health History	Nurses' Notes	Imaging Studies	Lab Results

1935: Reports was unable to ambulate this evening because of sharp chest pain that hurts worse when taking a deep breath. States has been "belching" since dinner because of eating onions and peppers on a steak. Restless and anxious about pain, but no acute confusion. T = 100°F (37.8°C); HR = 104 BPM; RR = 20 bpm with dyspnea; BP = 114/62 mm Hg; SpO₂ = 90% on RA. Right THA incision dry and intact without redness. Right pedal pulse nonpalpable but detected on Doppler; foot warm and not swollen. Posterior tibial and popliteal pulses +2 bilaterally. Able to flex both feet equally; cap refill <3 seconds.

For each client assessment finding, click or indicate with an X which finding is associated with which potential client condition. Some findings may be consistent with more than one condition.

Client Finding	PE	GERD	Respiratory Infection
Chest pain	☒	☒	☒
Belching	☐	☒	☐
Restlessness	☒	☐	☒
Anxiety	☒	☐	☒
T 100°F (37.8°C)	☐	☐	☒
HR 104 BPM	☒	☐	☒
RR 20 bpm with dyspnea	☒	☐	☒
SpO₂ 90% on RA	☒	☐	☒

Rationale: The client is at risk for postoperative complications including VTE and respiratory infection because of age, decreased mobility, smoking history, DVT history, and obesity. The client has a history of GERD, which can cause eructation (belching) and chest discomfort or pain after eating foods that are spicy or highly seasoned. However, none of the other client findings are associated with GERD. Chest pain can also occur in clients who are experiencing PE or respiratory infection such as pneumonia. PE can be massive or small, but most often results when a piece of clot dislodges from a DVT and occludes one or more pulmonary blood vessels. In many cases the DVT is undetected or not diagnosed. The results of a PE typically include an obstructed pulmonary blood flow, which leads to hypoxia. This hypoxia may manifest with tachypnea, dyspnea, restlessness, anxiety, and decreased oxygen saturation. As a compensatory mechanism, the HR increases (tachycardia) to circulate blood more rapidly throughout the body. These same pulmonary and cardiac findings may be seen in clients with a respiratory infection. Infection is also usually accompanied by a fever, which increases the body's metabolic rate. Anxiety may be present in clients with PE and respiratory infection because of dyspnea and chest pain. Increased temperature in clients with respiratory infection occurs as the body attempts to reduce or destroy the microorganisms that are causing the infection. Fever is not common in clients who have either a PE or GERD.

Test-Taking Strategy: To answer this test item you need to recall the pathophysiology and typical clinical manifestations associated with three health problems—PE, GERD, and respiratory infection, such as pneumonia. To help organize the information you will need to *Analyze Cues,* develop a table such as the one shown here. Review each client finding and decide if it provides supporting evidence for a PE, GERD, and/or respiratory infection.

Test-Taking Strategy

Client Finding (Assessment Data)	Supporting Evidence for PE? Yes or No	Supporting Evidence for GERD? Yes or No	Supporting Evidence for Respiratory Infection? Yes or No
Chest pain	Yes	Yes	Yes
Belching	No	Yes	No
Restlessness	Yes	No	Yes
Anxiety	Yes	No	Yes
T 100°F (37.8°C)	No	No	Yes
HR 104 BPM	Yes	No	Yes
RR 20 bpm with dyspnea	Yes	No	Yes
SpO$_2$ 90% on RA	Yes	No	Yes

As you will note, some client findings such as chest pain support several client conditions or health problems. In other cases the client finding supports only one of the client conditions. For example, belching (also called eructation) supports only GERD. This GI symptom is not associated with pulmonary problems. An elevated temperature can occur in clients with infection but is not associated with PE or GERD.

CJ Cognitive Skill: Analyze Cues

Practice Question 10.9   Unfolding Case Study 2

The nurse is assigned to care for a 68-year-old client who had a right THA 2 days ago. The client's pain is being managed with oral opioids and gabapentin. The client is preparing for possible discharge tomorrow. The client has been on apixaban 5 mg orally once a day and has ambulated at least 4 times each day in the hall with a walker. The nurse performs a shift assessment and documents the following Nurses' Notes.

Health History	Nurses' Notes	Imaging Studies	Lab Results

1935: Reports was unable to ambulate this evening because of sharp chest pain that hurts worse when taking a deep breath. States has been "belching" since dinner because of eating onions and peppers on a steak. Restless and anxious about pain, but no acute confusion. T = 100°F (37.8°C); HR = 104 BPM; RR = 20 bpm with dyspnea; BP = 114/62 mm Hg; SpO$_2$ = 90% on RA. Right THA incision dry and intact without redness. Right pedal pulse nonpalpable but detected on Doppler; foot warm and not swollen. Posterior tibial and popliteal pulses +2 bilaterally. Able to flex both feet equally; cap refill <3 seconds.

Based on the information in the Nurses' Notes, complete the following sentences from the lists of options provided.

The client **most likely** has **PE** as the *priority* condition as evidenced by **chest pain** and **dyspnea**.

Options for 1	Options for 2	Options for 3
Right leg neurovascular compromise	Chest pain	Tachypnea
	Hypotension	Belching
	Bradycardia	Decreased
PE	Nonpalpable right	capillary refill
Pneumonia	pedal pulse	Dyspnea
GERD		

Rationale: The client had orthopedic surgery 2 days ago and is at risk for a number of postoperative complications. The risk is further increased by obesity and a smoking history. Although the client may be at risk for or have findings associated with the four client conditions listed for Option 1, the potentially life-threatening condition is PE, which would therefore be the *priority* client problem. A respiratory infection such as pneumonia could possibly be life-threatening if not treated, but neurovascular compromise in the surgical leg and GERD are not life-threatening unless they progress over time. A long-term diagnosis of GERD that is not well managed can cause Barrett esophageal cell changes, which can predispose the client to esophageal or gastric cancer. Neurovascular compromise may result in compartment syndrome, which can cause irreversible tissue damage due to impaired perfusion.

The classic manifestations of a PE are a sudden onset of chest pain and dyspnea, which the client has according to the Nurses' Notes. Clients who have pneumonia may also have chest discomfort, but it tends to be more gradual in onset and may be described as discomfort rather than sharp pain. The client does not have hypotension, bradycardia, or tachypnea, but does have dyspnea, which can be associated with a PE or pneumonia. A nonpalpable pedal pulse may not be significant as long as there are other indicators of adequate perfusion. The client has adequate capillary refill and her affected foot is warm, indicating that there is no problem with perfusion. Therefore there is no evidence that she has neurovascular compromise.

Test-Taking Strategy

Test-Taking Strategy: This test item requires you to determine the priority client condition and the client findings that provide the supporting evidence for your answer. First you want to determine the priority client condition. Recall from Chapter 5 that factors such as complexity, urgency, risk, and difficulty affect how you decide on the client's priority problem. In this client's case, the amount of risk is the key factor in deciding the priority because one of the four choices is potentially immediately life-threatening and the others are not immediately life-threatening. Therefore PE is the client condition that takes *priority* over the other problems, because it affects perfusion and causes hypoxia.

Once you make that decision, you need to determine which findings are present in this client that provide supporting evidence for the condition you selected. Use the table to help make those decisions.

Client Finding Option	Supporting Evidence for PE? Yes or No	Finding Present in This Client? Yes or No
Chest pain	Yes	Yes
Hypotension	Yes	No
Bradycardia	No	No
Nonpalpable right pedal pulse	No	Yes
Tachypnea	Yes	No
Belching	No	Yes
Decreased capillary refill	No	No
Dyspnea	Yes	Yes

As you can see, there are four options for supporting evidence that could be associated with a PE. However, only two of those four findings are present in this client scenario—chest pain and dyspnea. The client does not have tachypnea at this point because her RR is within the normal range of 16 to 20 bpm. The client does report belching, but that is not a client finding associated with PE. Therefore you would select the client findings for which there is supporting evidence *and* that are present in this client scenario to *Prioritize Hypotheses.*

CJ Cognitive Skill: Prioritize Hypotheses

Practice Question 10.10   **Unfolding Case Study 2**

The nurse is assigned to care for a 68-year-old client who had a right THA 2 days ago. The client's pain is being managed with oral opioids and gabapentin. The client is preparing for possible discharge tomorrow. The client has been on apixaban 5 mg orally once a day and has ambulated at least 4 times each day in the hall with a walker. The nurse performs a shift assessment and documents the following Nurses' Notes.

Health History	Nurses' Notes	Imaging Studies	Lab Results

1935: Reports was unable to ambulate this evening because of sharp chest pain that hurts worse when taking a deep breath. States has been "belching" since dinner because of eating onions and peppers on a steak. Restless and anxious about pain, but no acute confusion. T = 100°F (37.8°C); HR = 104 BPM; RR = 20 bpm with dyspnea; BP = 114/62 mm Hg; SpO$_2$ = 90% on RA. Right THA incision dry and intact without redness. Right pedal pulse nonpalpable but detected on Doppler; foot warm and not swollen. Posterior tibial and popliteal pulses +2 bilaterally. Able to flex both feet equally; cap refill <3 seconds.

The nurse develops a plan of care to manage the client's suspected condition. Select six actions that would be appropriate for the nurse to include in the plan of care at this time.

- ☒ Obtain venous access.
- ☐ Place the client in a flat supine position.
- ☒ Connect the client to a continuous cardiac monitor.
- ☒ Prepare the client for computed tomography pulmonary angiography (CTPA).
- ☒ Apply oxygen by NC or mask.
- ☐ Increase the client's oral apixaban dosage from 5 mg to 10 mg.
- ☒ Draw blood for laboratory testing, including complete blood count (CBC) and coagulation studies.
- ☒ Place the client on continuous oxygen saturation monitoring.

Rationale: The client most likely has PE with one or more emboli obstructing pulmonary blood flow. To confirm this probable health problem, the client usually has a CTPA or helical CT. In some settings, magnetic resonance angiography (MRA) may be used instead of either CT scan procedure. As a result of PE, the client develops hypoxia with either normal breath sounds or adventitious sounds such as crackles and wheezes. Therefore the nurse would place the client in a sitting (high-Fowler) position rather than a flat supine position to facilitate breathing and would apply oxygen therapy and continuous pulse oximetry to monitor SpO_2. If the PE is not treated or is large, cardiac symptoms such as hypotension and tachycardia can occur owing to decreased tissue perfusion. Electrocardiography changes such as transient T-wave and ST-segment changes can also occur, so the nurse ensures that the client has continuous cardiac monitoring. Venous access is needed for administering drug therapy or fluids as indicated. The client needs IV anticoagulant therapy if PE is confirmed to prevent the clot(s) from becoming larger. Laboratory testing to check her platelet count, serum creatinine, CBC, and coagulation studies provide a baseline before drug therapy is initiated. Increasing the dosage of her oral anticoagulant, apixaban, would not be effective in managing this potentially life-threatening condition because it does not act immediately or prevent a clot from becoming larger.

Test-Taking Strategy

Test-Taking Strategy: To help you decide on possible actions to include in the client's care, first recall the pathophysiology of PE. This acute health problem causes respiratory and cardiovascular compromise, which can be potentially life-threatening. Therefore, nursing interventions would be planned to provide respiratory and/or cardiovascular assessment data or support. Use the table to help decide which actions would be indicated for this client:

Potential Nursing Action	Action Provides Respiratory Assessment Data or Support? Yes or No	Action Provides Cardiovascular Assessment Data or Support? Yes or No
Obtain venous access.	No	Yes
Place the client in a flat supine position.	No	No
Connect the client to a continuous cardiac monitor.	No	Yes
Prepare the client for computed tomography pulmonary angiography (CTPA).	Yes	Yes
Apply oxygen by NC or mask.	Yes	Yes
Increase the client's oral apixaban dosage from 5 mg to 10 mg.	No	No
Draw blood for laboratory testing including CBC and coagulation studies.	No	Yes
Place the client on continuous oxygen saturation monitoring.	Yes	Yes

Once you review the table, select all of the nursing actions that provide assessment data regarding the status of the client's cardiopulmonary system *and/or* support the function of the cardiopulmonary system to *Generate Solutions.*

CJ Cognitive Skill: Generate Solutions

Practice Question 10.11   Unfolding Case Study 2

The nurse is assigned to care for a 68-year-old client who had a right THA 2 days ago. During shift assessment, the nurse documents new onset of symptoms including chest pain and dyspnea. Computed tomography pulmonary angiography (CTPA) confirmed the diagnosis of a submassive PE. The orthopedic surgeon enters the following orders:

| Nurses' Notes | Physician Orders | Imaging Studies | Lab Results |

1020:
- Fondaparinux 7.5 mg subcutaneously once daily
- Warfarin 5 mg orally once daily
- Supplemental oxygen per NC at 5 L/min
- Continuous pulse oximetry monitoring

The nurse revises the plan of care for the client with confirmed diagnosis of PE. Click or place an X to specify nursing actions that are **Indicated** *(appropriate or necessary) and those that are* **Contraindicated** *(not useful and could be harmful) related to drug therapy for this client.*

Potential Nursing Action	Indicated	Contraindicated
Monitor the client's platelet count.	X	☐
Monitor the client's activated partial thromboplastin time (aPTT).	☐	X
Assess the client for bleeding or excessive bruising.	X	☐
Monitor the client's international normalized ratio (INR).	X	☐
Monitor the client's hematocrit.	X	☐
Check for availability of protamine sulfate.	☐	X
Check for availability of phytonadione (vitamin K).	X	☐

Rationale: Fondaparinux is a synthetic anticoagulant that increases the activity of antithrombin to cause selective inhibition of factor Xa. Unlike heparin, this drug does not affect thrombin and therefore has no effect on prothrombin time or aPTT. However, it can lower platelet counts. Warfarin affects multiple vitamin K–dependent clotting factors in the liver. The drug's effectiveness is measured by monitoring the INR. Therefore the nurse would monitor the client's platelets (for fondaparinux) and INR (for warfarin), but there is no need to monitor the aPTT. Both drugs can cause bleeding, and therefore the nurse would monitor the client for bleeding and excessive bruising. The client's hematocrit would decrease if the client experiences internal bleeding and would also need to be monitored. Unlike heparin, the antidote for fondaparinux is not protamine sulfate, but vitamin K is the antidote for warfarin overdose. The nurse would ensure that vitamin K is readily available if needed.

Test-Taking Strategy: To correctly answer this test item, you'll need to differentiate fondaparinux from heparin, although both drugs are fast-acting anticoagulants used for DVT and PE and given parenterally to prevent clots from enlarging. Fondaparinux is administered as a fixed dose, but IV heparin must be titrated based on the client's lab values. Warfarin is an oral anticoagulant that works slowly in the liver and takes several days to begin its effectiveness. Both drugs that are ordered for the client can cause bleeding. There is no antidote for fondaparinux, but vitamin K is the antidote for warfarin. The remaining nursing actions are primarily focused on laboratory test monitoring. Use the table to help decide which lab tests are appropriate based on the mechanism of drug actions.

Test-Taking Strategy

Laboratory Test	Appropriate to Monitor When Client Receives Fondaparinux? Yes or No	Appropriate to Monitor When Client Receives Warfarin? Yes or No?
aPTT	No	No
Prothrombin time	No	Yes
INR	No	Yes
Hematocrit	Yes	Yes
Platelet count	Yes	No

Review the table to determine which lab tests are appropriate to monitor for each of the two drugs and select those lab tests that match the choices provided in the test item to measure *Take Action.*

CJ Cognitive Skill: Take Action

Practice Question 10.12 **Unfolding Case Study 2**

A 68-year-old client who had a right THA is returning to the orthopedic surgeon's office for a 6-week follow-up visit. While in the hospital recovering from surgery, the client experienced a PE, which was successfully treated. Today the office nurse conducts a brief assessment before the client is examined by the surgeon and documents the following note.

Health History	Nurses' Notes	Imaging Studies	Lab Results

1015: Walking independently with a cane with full weight bearing; states is able to perform ADLs without assistance. Right hip incision healed with hairline scar and slight distal bruising. Taking warfarin as prescribed and following up on INR testing, but depends mostly on family friends for transportation to the lab. Right arm badly bruised but reports no other bleeding. T = 97.9°F (36.6°C); HR = 86 BPM; RR = 18 bpm; BP = 126/74 mm Hg; SpO$_2$ = 95% on RA. No adventitious breath sounds; no new report of shortness of breath or chest pain. States a loss of 27 lb since hospitalization as part of a new weight loss program. Also reports that left nonsurgical hip is increasingly painful and may soon need to be replaced.

Based on the nurse's brief assessment, which findings indicate that the client is improving or progressing? **Select all that apply.**

- ☒ No new report of shortness of breath or chest pain
- ☒ Hip incision healed with hairline scar
- ☒ SpO$_2$ of 95% on RA
- ☐ Right arm badly bruised
- ☒ Recent weight loss of 27 lb
- ☐ Left hip is becoming more painful
- ☒ Walking independently with cane
- ☒ Performing ADLs without assistance

Rationale: The client was treated for PE on the second postoperative day while recovering from hip surgery 6 weeks ago. At that time, the client was able to ambulate with assistance and a walker, and likely needed help with selected ADLs. Today the client is independent in both ADLs and ambulation and has progressed from walking with a walker to walking with a cane, which provides less support for the client. The client does not currently have chest pain or dyspnea, and the SpO$_2$ has increased from 90% to 95%. The desired SpO$_2$ is 95% or greater for adults without chronic pulmonary problems.

The client's incision has healed normally with minimal bruising or scarring, which is a desired outcome. However, the client's right arm is badly bruised, which is an adverse effect of warfarin therapy. When admitted for hip arthroplasty, the client's BMI was 30.1, indicating that the client was obese. Obesity likely contributed to hip arthritis and PE. The increased pain in the client's left hip demonstrates that the arthritis is worsening rather than improving. After discharge, the client apparently entered a new weight loss program and has already lost 27 lb in about 6 weeks. This weight loss will help the client continue to become more mobile, decrease left hip pain, and place the client at less risk for additional medical complications.

Test-Taking Strategy: To correctly answer this test item, you'll need to compare the client assessment findings in the most recent Nurses' Notes with those documented in the hospital Nurses' Notes. Use a table like the one shown here to make this comparison, and then determine if the most current findings show improvement in the client's condition, in order to *Evaluate Outcomes.*

Test-Taking Strategy

Client Finding During Hospitalization	Current Client Finding	Client Condition Improving or Progressing? Yes or No
Acute onset of dyspnea and chest pain	No new report of shortness of breath or chest pain	Yes
Incision only a few days old and likely not healed	Hip incision healed with hairline scar	Yes
Oxygen saturation of 90% on RA	SpO$_2$ of 95% on RA	Yes
No noted arm bruising	Right arm badly bruised	No
Weight not noted but client obese as evidenced by BMI over 30	Recent weight loss of 27 lb	Yes
Right hip pain was worse than left and was therefore replaced first during THA	Left hip is becoming more painful	No
Ambulated with walker 4 times a day until onset of chest pain and dyspnea	Walking independently with cane	Yes
Was receiving drug therapy to manage pain and likely needed assistance with selected ADLs such as dressing or bathing lower extremities	Performing ADLs without assistance	Yes

To answer the test item, review the table and select all of the findings for which you indicated "yes" for improvement in the client's condition in the right column.

CJ Cognitive Skill: Evaluate Outcomes

Unfolding Case Study 3

CJ Cognitive Skill: Medical-Surgical Nursing
Priority Concept: Glucose Regulation
Reference(s): Ignatavicius et al., 2021, pp. 226, 568–570, 721, 1250, 1292–1298; Pagana et al., 2021, pp. 104, 157, 302, 304, 307, 325, 464, 721, 824, 877, 901, 933, 973; Pagana et al., 2019, pp. 121,199, 201, 205, 217, 269, 420, 479, 500, 531, 534, 549, 824, 991; Centers for Disease Control and Prevention (CDC), 2021; National Institutes of Health (NIH), 2021

Practice Question 10.13   Unfolding Case Study 3

A 64-year-old client presents to the ED and reports a 2-week history of fever and chills, nausea and abdominal pain, sore throat, cough, fatigue and lethargy, and muscle aches. An initial nursing assessment reveals the following:

Health History	Nurses' Notes	Lab Tests	Diagnostic Tests

1000: History of diabetes type 1, hypertension, hyperlipidemia, hypothyroidism. Denies chest pain or shortness of breath. Nonproductive cough, coarse crackles heard in lower lobes bilaterally. Blood glucose levels have been well controlled, but this morning the client reports a level of 375 mg/dL (20.8 mmol/L), prompting the visit to the ED. States recent glycated hemoglobin (A1c) level done 2 months ago was 7.0%. Unable to eat and reports stopping medications 3 days ago because of the nausea and abdominal pain. States has had increased urination despite the inability to tolerate food or fluids. Reports weakness and muscle aches and being confined to bed for the past 3 weeks. Fruity breath odor noted. POC glucose 400 mg/dL (22.2 mmol/L).
VS: T = 100.4°F (38.0°C); HR = 96 BPM; RR = 24 bpm; BP = 142/90 mm Hg; SpO₂ = 91% on RA.
Weight 175 lb (79.37 kg), height 5 feet 9 inches (stated).
Voided: 250 mL.

Medications:
Levothyroxine 125 mcg oral daily
Lisinopril 2.5 mg oral daily
Simvastatin 20 mg oral daily
Insulin glargine 28 units subcutaneous daily
Semaglutide 1 mg subcutaneous weekly

1120: The nurse reviews the recent laboratory and diagnostic test results, which include the following:

Health History	Nurses' Notes	Lab Tests	Diagnostic Tests

Laboratory Test	Results	Normal Reference Range
Glucose	440 mg/dL (24.4 mmol/L) H	74–106 mg/dL (3.9–6.1 mmol/L)
Ketones	86.4 mg/dL (4.8 mmol/L) H	<0 mg/dL (0.0–0.27 mmol/L)
White blood cells (WBCs)	9900/mm³ (6.3 × 10⁹/L)	5000–10,000/mm³ (3.5–12 × 10⁹/L)
Blood urea nitrogen (BUN)	22 mg/dL (9.0 mmol/L) H	10-20 mg/dL (2.9–8.2 mmol/L)
Creatinine (Cr)	1.0 mg/dL (88.3 mcmol/L)	0.6–1.2 mg/dL (53–106 mcmol/L)
Potassium (K)	5.9 mEq/L (5.9 mmol/L) H	3.5-5.0 mEq/L (3.5–5.1 mmol/L)
Sodium (Na)	150 mEq/L (150 mmol/L) H	136-145 mEq/L (136–145 mmol/L)
Thyroid-stimulating hormone (TSH)	4.0 mIU/mL (4.0 mIU/L)	2-10 mIU/mL (0.4–4.8 mIU/L)
D-dimer	15 mcg/mL (112.5 nmol/L) H	<250 ng/mL or <0.4 mcg/mL (<3 nmol/L)
Creatine kinase (CK)	140 U/L (150.5 U/L)	20–200 U/L (20–215 U/L)
C-reactive protein (CRP)	10.2 mg/dL (102 mg/L) H	<1 mg/dL (<10.0 mg/L)
Troponin I	0.01 ng/mL (0.17 mcg/L)	<0.03 ng/mL (<0.35 mcg/L)
Blood culture	Pending	No growth

Urinalysis
  WBCs
  Ketones
	
	0 (0)
	Positive H
		
		0–4 low-power field
		None

Urine culture	Pending	No growth
Arterial blood gases (ABGs)	pH 7.30 L Pco₂ 27 mm Hg L HCO₃ 14 mEq/L L Po₂ 85 mm Hg	pH 7.35–7.45 (7.35–7.45) Pco₂ 35–45 mm Hg (35–45 mm Hg) HCO₃ 21–28 mEq/L (23–29 mEq/L) Po₂ 80–100 mm Hg (80–100 mm Hg)
SARS-CoV-2 PCR	Positive	Negative

Practice Question 10.13   Unfolding Case Study 3—cont'd

| Health History | Nurses' Notes | Lab Tests | Diagnostic Tests |

Diagnostic Test	Results
Chest x-ray	Bilateral pulmonary infiltrates compatible with COVID-19 pneumonitis
ECG	NSR

*Which four laboratory findings require **immediate** follow-up?*
- ☐ A1c
- ☐ BUN
- ☐ Sodium
- ☒ Glucose
- ☒ D-dimer
- ☒ Potassium
- ☐ C-reactive protein
- ☒ Arterial blood gases

Rationale: DKA is a complication of DM and is characterized by uncontrolled hyperglycemia, metabolic acidosis, and increased production of ketones. This condition results from the combination of insulin deficiency and an increase in hormone release that leads to increased liver and kidney glucose production. The most common precipitating factor for DKA is infection. Other precipitating factors include an inadequate insulin dose. COVID-19 is a viral infection, and this client demonstrates manifestations of COVID in addition to a positive test for the virus. This is one of the client's precipitating factors for DKA. The client also reports being unable to eat and stopping medications 3 days ago because of the nausea and abdominal pain and inability to tolerate food or fluids. This lack of insulin is also a precipitating factor for DKA. DKA is a life-threatening complication of DM. The nurse needs to recognize manifestations of this event early so that interventions can be performed immediately. Classic symptoms of DKA include hyperglycemia, polyuria, polydipsia, polyphagia, a rotting citrus fruit odor to the breath, nausea or vomiting, abdominal pain, dehydration, weakness, and confusion. Shock and coma can result. From the laboratory tests listed in the options, the nurse would be most concerned with the glucose, D-dimer, potassium, and ABG results. The glucose level is extremely elevated at 440 mg/dL (24.4 mmol/L), which is significant, indicating hyperglycemia. This result along with the serum and urinary ketone results is an additional indication of DKA. Arterial blood gas results also indicate metabolic acidosis, another indication of DKA. The pH is low and the HCO_3 is low—other indicators of DKA. The potassium level is elevated, and although this will return to normal once treatment begins, it is an immediate concern because of the risk associated with life-threatening dysrhythmias when the potassium level is outside of the normal range. Coagulopathy and thromboembolism are complications of COVID. The D-dimer is a test that helps to confirm coagulopathy; because this level is elevated, it is an immediate concern because of the risk for thromboembolism. The A1c is 7%; although a value of <7% indicates good diabetic control, the test is a long-term index of the client's average glucose level and is not an immediate concern. The sodium (Na^+) level is elevated, and although this is an abnormal value, it is not of immediate concern. This increase is expected because of the dehydration that occurs with illness. Once treatment begins and hydration is provided, the Na^+ level will likely return to a normal level. The slightly elevated BUN is expected because of the dehydration and is not an indication of renal involvement, especially as the Cr is normal and there are no other manifestations of kidney injury. The C-reactive protein is elevated; this is a finding that is noted in the client with COVID owing to the infection and inflammation that occur. Elevated levels also occur in the client with hypertension, metabolic syndrome, or DM.

Test-Taking Strategy: First, note that this question is asking for the laboratory results that require *immediate* follow-up by the nurse. This indicates that there may be other results that are abnormal but not of immediate concern. Remember to first identify normal/usual or abnormal but expected results. These results would *not* require immediate follow-up by the nurse. Next, identify abnormal/not expected results to determine which results require immediate follow-up by the nurse. The laboratory results in the medical record can be categorized as shown in the table to help *Recognize Cues.*

Laboratory Results	Normal/Usual or Abnormal/ Expected Not Requiring Immediate Follow-up	Abnormal/ Not Expected Requiring Immediate Follow-up	Acute or Chronic Safety Implication if Not Addressed Immediately/Requires Immediate Follow-up? Yes or No
A1c 7.0% H	☒	☐	Chronic No
BUN	☒	☐	Acute No
Sodium 150 mEq/L (150 mmol/L) H	☒	☐	Acute No
Glucose 440 mg/dL (24.4 mmol/L) H	☐	☒	Acute/Chronic Yes
D-dimer 15 mcg/mL (112.5 nmol/L) H	☐	☒	Acute Yes
Potassium 5.9 mEq/L (5.9 mmol/L) H	☐	☒	Acute Yes
CRP	☒	☐	Acute No
Arterial blood gases pH 7.30 L Pco$_2$ 27 mm Hg L HCO$_3$ 14 mEq/L L Po$_2$ 85 mm Hg	☐	☒	Acute Yes

Note that the question asks you to select the four options requiring immediate follow-up. Of all the options, the four options that are most concerning are the glucose, D-dimer, potassium, and arterial blood gas levels. These results could have immediate safety implications and acute findings and therefore need to be addressed immediately. The other results, although they could be relevant in some way to the acute condition or be abnormal, do not require immediate follow-up and could be safely addressed at a later time. They may also be related to a chronic condition and therefore do not require immediate follow-up.

CJ Cognitive Skill: Recognize Cues

Practice Question 10.14   Unfolding Case Study 3

A 64-year-old client presents to the ED and reports a 2-week history of fever and chills, nausea and abdominal pain, sore throat, cough, fatigue and lethargy, and muscle aches. An initial nursing assessment reveals the following:

Health History	Nurses' Notes	Lab Tests	Diagnostic Tests

1000: History of diabetes type 1, hypertension, hyperlipidemia, hypothyroidism. Denies chest pain or shortness of breath. Nonproductive cough, coarse crackles heard in lower lobes bilaterally. Blood glucose levels have been well controlled, but this morning the client reports a level of 375 mg/dL (20.8 mmol/L), prompting the visit to the ED. States recent glycated hemoglobin (A1c) level done 2 months ago was 7.0%. Unable to eat and reports stopping medications 3 days ago because of the nausea and abdominal pain. States has had increased urination despite the inability to tolerate food or fluids. Reports weakness and muscle aches and being confined to bed for the past 3 weeks. Fruity breath odor noted. POC glucose 400 mg/dL (22.2 mmol/L).
VS: T = 100.4°F (38.0°C); HR = 96 BPM; RR = 24 bpm; BP = 142/90 mm Hg; SpO$_2$ = 91% on RA.
Weight 175 lb (79.37 kg), height 5 feet 9 inches (stated).
Voided: 250 mL.

Medications:
Levothyroxine 125 mcg oral daily
Lisinopril 2.5 mg oral daily
Simvastatin 20 mg oral daily
Insulin glargine 28 units subcutaneous daily
Semaglutide 1 mg subcutaneous weekly

1120: The nurse reviews the recent laboratory and diagnostic test results, which include the following:

Health History	Nurses' Notes	Lab Tests	Diagnostic Tests

Laboratory Test	Results	Normal Reference Range
Glucose	440 mg/dL (24.4 mmol/L) H	74–106 mg/dL (3.9–6.1 mmol/L)
Ketones	86.4 mg/dL (4.8 mmol/L) H	<0 mg/dL (0.0–0.27 mmol/L)
White blood cells (WBCs)	9900/mm³ (6.3 × 10⁹/L)	5000–10,000/mm³ (3.5–12 × 10⁹/L)
Blood urea nitrogen (BUN)	22 mg/dL (9.0 mmol/L) H	10–20 mg/dL (2.9–8.2 mmol/L)
Creatinine (Cr)	1.0 mg/dL (88.3 mcmol/L)	0.6–1.2 mg/dL (53–106 mcmol/L)
Potassium (K)	5.9 mEq/L (5.9 mmol/L) H	3.5–5.0 mEq/L (3.5–5.1 mmol/L)
Sodium (Na)	150 mEq/L (150 mmol/L) H	136–145 mEq/L (136–145 mmol/L)
Thyroid-stimulating hormone (TSH)	4.0 mIU/mL (4.0 mIU/L)	2–10 mIU/mL (0.4–4.8 mIU/L)
D-dimer	15 mcg/mL (112.5 nmol/L) H	<250 ng/mL or <0.4 mcg/mL (<3 nmol/L)
Creatine kinase (CK)	140 U/L (150.5 U/L)	20–200 U/L (20–215 U/L)
C-reactive protein (CRP)	10.2 mg/dL (102 mg/L) H	<1 mg/dL (<10.0 mg/L)
Troponin I	0.01 ng/mL (0.17 mcg/L)	<0.03 ng/mL (<0.35 mcg/L)
Blood culture	Pending	No growth

Urinalysis
  WBCs
  Ketones
	
	0 (0)
	Positive H
		
		0–4 low-power field
		None

Urine culture	Pending	No growth
Arterial blood gases (ABGs)	pH 7.30 L Pco$_2$ 27 mm Hg L HCO$_3$ 14 mEq/L L Po$_2$ 85 mm Hg	pH 7.35–7.45 (7.35–7.45) Pco$_2$ 35–45 mm Hg (35–45 mm Hg) HCO$_3$ 21–28 mEq/L (23–29 mEq/L) Po$_2$ 80–100 mm Hg (80–100 mm Hg)
SARS-CoV-2 PCR	Positive	Negative

Continued

Practice Question 10.14   **Unfolding Case Study 3—cont'd**

| Health History | Nurses' Notes | Lab Tests | Diagnostic Tests |

Diagnostic Test	Results
Chest x-ray	Bilateral pulmonary infiltrates compatible with COVID-19 pneumonitis
ECG	NSR

For each client finding below, click or check to specify if the finding is consistent with the disease process of DKA or COVID-19. Each finding may support more than one disease process.

Client Findings	DKA	COVID-19
Fever and chills	☐	☒
Nausea	☒	☒
Abdominal pain	☒	☒
Increased urination	☒	☐
Cough	☐	☒
Lung crackles	☐	☒
High C-reactive protein level	☒	☒
High glucose level	☒	☐
Abnormal ABGs	☒	☐

Rationale: The signs and symptoms of COVID-19 that present at illness onset vary, but over the course of the disease, most individuals experience fever and chills, cough, shortness of breath or difficulty breathing, fatigue, muscle or body aches, headache, new loss of taste or smell, sore throat, congestion or a runny nose, nausea or vomiting, abdominal pain, and diarrhea. Fine or coarse crackles are heard in the lungs, and a chest x-ray reveals pulmonary infiltrates characteristic of COVID-19 pneumonitis. In addition to a positive SARS-CoV-2 PCR test, other findings include, depending on the severity of the disease, lymphopenia, neutropenia, elevated liver enzyme levels, high CRP, high ferritin levels, and elevated D-dimer levels. Respiratory failure is a concern in COVID. If the client's condition deteriorates, ABGs would show values indicative of respiratory acidosis. The ABG values for this client are not indicative of respiratory acidosis. Classic symptoms of DKA include hyperglycemia, polyuria, polydipsia, polyphagia, a fruity odor to the breath, nausea or vomiting, abdominal pain, dehydration, weakness, and confusion. An elevated C-reactive protein is a normal finding in DM. Arterial blood gas results also indicate metabolic acidosis.

Test-Taking Strategy

Test-Taking Strategy: Considering the two conditions, DKA and COVID, think about the pathophysiology that occurs with each of these conditions. The client's findings in the medical record can be categorized, as shown in the table, to help *Analyze Cues.* Remember that with *Analyze Cues,* you are thinking about what could be happening to the client based on the information in the clinical scenario.

Client Finding	Pathophysiology
Fever and chills: COVID-19	COVID-19: Immune response related to infectious process
Nausea: Both	DKA: Metabolic decompensation COVID-19: Virus in GI tract
Abdominal pain: Both	DKA: Metabolic decompensation COVID-19: Virus in GI tract
Increased urination: DKA	DKA: Kidneys remove excess glucose, and water is excreted along with the glucose
Cough: COVID-19	COVID-19: Cough as a compensatory mechanism to respiratory injury and infection
Lung crackles: COVID-19	COVID-19: Fluid develops as part of the immune response and compensatory mechanism to respiratory injury and infection
C-reactive protein level: Both	DKA: Inflammation from metabolic imbalance COVID-19: Inflammation from infectious process
Glucose level: DKA	DKA: Insulin deficiency leading to hyperglycemia
ABG levels: DKA	DKA: Buildup of ketone bodies when diabetes is uncontrolled

Think about DKA primarily as a metabolic process and COVID-19 primarily as a respiratory process. Remember that absolute insulin deficiency is the main cause of DKA. Recall that metabolic decompensation and acidosis occur, causing a number of signs and symptoms including nausea, abdominal pain, increased urination, inflammation, and elevated glucose levels. With COVID-19, remember that respiratory infection and subsequent injury is the main manifestation; however, other bodily processes are also affected. Fever and chills, nausea, abdominal pain, cough, lung crackles, and elevated CRP are all common possible findings associated with COVID-19. Thinking about the pathophysiology of each condition and considering all of the data available to you will help you *Analyze Cues* and direct you to the correct options.

CJ Cognitive Skill: Analyze Cues

Practice Question 10.15   Unfolding Case Study 3

A 64-year-old client presents to the ED and reports a 2-week history of fever and chills, nausea and abdominal pain, sore throat, cough, fatigue and lethargy, and muscle aches. An initial nursing assessment reveals the following:

Health History	Nurses' Notes	Lab Tests	Diagnostic Tests

1000: History of diabetes type 1, hypertension, hyperlipidemia, hypothyroidism. Denies chest pain or shortness of breath. Nonproductive cough, coarse crackles heard in lower lobes bilaterally. Blood glucose levels have been well controlled, but this morning the client reports a level of 375 mg/dL (20.8 mmol/L), prompting the visit to the ED. States recent glycated hemoglobin (A1c) level done 2 months ago was 7.0%. Unable to eat and reports stopping medications 3 days ago because of the nausea and abdominal pain. States has had increased urination despite the inability to tolerate food or fluids. Reports weakness and muscle aches and being confined to bed for the past 3 weeks. Fruity breath odor noted. POC glucose 400 mg/dL (22.2 mmol/L).

VS: T = 100.4°F (38.0°C); HR = 96 BPM; RR = 24 bpm; BP = 142/90 mm Hg; SpO_2 = 91% on RA.

Weight 175 lb (79.37 kg), height 5 feet 9 inches (stated). Voided: 250 mL.

Medications:
Levothyroxine 125 mcg oral daily
Lisinopril 2.5 mg oral daily
Simvastatin 20 mg oral daily
Insulin glargine 28 units subcutaneous daily
Semaglutide 1 mg subcutaneous weekly

1120: The nurse reviews the recent laboratory and diagnostic test results, which include the following:

Health History	Nurses' Notes	Lab Tests	Diagnostic Tests

Laboratory Test	Results	Normal Reference Range
Glucose	440 mg/dL (24.4 mmol/L) **H**	74–106 mg/dL (3.9–6.1 mmol/L)
Ketones	86.4 mg/dL (4.8 mmol/L) **H**	<0 mg/dL (0.0–0.27 mmol/L)
White blood cells (WBCs)	9900/mm³ (6.3 × 10⁹/L)	5000–10,000/mm³ (3.5–12 × 10⁹/L)
Blood urea nitrogen (BUN)	22 mg/dL (9.0 mmol/L) **H**	10-20 mg/dL (2.9–8.2 mmol/L)
Creatinine (Cr)	1.0 mg/dL (88.3 mcmol/L)	0.6–1.2 mg/dL (53–106 mcmol/L)
Potassium (K)	5.9 mEq/L (5.9 mmol/L) **H**	3.5-5.0 mEq/L (3.5–5.1 mmol/L)
Sodium (Na)	150 mEq/L (150 mmol/L) **H**	136-145 mEq/L (136–145 mmol/L)
Thyroid-stimulating hormone (TSH)	4.0 mIU/mL (4.0 mIU/L)	2-10 mIU/mL (0.4–4.8 mIU/L)
D-dimer	15 mcg/mL (112.5 nmol/L) **H**	<250 ng/mL or <0.4 mcg/mL (<3 nmol/L)
Creatine kinase (CK)	140 U/L (150.5 U/L)	20–200 U/L (20–215 U/L)
C-reactive protein (CRP)	10.2 mg/dL (102 mg/L) **H**	<1 mg/dL (<10.0 mg/L)
Troponin I	0.01 ng/mL (0.17 mcg/L)	<0.03 ng/mL (<0.35 mcg/L)
Blood culture	Pending	No growth
Urinalysis WBCs Ketones	0 (0) Positive **H**	0–4 low-power field None
Urine culture	Pending	No growth
Arterial blood gases (ABGs)	pH 7.30 **L**	pH 7.35–7.45 (7.35–7.45)
	Pco_2 27 mm Hg **L**	Pco_2 35–45 mm Hg (35–45 mm Hg)
	HCO_3 14 mEq/L **L**	HCO_3 21–28 mEq/L (23–29 mEq/L)
	Po_2 85 mm Hg	Po_2 80–100 mm Hg (80–100 mm Hg)
SARS-CoV-2 PCR	Positive	Negative

Health History	Nurses' Notes	Lab Tests	Diagnostic Tests

Diagnostic Test	Results
Chest x-ray	Bilateral pulmonary infiltrates compatible with COVID-19 pneumonitis
ECG	NSR

Complete the following sentence by choosing from the lists of options provided.

The client is at **highest** risk for developing <u>thromboembolism</u>, as evidenced by <u>D-dimer level</u> and <u>immobility</u>.

Options for 1	Options for 2	Options for 3
Seizures	BUN	Chills
Acute renal injury	Fever	Creatinine levels
Myxedema coma	D-dimer level	Chest x-ray result
Respiratory failure	Lung crackles	TSH level
Thromboembolism	History of hypothyroidism	Immobility

Rationale: Thrombus formation has been associated with stasis of blood, endothelial injury, and/or hypercoagulability, known as the Virchow triad. Immobility is one condition that can promote thrombus formation. COVID-19 can cause severe inflammation, which can trigger alteration of the clotting mechanism. Older adults and those individuals who have underlying medical conditions such as heart or lung disease or diabetes seem to be at higher risk for developing more serious complications from COVID-19 illness. In severe cases of COVID-19, these individuals may develop abnormal blood clots—from PE in the lungs and DVT in the legs to clots that lead to strokes or heart attacks. This client is at highest risk for developing thromboembolism because of the report of immobility for the last 3 weeks and the elevated D-dimer level. The client is experiencing chills and has a temperature of 100.4°F (38.0°C). However, it is unlikely for the client to experience seizures related to this temperature reading; seizures are most likely to occur with a sustained high fever. There is no evidence of renal injury. Although the BUN level is elevated, this elevation is most likely due to the dehydration that occurs in DKA. In addition, the Cr is normal. Myxedema coma, sometimes called hypothyroid crisis, is a serious complication of untreated or poorly treated hypothyroidism. This client has a history of hypothyroidism, but the TSH level is within a normal reference range, indicating that the condition is controlled. There is no evidence of respiratory failure. Although the client has lung crackles bilaterally and the chest x-ray shows pneumonitis, the client is not experiencing difficulty breathing or shortness of breath. The ABGs show evidence of metabolic acidosis and not a respiratory condition.

Test-Taking Strategy

Test-Taking Strategy: Note the strategic word *highest* in this question. The ability to use judgment and prioritize potential complications and associated evidence is needed in order to *Prioritize Hypotheses.* Considering the possible complications in the context of the clinical scenario and deciding which definitive evidence would support and apply to each complication listed can direct you to the correct options. Using a thinking process as illustrated in the table may help you *Prioritize Hypotheses.*

Potential Complication	Definitive Evidence/Supportive or Not Supportive of Complication?
Seizures	Fever, chills; not supportive
Acute renal injury	BUN, Cr normal; not supportive
Myxedema coma	History of hypothyroidism, TSH level is normal; not supportive
Respiratory failure	Lung crackles, chest x-ray result; not supportive
Thromboembolism	D-dimer level, immobility; supportive: D-dimer level is highly suggestive of this risk, and immobility is a major risk factor

Remember that in order to *Prioritize Hypotheses,* you need to decide on the potential complication that is of *highest* priority first, and then decide on the definitive evidence that is supportive of the complication. For each condition, there are risk factors present, but the only option that has definitive evidence of risk is thromboembolism, with an elevated D-dimer level and immobility as a major risk factor for this complication.

CJ Cognitive Skill: Prioritize Hypotheses

Practice Question 10.16   Unfolding Case Study 3

1145: The ED physician documents orders for the client and the nurse is planning care. The nurse rechecks VS and obtains a POC glucose reading. VS: T = 100.4°F (38.0°C); HR = 98 BPM; RR = 24 bpm; BP = 146/92 mm Hg; SpO₂ = 89% on RA. POC glucose reading is 500 mg/dL (27.7 mmol/L). The client is alert but lethargic yet arousable. Voiding 200 mL/hr. Dry cough. No shortness of breath. Coarse crackles heard in lower lobes bilaterally. Hospital admission is planned.

Health History	Nurses' Notes	Lab Tests	Diagnostic Tests

1000: History of diabetes type 1, hypertension, hyperlipidemia, hypothyroidism. Denies chest pain or shortness of breath. Nonproductive cough, coarse crackles heard in lower lobes bilaterally. Blood glucose levels have been well controlled, but this morning the client reports a level of 375 mg/dL (20.8 mmol/L), prompting the visit to the ED. States recent glycated hemoglobin (A1c) level done 2 months ago was 7.0%. Unable to eat and reports stopping medications 3 days ago because of the nausea and abdominal pain. States has had increased urination despite the inability to tolerate food or fluids. Reports weakness and muscle aches and being confined to bed for the past 3 weeks. Fruity breath odor noted. POC glucose 400 mg/dL (22.2 mmol/L).

VS: T = 100.4°F (38.0°C); HR = 96 BPM; RR = 24 bpm; BP = 142/90 mm Hg; SpO₂ = 91% on RA.
Weight 175 lb (79.37 kg), height 5 feet 9 inches (stated).
Voided: 250 mL.

Medications:
Levothyroxine 125 mcg oral daily
Lisinopril 2.5 mg oral daily
Simvastatin 20 mg oral daily
Insulin glargine 28 units subcutaneous daily
Semaglutide 1 mg subcutaneous weekly

1120: The nurse reviews the recent laboratory and diagnostic test results, which include the following:

Health History	Nurses' Notes	Lab Tests	Diagnostic Tests

Laboratory Test	Results	Normal Reference Range
Glucose	440 mg/dL (24.4 mmol/L) H	74–106 mg/dL (3.9–6.1 mmol/L)
Ketones	86.4 mg/dL (4.8 mmol/L) H	<0 mg/dL (0.0–0.27 mmol/L)
White blood cells (WBCs)	9900/mm³ (6.3 × 10⁹/L)	5000–10,000/mm³ (3.5–12 × 10⁹/L)
Blood urea nitrogen (BUN)	22 mg/dL (9.0 mmol/L) H	10-20 mg/dL (2.9–8.2 mmol/L)
Creatinine (Cr)	1.0 mg/dL (88.3 mcmol/L)	0.6–1.2 mg/dL (53–106 mcmol/L)
Potassium (K)	5.9 mEq/L (5.9 mmol/L) H	3.5-5.0 mEq/L (3.5–5.1 mmol/L)
Sodium (Na)	150 mEq/L (150 mmol/L) H	136-145 mEq/L (136–145 mmol/L)
Thyroid-stimulating hormone (TSH)	4.0 mIU/mL (4.0 mIU/L)	2-10 mIU/mL (0.4–4.8 mIU/L)
D-dimer	15 mcg/mL (112.5 nmol/L) H	<250 ng/mL or <0.4 mcg/mL (<3 nmol/L)
Creatine kinase (CK)	140 U/L (150.5 U/L)	20–200 U/L (20–215 U/L)
C-reactive protein (CRP)	10.2 mg/dL (102 mg/L) H	<1 mg/dL (<10.0 mg/L)
Troponin I	0.01 ng/mL (0.17 mcg/L)	<0.03 ng/mL (<0.35 mcg/L)
Blood culture	Pending	No growth

Urinalysis
  WBCs
  Ketones
	
	0 (0)
	Positive H
		
		0–4 low-power field
		None

Urine culture	Pending	No growth
Arterial blood gases (ABGs)	pH 7.30 L Pco₂ 27 mm Hg L HCO₃ 14 mEq/L L Po₂ 85 mm Hg	pH 7.35–7.45 (7.35–7.45) Pco₂ 35–45 mm Hg (35–45 mm Hg) HCO₃ 21–28 mEq/L (23–29 mEq/L) Po₂ 80–100 mm Hg (80–100 mm Hg)
SARS-CoV-2 PCR	Positive	Negative

Practice Question 10.16	Unfolding Case Study 3—cont'd

Health History	Nurses' Notes	Lab Tests	Diagnostic Tests

Diagnostic Test	Results
Chest x-ray	Bilateral pulmonary infiltrates compatible with COVID-19 pneumonitis
ECG	NSR

Click or check to indicate whether each potential intervention listed below is either **Anticipated** (appropriate or necessary) or **Contraindicated** (could be harmful)/**Not Helpful** for the client's plan of care at this time.

Potential Intervention	Anticipated	Contraindicated/ Not Helpful
O_2 per NC	☒	☐
0.45% normal saline infusion	☒	☐
Insulin glargine bolus	☐	☒
Continuous infusion of regular insulin diluted in normal saline	☒	☐
IV potassium	☐	☒
Continuous cardiac monitoring	☒	☐
Enoxaparin subcutaneously daily	☒	☐
Tocilizumab and dexamethasone	☒	☐
Ceftriaxone	☐	☒

Rationale: DKA is a complication of DM and is characterized by hyperglycemia, metabolic acidosis, and increased production of ketones. The hyperglycemia leads to osmotic diuresis and electrolyte loss. Fluid therapy and the administration of regular insulin are needed to treat this condition. The first outcome of fluid therapy is to restore blood volume and maintain perfusion to vital organs. Dehydration will be treated with IV infusions of 0.9% or 0.45% normal saline as prescribed. Hyperglycemia will be treated with regular insulin as prescribed. An IV bolus dose of regular insulin is prescribed, followed by a continuous infusion of regular insulin mixed in 0.9% or 0.45% normal saline. Insulin glargine is a long-acting insulin that works slowly over 24 hours. Thus it is not helpful in treating DKA when blood glucose levels are critically high and need to be lowered. When treating DKA, the electrolyte levels are monitored closely. This client's potassium level is 5.9 mEq/L (5.9 mmol/L), which is elevated above the normal reference range, so administering potassium would be contraindicated at this time. In addition, continuous cardiac monitoring is necessary because of the risk of dysrhythmias associated with an elevated potassium level. This client also tests positive for COVID-19 and exhibits signs of the viral infection. Although the client has no shortness of breath or difficulty breathing, the SpO_2 reading is 89% on RA, which warrants the need for oxygen. COVID-19 is a viral infection; therefore there is no need for ceftriaxone, an antibiotic that treats bacterial infections. An antibiotic is not helpful and could actually be harmful in treating a viral infection because of its effect on the immune system, and could lead to a superinfection. Although the blood culture is pending, there is no evidence of bacterial infection warranting the use of an antibiotic. Older adults and those individuals who have underlying medical conditions such as diabetes seem to be at higher risk for developing more serious complications from COVID-19 illness. In severe cases of COVID-19, these individuals may develop abnormal blood clots. This client is at high risk for developing VTE because of the report of immobility for the last 3 weeks and the elevated D-dimer level. Therefore prophylaxis with enoxaparin, a low-molecular-weight anticoagulant, is warranted. Tocilizumab, a monoclonal antibody, is currently used to treat hospitalized clients with COVID-19 who show signs of inflammation and experience hypoxemia. This client has an elevated C-reactive protein, indicating the presence of inflammation, and an SpO_2 of 89% on RA. Dexamethasone, a corticosteroid, may also be prescribed to treat inflammation and reduce mortality in COVID.

Test-Taking Strategy: Note that the question is asking for potential interventions that are either anticipated or contraindicated/not helpful to the client with DKA complicated by COVID-19 infection. Think about the clinical scenario and what each of the listed interventions would do for this client. Look at each option provided, and think about the potential effect of that information and how that relates to promoting safe client care. Organize your thought process as illustrated in the table.

Intervention	Potential Effect	Promotes/Inhibits Safety/Neither
O₂ per NC	Treat hypoxemia related to respiratory infection	Promotes
0.45% normal saline infusion	Hypotonic, does not add to the glucose load; administered with regular IV insulin	Promotes
Insulin glargine bolus	Long-acting insulin, not useful in treating acutely elevated blood glucose levels	Inhibits
Continuous infusion of regular insulin diluted in normal saline	Treat elevated blood glucose levels associated with DKA	Promotes
IV potassium	Currently hyperkalemic	Inhibits
Continuous cardiac monitoring	Help detect complications of condition and need for treatment	Promotes
Enoxaparin subcutaneously daily	Help prevent VTE	Promotes
Tocilizumab and dexamethasone	Treat inflammation associated with COVID-19 infection	Promotes
Ceftriaxone	Antibiotic: not necessary because infection is viral; may contribute to superinfection risk	Inhibits

Consider the rationale behind each of the actions in the context of whether it would promote or inhibit safety, or if the action would not make a difference either way. Each intervention that you categorize as promoting safety should be an anticipated action, whereas the interventions categorized as inhibiting safety or doing neither would be chosen as contraindicated or not helpful actions. Remember that in order to *Generate Solutions,* you need think about expected outcomes and use your hypotheses to define a set of interventions that will enable the client to achieve the expected outcomes.

CJ Cognitive Skill: Generate Solutions

Practice Question 10.17   Unfolding Case Study 3

1345: The ED physician orders are initiated and the client with DKA and COVID-19 is transferred to the acute care medical unit for hospital admission. The client is alert and oriented on admission. VS: T = 99.4°F (37.4°C); HR = 88 BPM; RR = 20 bpm; BP = 138/90 mm Hg; SpO$_2$ = 90% on RA. The admitting physician prescribes laboratory studies, and the nurse contacts the laboratory for the tests.

1415: The laboratory results are reported, and the nurse reviews the results and subsequent physician prescriptions.

Health History	Nurses' Notes	Vital Signs	Lab Tests

Laboratory Test	Current Results	Normal Reference Range
Glucose	240 mg/dL (12.6 mmol/L) **H**	74–106 mg/dL (3.9–6.1 mmol/L)
BUN	18 mg/dL (5.22 mmol/L)	10–20 mg/dL (2.9–8.2 mmol/L)
Cr	1.2 mg/dL (106 mcmol/L)	0.6–1.2 mg/dL (53–106 mcmol/L)
K	4.0 mEq/L (4.0 mmol/L)	3.5–5.0 mEq/L (3.5–5.1 mmol/L)
Na	150 mEq/L (150 mmol/L) **H**	136–145 mEq/L (136–145 mmol/L)

Based on the client assessment and laboratory findings, which three actions would be the priority?

- ☒ Administer IV potassium.
- ☐ Offer a sports drink for sipping.
- ☒ Check hourly output measurements.
- ☐ Teach about the ways to prevent dehydration.
- ☒ Administer 5% dextrose in 0.45% normal saline.

Rationale: During treatment for DKA, it is critical for the nurse to monitor the fluid and electrolyte status of the client along with the glucose levels. When treating dehydration, 0.9% or 0.45% normal saline solution is infused. A continuous infusion of regular insulin is administered to lower the blood glucose level. During the first hour of treatment, the potassium level will fall rapidly as the dehydration and acidosis are treated. To prevent hypokalemia, potassium replacement is initiated after the potassium level falls below 5.0 mEq/L (5.0 mmol/L). This client's potassium level has decreased from 5.9 mEq/L (5.9 mmol/L) to 4.0 mEq/L (4.0 mmol/L), warranting the need for potassium. Therefore this would be a first action by the nurse. Because potassium is excreted through the kidneys, adequate renal function is ensured before potassium is administered; therefore another first action is to check hourly urine outputs to ensure that the client is urinating a minimum of 30 mL/hr. This is another important intervention because if renal function is altered, potassium accumulation could occur, leading to life-threatening dysrhythmias. The blood glucose level is monitored closely. When the blood glucose level reaches 250 mg/dL (13.8 mmol/L), 5% dextrose in 0.45% normal saline is administered to help prevent hypoglycemia and cerebral edema, which can occur when serum osmolarity declines too rapidly. If the blood glucose level falls too far or too fast before the brain has time to equilibrate, water is pulled from the blood to the cerebrospinal fluid and the brain, causing cerebral edema and increased ICP. Teaching the client about self-care is important, but this would not be a first action and can wait until the emergent situation is stabilized. The client needs to be taught ways to prevent dehydration because dehydration can precipitate DKA. The client should be taught that when nausea is present, liquids containing both glucose and electrolytes, such as a sports drink, should be consumed. The client is also taught not to stop taking medications for diabetes when ill.

Test-Taking Strategy

Test-Taking Strategy: Note that this question is asking you about the actions the nurse will take based on updated assessment findings and laboratory results.

Intervention	Related to New Finding	Correct First Action?
Administer IV potassium.	Yes—decreased K level	Yes
Offer a sports drink for sipping.	Yes—decreased K level	No
Check hourly urine output amounts.	Yes—assess renal function, which can be affected by condition and treatment	Yes
Teach about the ways to prevent dehydration.	No—being managed with IV fluids	No
Administer 5% dextrose in 0.45% normal saline.	Yes—decreased blood glucose level, IV insulin	Yes

Once you determine which interventions are specifically related to a new finding (which could be related to the condition itself or to the treatment for the condition), then you want to think about whether it would be a correct *first* action. Administering IV potassium is needed because of the decreased K level and would be a correct first action to prevent hypokalemia from IV insulin therapy. Hourly urine output measurements are important to ensure adequate renal function, as the conditions and the treatments can both cause renal impairment leading to additional complications. A sports drink may be helpful is treating dehydration, but the question asks for the three priority actions; considering the options provided, this would not be a priority but could be an intervention once the others have been implemented. Teaching about ways to prevent dehydration may be important at some point in time but not as a first action. The client's condition is being treated with IV fluids, and ultimately this measure could wait until a later time once the acute issues have been resolved. Administering 5% dextrose in 0.45% normal saline is important to prevent hypoglycemia from the treatment. Because the blood glucose level has decreased, this is an important action to prevent complications of the insulin therapy. Remember that in order to *Take Action,* you need to think about the solutions that address the highest priorities and relevant problems. In this scenario the actions are focused on managing the acute condition and preventing complications related to treatment.

CJ Cognitive Skill: Take Action

Practice Question 10.18 Unfolding Case Study 3

0700: Hand-off report from the night nurse to the day nurse has been completed. The night nurse reports that the client prescriptions to treat DKA were implemented on the previous evening shift. The client also reports that the client had a comfortable night. Laboratory tests and VS were checked every 4 hours during the night and remained stable. The day nurse assesses the client and reviews the most current laboratory results.

1415: The laboratory results are reported, and the nurse reviews the results and subsequent physician prescriptions.

Health History	Nurses' Notes	Vital Signs	Lab Tests

Laboratory Test	Current Results	Normal Reference Range
Glucose	240 mg/dL (12.6 mmol/L) H	74–106 mg/dL (3.9–6.1 mmol/L)
BUN	18 mg/dL (5.22 mmol/L)	10–20 mg/dL (2.9–8.2 mmol/L)
Cr	1.2 mg/dL (106 mcmol/L)	0.6–1.2 mg/dL (53–106 mcmol/L)
K	4.0 mEq/L (4.0 mmol/L)	3.5–5.0 mEq/L (3.5–5.1 mmol/L)
Na	150 mEq/L (150 mmol/L) H	136–145 mEq/L (136–145 mmol/L)

Which findings indicate that the treatment plan is effective? For each client finding, click or place an X to specify if the finding indicates that the treatment plan is **Effective** or **Ineffective**.

Previous Client Finding	Current Client Finding	Effective	Ineffective
Glucose 240 mg/dL (12.6 mmol/L)	Glucose 190 mg/dL (10.64 mmol/L)	X	☐
Potassium 4.0 mEq/L (4.0 mmol/L)	Potassium 4.0 mEq/L (4.0 mmol/L)	X	☐
Urine output 200 mL/hr	Urine output 45 mL/hr	X	☐
Na 150 mEq/L (150 mmol/L)	Na 150 mEq/L (150 mmol/L)	☐	X

Rationale: In DKA, the priority is treating the dehydration with fluids, managing the electrolyte imbalances, and treating the hyperglycemia. DKA is considered resolved when the blood glucose is less than 200 mg/dL (11.2 mmol/L); therefore a blood glucose level of 190 mg/dL (10.64 mmol/L) indicates resolution and effectiveness of the treatment. The client's initial potassium level was 5.9 mEq/L (5.9 mmol/L), and it decreased to 4.0 mEq/L (4.0 mmol/L), which indicates a normal level. Although the nurse needs to continue to monitor the potassium level closely and for signs of an imbalance, the normal level indicates effectiveness of treatment. A manifestation of DKA is polyuria, which was an initial complaint for this client, and urine output has been 200 mL/hr. Once the dehydration and acidosis are treated, the urine output will return to normal. An output of 45 mL/hr is within the range, indicating effectiveness of treatment. The Na$^+$ level of 150 mEq/L (150 mmol/L) could indicate that further resolution of the dehydration status is necessary. The nurse would report this finding to the physician to further investigate the reason it remains elevated and to determine further necessary treatment measures.

258   Answers to Practice Questions

Test-Taking Strategy: This question is asking you to evaluate treatment effectiveness for DKA. Remember that treatments for this condition may result in a number of other effects that need to be monitored for and addressed if they occur. Think about each assessment finding and determine how it has changed and then decide whether that is in line with improvement or worsening of the condition or if the condition remains unchanged. If the result is evidence of improvement, then it would be considered effective; however, if it is evidence of worsening or is unchanged, then it would be considered ineffective. Use a thinking process as illustrated in the table.

Assessment Finding	Improvement/Worsening or Unchanged
Glucose 190 mg/dL (10.64 mmol/L)	Improvement—indicates resolution of DKA
Potassium 4.0 mEq/L (4.0 mmol/L)	Improvement—indicates resolution of hyperkalemia and avoidance of hypokalemia owing to insulin therapy
Urine output 45 mL/hr	Improvement—indicates stable renal function despite acute condition and treatment measures
Na 150 mEq/L (150 mmol/L)	Unchanged—indicates hypernatremia and possible continued dehydration; could lead to neurologic problems and needs to be reported

Remember that in order to *Evaluate Outcomes,* you need compare observed outcomes against expected outcomes, and look for evidence that the interventions were effective. In this case, you need to determine whether the assessment findings demonstrate improvement or worsening or no change with regard to DKA treatment.

CJ Cognitive Skill: Evaluate Outcomes

Unfolding Case Study 4

Content Area: Medical-Surgical Nursing
Priority Concept: Perfusion
Reference(s): Ignatavicius et al., 2021, pp. 657–658, 772–774, 781, 790; The Joint Commission (TJC), n.d.

Practice Question 10.19   Unfolding Case Study 4

A 70-year-old client arrived at the ED for chest heaviness and difficulty breathing. The nurse documents the admission assessment.

*Highlight the client findings in the medical record below that are of **immediate** concern to the nurse.*

Health History	Physical Assessment	Vital Signs	Test Results

70-year-old client admitted to the ED reporting chest heaviness and difficulty breathing for 2 days. Symptoms are noticed more with activity and subside with rest after a few minutes. Past medical history of type 2 DM, hypertension, hyperlipidemia, hypothyroidism, osteoarthritis. Currently smokes 1 pack cigarettes per day × 20 years. Medications include sliding scale insulin aspart prior to meals and at bedtime, insulin glargine at bedtime, lisinopril, atorvastatin, levothyroxine, and naproxen.

Health History	Physical Assessment	Vital Signs	Test Results

General: Appears nontoxic, well nourished, well hydrated.
Integumentary: Warm, dry, intact.
Respiratory: Lungs clear to auscultation bilaterally, no adventitious sounds. No use of accessory muscles.
Cardiovascular: HR irregularly irregular. S1 and S2 noted, no S3 or S4, no murmurs, rubs, gallops. No peripheral edema.
GI: Abdomen soft, nontender, nondistended. BS present × 4 quads.
Neurologic: Cranial nerves II–XII grossly intact.

Health History	Physical Assessment	Vital Signs	Test Results

1200: VS: T = 36.4°C (97.5°F) oral; HR = 130 BPM; RR = 20 bpm; BP = 108/59 mm Hg; SpO$_2$ = 95% on RA
Height: 165 cm (5 feet 5 inches)
Weight: 81.6 kg (180 lb)
BMI: 30.0
1200: I: 120 mL water (oral)
1230: O: 140 mL clear yellow urine

Health History	Physical Assessment	Vital Signs	Test Results

ECG:
Atrial fibrillation with rapid ventricular response, rate 130 BPM
Acute anterior and lateral MI
Intraventricular conduction delay
No ST elevation

Laboratory Test	Results	Normal Reference Range
Sodium (Na)	136 mEq/L (136 mmol/L)	136–145 mEq/L (136–145 mmol/L)
Potassium (K)	3.8 mEq/L (3.8 mmol/L)	3.5–5.0 mEq/L (3.5–5.1 mmol/L)
Calcium (Ca)	9.2 mg/dL (2.4 mmol/L)	9–10.5 mg/dL (2.25–2.62 mmol/L)
Chloride (Cl)	98 mEq/L (98 mmol/L)	98–106 mEq/L (98–106 mmol/L)
Glucose level	212 mg/dL (11.8 mmol/L) H	74–106 mg/dL (3.9–6.1 mmol/L)
Blood urea nitrogen (BUN)	22 mg/dL (7.8 mmol/L) H	10–20 mg/dL (2.9–8.2 mmol/L)
Creatinine (Cr)	1.0 mg/dL (88.3 mcmol/L)	0.6–1.2 mg/dL (53–106 mcmol/L)
Glomerular filtration rate (eGFR)	70 mL/min/1.73 m²	>60 mL/min/1.73 m²

Complete Blood Count (CBC)

White blood cells (WBC)	6000/mm³ (6.0 × 10⁹/L)	5000–10,000/mm³ (3.5–12 × 10⁹/L)
Red blood cells (RBCs)	4.6 × 10¹²/L (4.6 × 10¹²/L)	4.2–6.1 × 10¹²/L (4.2–6.2 × 10¹²/L)
Hemoglobin (Hgb)	Hgb: 13 g/dL (130 g/L)	12–18 g/dL (120–180 g/L)
Hematocrit (Hct)	38% (0.38 volume fraction)	37%–52% (0.37–0.54 volume fraction)

Cardiac Markers

Troponin T	0.8 ng/mL (0.8 mcg/L) H	<0.1 ng/mL (0.1 mcg/L)

Rationale: Client findings that are of immediate concern to the nurse include reports of chest heaviness, difficulty breathing for the last 2 days, irregularly irregular HR at 130 BPM, atrial fibrillation with rapid ventricular response, acute anterior and lateral MI, intraventricular conduction delay on the ECG, and the troponin T level of 0.8 ng/mL (0.8 mcg/L). These findings support an acute problem with the cardiovascular system and confirm that the client had an MI. In order to promote optimal outcomes, the nurse would need to follow up on these findings immediately. Other items in the health history, such as the past medical history, social history, and medications, are important and may relate to the acute condition, but are not of *immediate* concern to the nurse. The findings in the physical assessment that are of immediate concern would be the cardiovascular and respiratory findings. An irregularly irregular elevated HR is consistent with atrial fibrillation with rapid ventricular response, which is a potentially life-threatening dysrhythmia. Physical assessment findings in all other body systems are normal or stable. The troponin T level is elevated, with a normal level being <0.1 ng/mL (<0.1 mcg/L), which indicates cardiac muscle damage and is consistent with myocardial ischemia and MI. All other laboratory results are normal or only slightly out of range.

Test-Taking Strategy

Test-Taking Strategy: First, note that this question is asking which findings are of *immediate* concern to the nurse. This indicates that there may be findings that are abnormal but not of immediate concern. Remember to first identify normal/usual or abnormal/expected client findings. These findings would *not* be of immediate concern to the nurse. Next, identify abnormal/not expected findings to determine which findings are of immediate concern to the nurse. The client's findings in the medical record can be categorized as shown in the table, in order to help *Recognize Cues*.

Client Finding	Normal/Usual or Abnormal/Expected Not of Immediate Concern	Abnormal/Not Expected and of Immediate Concern
Chest heaviness	☐	☒
Difficulty breathing	☐	☒
Past medical history	☒	☐
Current smoker	☒	☐
Current medications	☒	☐
Physical assessment: General	☒	☐
Physical assessment: Integumentary	☒	☐
Physical assessment: Respiratory	☐	☒
Physical assessment: Cardiovascular	☐	☒
Physical assessment: GI	☒	☐
Physical assessment: Neurologic	☒	☐
T 36.4°C (97.5°C)	☒	☐
HR 130 BPM	☐	☒
RR 20 bpm	☒	☐
BP 108/59 mm Hg	☒	☐
SpO$_2$ 95% on RA	☒	☐

Client Finding	Normal/Usual or Abnormal/Expected Not of Immediate Concern	Abnormal/Not Expected and of Immediate Concern
I & O	☒	☐
Atrial fibrillation with rapid ventricular response, rate 130 BPM	☐	☒
Acute anterior and lateral MI	☐	☒
Intraventricular conduction delay	☐	☒
No ST elevation	☒	☐
Sodium: 136 mEq/L (136 mmol/L)	☒	☐
Potassium 3.8 mEq/L (3.8 mmol/L)	☒	☐
Calcium: 9.2 mg/dL (2.4 mmol/L)	☒	☐
Chloride: 98 mEq/L (98 mmol/L)	☒	☐
Glucose level: 212 mg/dL (11.8 mmol/L)	☒	☐
BUN: 22 mg/dL (7.8 mmol/L)	☒	☐
Cr: 1.0 mg/dL (88.3 mcmol/L)	☒	☐
eGFR 70 mL/min (2 m²)	☒	☐
WBCs: 6000/mm³ (6.0 × 10⁹/L)	☒	☐
RBCs: 4.6 × 10¹²/L (4.6 × 10¹²/L)	☒	☐
Hgb: 13 g/dL (130 g/L)	☒	☐
Hct: 38% (0.38 volume fraction)	☒	☐
Troponin T 0.8 ng/mL (0.8 mcg/L)	☐	☒

Chest heaviness; difficulty breathing; cardiovascular assessment findings (specifically the HR and rhythm); ECG findings indicating dysrhythmia, MI, and conduction delay; and the troponin T level are all findings that are of immediate concern to the nurse because they are specifically related to a life-threatening condition and require immediate follow-up to promote optimal outcomes. The other options, although they could be relevant in some way to the acute condition or abnormal, are not of immediate concern and could be safely addressed at a later time.

CJ Cognitive Skill: Recognize Cues

Practice Question 10.20   Unfolding Case Study 4

A 70-year-old client arrived at the ED for chest heaviness and difficulty breathing. The nurse is conducting the admission assessment.

Health History	Physical Assessment	Vital Signs	Test Results

1200: 70-year-old client admitted to the ED reporting chest heaviness and difficulty breathing for 2 days. Symptoms are noticed more with activity and subside with rest after a few minutes. Past medical history of type 2 DM, hypertension, hyperlipidemia, hypothyroidism, osteoarthritis. Currently smokes 1 pack cigarettes per day × 20 years. Medications include sliding scale insulin aspart prior to meals and at bedtime, insulin glargine at bedtime, lisinopril, atorvastatin, levothyroxine, and naproxen.

Health History	Physical Assessment	Vital Signs	Test Results

General: Appears nontoxic, well nourished, well hydrated.
Integumentary: Warm, dry, intact.
Respiratory: Lungs clear to auscultation bilaterally, no adventitious sounds. No use of accessory muscles.
Cardiovascular: HR irregularly irregular. S1 and S2 noted, no S3 or S4, no murmurs, rubs, gallops. No peripheral edema.
GI: Abdomen soft, nontender, nondistended. BS present × 4 quads.
Neurologic: Cranial nerves II–XII grossly intact.

Health History	Physical Assessment	Vital Signs	Test Results

1200: VS: T = 36.4°C (97.5°F) oral; HR = 130 BPM; RR = 20 bpm; BP = 108/59 mm Hg; SpO_2 = 95% on RA
Height: 165 cm (5 feet 5 inches)
Weight: 81.6 kg (180 lb)
BMI: 30.0
1200: I: 120 mL water (oral)
1230: O: 140 mL clear yellow urine

Health History	Physical Assessment	Vital Signs	Test Results

ECG:
Atrial fibrillation with rapid ventricular response, rate 130 BPM
Acute anterior and lateral MI
Intraventricular conduction delay
No ST elevation

Laboratory Test	Results	Normal Reference Range
Sodium (Na)	136 mEq/L (136 mmol/L)	136–145 mEq/L (136–145 mmol/L)
Potassium (K)	3.8 mEq/L (3.8 mmol/L)	3.5–5.0 mEq/L (3.5–5.1 mmol/L)
Calcium (Ca)	9.2 mg/dL (2.4 mmol/L)	9–10.5 mg/dL (2.25–2.62 mmol/L)
Chloride (Cl)	98 mEq/L (98 mmol/L)	98–106 mEq/L (98–106 mmol/L)
Glucose level	212 mg/dL (11.8 mmol/L) **H**	74–106 mg/dL (3.9–6.1 mmol/L)
Blood urea nitrogen (BUN)	22 mg/dL (7.8 mmol/L) **H**	10–20 mg/dL (2.9–8.2 mmol/L)
Creatinine (Cr)	1.0 mg/dL (88.3 mcmol/L)	0.6–1.2 mg/dL (53–106 mcmol/L)
Glomerular filtration rate (eGFR)	70 mL/min/1.73 m²	>60 mL/min/1.73 m²
Complete Blood Count (CBC)		
White blood cells (WBC)	6000/mm³ (6.0 × 10⁹/L)	5000–10,000/mm³ (3.5–12 × 10⁹/L)
Red blood cells (RBCs)	4.6 × 10¹²/L (4.6 × 10¹²/L)	4.2–6.1 × 10¹²/L (4.2–6.2 × 10¹²/L)
Hemoglobin (Hgb)	Hgb: 13 g/dL (130 g/L)	12–18 g/dL (120–180 g/L)
Hematocrit (Hct)	38% (0.38 volume fraction)	37%–52% (0.37–0.54 volume fraction)
Cardiac Markers		
Troponin T	0.8 ng/mL (0.8 mcg/L) **H**	<0.1 ng/mL (0.1 mcg/L)

Based on the assessment findings, the nurse monitors for complications. Complete the following sentence by choosing from the lists of options provided.

The client is at **highest** risk for developing <u>diminished cardiac output</u> as evidenced by <u>cardiovascular assessment</u>.

Options for 1	Options for 2
Fluid volume overload	I&O
Diminished cardiac output	Respiratory assessment
Decreased renal perfusion	Neurologic assessment
VTE	Cardiovascular assessment

Rationale: Atrial fibrillation is a cardiac dysrhythmia in which the atria quiver as a result of chaotic electrical signals. This dysrhythmia is often accompanied by a rapid ventricular response, causing a rapid HR. Owing to the ineffectiveness of this rhythm, there is a risk for diminished cardiac output. In addition, the ECG results indicate MI, which is tissue necrosis of the heart muscle. This can also contribute to diminished cardiac output. The cardiovascular assessment findings are characteristic of diminished cardiac output. Fluid volume overload, decreased renal perfusion, and VTE could also occur as potential complications for someone experiencing atrial fibrillation and MI; however, the highest risk complication would be diminished cardiac output. Diminished cardiac output would be a predisposing factor to these other complications and can affect all body organ systems.

Test-Taking Strategy: Looking at each complication listed in the first set of options, determine the supportive data from the clinical scenario for each condition. The client's findings in the medical record can be categorized as shown in the table to help *Analyze Cues.* Remember that with *Analyze Cues* you are thinking about what could be happening to the client based on the information in the clinical scenario.

Test-Taking Strategy

Complication	Supportive Data
Fluid volume overload	Chest heaviness Difficulty breathing Past medical history Cardiovascular assessment (although there is no peripheral edema, which is usually noted) VS (HR specifically)
Diminished cardiac output	Chest heaviness Difficulty breathing Past medical history Cardiovascular assessment VS (HR and BP) ECG results
Decreased renal perfusion	Past medical history BUN level (although creatinine is not elevated and eGFR is not low)
VTE	Chest heaviness Difficulty breathing Past medical history ECG results

The complication with the most supportive data would be the one that is the highest risk. Chest heaviness and difficulty breathing could both be present with fluid volume overload, diminished cardiac output, and VTE. The client's past medical history could also predispose the client to any of these complications. The VS and cardiovascular assessment, which shows a rapid irregular HR and atrial fibrillation, could potentially lead to fluid overload and diminished cardiac output. In fluid overload, however, it is very common to see peripheral edema, and this is not present, making this complication less likely in comparison to diminished cardiac output. The laboratory results show an elevated BUN, but the Cr and eGFR are both normal; therefore decreased renal perfusion would be less likely compared with diminished cardiac output. Although the ECG shows evidence of atrial fibrillation, there are no findings on the physical assessment that elevate the suspicion of VTE, such as redness, swelling, and pain in an extremity, and therefore this is less likely than diminished cardiac output. Thinking about the pathophysiology of each of the listed complications and considering all of the data available to you will assist in *Analyzing Cues* and will direct you to the correct options. Remember that in the Drop-Down Rationale item type, you need to select the correct potential complication first in order to select the correct evidence to support that complication.

CJ Cognitive Skill: Analyze Cues

Practice Question 10.21   Unfolding Case Study 4

A 70-year-old client arrived at the ED for chest heaviness and difficulty breathing. The nurse is conducting the admission assessment.

Health History	Physical Assessment	Vital Signs	Test Results

1200: 70-year-old client admitted to the ED reporting chest heaviness and difficulty breathing for 2 days. Symptoms are noticed more with activity and subside with rest after a few minutes. Past medical history of type 2 DM, hypertension, hyperlipidemia, hypothyroidism, osteoarthritis. Currently smokes 1 pack cigarettes per day × 20 years. Medications include sliding scale insulin aspart prior to meals and at bedtime, insulin glargine at bedtime, lisinopril, atorvastatin, levothyroxine, and naproxen.

Health History	Physical Assessment	Vital Signs	Test Results

General: Appears nontoxic, well nourished, well hydrated.
Integumentary: Warm, dry, intact.
Respiratory: Lungs clear to auscultation bilaterally, no adventitious sounds. No use of accessory muscles.
Cardiovascular: HR irregularly irregular. S1 and S2 noted, no S3 or S4, no murmurs, rubs, gallops. No peripheral edema.
GI: Abdomen soft, nontender, nondistended. BS + × 4 quads.
Neurologic: Cranial nerves II–XII grossly intact.

Health History	Physical Assessment	Vital Signs	Test Results

1200: VS: T = 36.4°C (97.5°F) oral; HR = 130 BPM; RR = 20 bpm; BP = 108/59 mm Hg; SpO$_2$ = 95% on RA
Height: 165 cm (5 feet 5 inches)
Weight: 81.6 kg (180 lb)
BMI: 30.0
1200: I: 120 mL water (oral)
1230: O: 140 mL clear yellow urine

Health History	Physical Assessment	Vital Signs	Test Results

ECG:
Atrial fibrillation with rapid ventricular response, rate 130 BPM
Acute anterior and lateral MI
Intraventricular conduction delay
No ST elevation

Laboratory Test	Results	Normal Reference Range
Sodium (Na)	136 mEq/L (136 mmol/L)	136–145 mEq/L (136–145 mmol/L)
Potassium (K)	3.8 mEq/L (3.8 mmol/L)	3.5–5.0 mEq/L (3.5–5.1 mmol/L)
Calcium (Ca)	9.2 mg/dL (2.4 mmol/L)	9–10.5 mg/dL (2.25–2.62 mmol/L)
Chloride (Cl)	98 mEq/L (98 mmol/L)	98–106 mEq/L (98–106 mmol/L)
Glucose level	212 mg/dL (11.8 mmol/L) H	74–106 mg/dL (3.9–6.1 mmol/L)
Blood urea nitrogen (BUN)	22 mg/dL (7.8 mmol/L) H	10–20 mg/dL (2.9–8.2 mmol/L)
Creatinine (Cr)	1.0 mg/dL (88.3 mcmol/L)	0.6–1.2 mg/dL (53–106 mcmol/L)
Glomerular filtration rate (eGFR)	70 mL/min/1.73 m²	>60 mL/min/1.73 m²
Complete Blood Count (CBC)		
White blood cells (WBCs)	6000/mm³ (6.0 × 10⁹/L)	5000–10,000/mm³ (3.5–12 × 10⁹/L)
Red blood cells (RBCs)	4.6 × 10¹²/L (4.6 × 10¹²/L)	4.2–6.1 × 10¹²/L (4.2–6.2 × 10¹²/L)
Hemoglobin (Hgb)	Hgb: 13 g/dL (130 g/L)	12–18 g/dL (120–180 g/L)
Hematocrit (Hct)	38% (0.38 volume fraction)	37%–52% (0.37–0.54 volume fraction)
Cardiac Markers		
Troponin T	0.8 ng/mL (0.8 mcg/L) H	<0.1 ng/mL (0.1 mcg/L)

The nurse has completed the admission assessment and is initiating the plan of care. The nurse notes that the cardiologist has been consulted and has ordered further diagnostic testing.
Based on the clinical scenario, complete the following sentence by dragging one answer from each list of options.

The **priority** and **most specific** diagnostic test would be cardiac catheterization to assess for blockages and narrowed vessels.

Options for 1	Options for 2
D-dimer level	Blood clots
Chest radiograph	Cardiomegaly
Cardiac catheterization	Hyperthyroidism
Trended electrolyte levels	Hypokalemia or hyperkalemia
Thyroid-stimulating hormone	Blockages and narrowed vessels

Rationale: For acute coronary syndrome, which includes acute MI, a number of diagnostic tests could be ordered to assess for various causes contributing to this health problem. The priority diagnostic test would be cardiac catheterization, as this is the most definitive test in diagnosing heart disease. Indications for cardiac catheterization include confirmation of suspected heart problems such as congenital abnormalities, coronary artery disease, myocardial disease, valvular disease, and valvular dysfunction. It is also done to determine the location and extent of the problem; determine the best therapeutic option, such as angioplasty, stenting, bypass graft, or valve replacement; and to evaluate the effects of medical or invasive treatment for cardiac problems. Because the ECG indicates MI, the client needs to undergo cardiac catheterization for further diagnostic determination of the extent of the problem as well as for treatment of the problem. The D-dimer level is helpful in evaluating for the presence of blood clots; however, this is a nonspecific test and the result can be elevated by several conditions, such as pregnancy, liver disease, inflammation, malignancy, and hypercoagulable states. Given the client's symptoms, a D-dimer would be helpful but would not be the priority diagnostic test. A chest-x-ray may be done to assess for cardiomegaly or other complications of ischemia such as pulmonary edema but will not determine further treatment measures for this client. This would not be the priority diagnostic test because it would not provide information needed to treat the causative factors. Trending electrolyte levels are important because electrolyte imbalances, particularly potassium, can result in cardiac dysrhythmias that may lead to myocardial ischemia or MI and diminished cardiac output. This client's electrolyte levels were all within normal range 1 hour ago, and so this would not be the priority diagnostic test at this time. That the client is already experiencing MI would make this laboratory test of lesser importance in comparison to the cardiac catheterization. A thyroid-stimulating hormone level may provide information on other, less common causes of MI, such as hyperthyroidism. This diagnostic test may be done especially if there are no blockages or narrowed vessels causing the ischemia or infarction. As with the other tests, in comparison with the cardiac catheterization, this test is of a lesser priority at this point in time.

Test-Taking Strategy: Note the strategic word *priority* in this question. The ability to use judgment and prioritize client needs is necessary to *Prioritize Hypotheses.* Considering the client's needs in the context of the current health problem she is experiencing can help you decide on priorities of care and the most important diagnostic test to further direct client care. Think about whether the test would be the *initial* step in determination of further treatment. Using a thinking process as illustrated in the table may be helpful to *Prioritize Hypotheses.*

Test-Taking Strategy

Diagnostic Test	Initial Step in Determining Further Treatment	Helpful but Not an Initial Step in Determining Further Treatment
D-dimer level	☐	☒
Chest radiograph	☐	☒
Cardiac catheterization	☒	☐
Trended electrolyte levels	☐	☒
Thyroid-stimulating hormone	☐	☒

Another way to look at this is whether the diagnostic test would address the *highest priority* problem for the client based on the clinical scenario, which would be narrowed or blocked cardiac blood vessels. Use this thinking process as illustrated in the table.

Diagnostic Test	Addresses Narrowed or Blocked Vessels
D-dimer level	No
Chest radiograph	No
Cardiac catheterization	Yes
Trended electrolyte levels	No
Thyroid stimulating hormone	No

Once you determine that cardiac catheterization is the *priority* diagnostic test because it is the *most important* in promoting optimal outcomes, you then need to choose the correct indication. Use your nursing knowledge of the indications for cardiac catheterization to assist in directing you to the correct option of assessing for blockages or narrowed cardiac vessels as the second answer. Remember that in order to *Prioritize Hypotheses,* you need to decide on the diagnostic test that is of *highest priority* first, and then decide on the correct indication.

CJ Cognitive Skill: Prioritize Hypotheses

Practice Question 10.22   Unfolding Case Study 4

The consulting cardiologist ordered cardiac catheterization for a 70-year-old client suspected of having an MI. Stents were placed, and blood flow was re-established to the affected areas of the heart. The procedure has been completed, and the nurse is monitoring the client on the intermediate care unit. The left femoral vein was used as the insertion site for the procedure.

Choose the interventions the nurse would plan in the care of this client following cardiac catheterization. **Select all that apply.**

- ☒ Assess for shortness of breath.
- ☐ Keep both extremities straight.
- ☐ Encourage activity as tolerated.
- ☒ Apply a soft knee brace to the left leg.
- ☒ Position the client in a supine position.
- ☒ Monitor the client for changes in mental status.
- ☒ Monitor the VS every 15 minutes initially.
- ☒ Assess the insertion site for bloody drainage or hematoma.
- ☐ Apply SCDs to both lower extremities.
- ☒ Assess circulation, sensation, and motion of the affected extremity.

Rationale: For a cardiac catheterization procedure, the client is taken to the catheterization laboratory ("cath lab") and positioned on the table securely. The cardiologist or technician injects a local anesthetic to the insertion site. A catheter is then inserted into the access site, usually through the femoral vein to the inferior vena cava or through the basilic vein to the superior vena cava. The catheter is advanced into the right atrium, through the right ventricle, and through the pulmonary artery if needed. Intracardiac pressures are measured, and blood samples are obtained. The contrast medium is injected to detect cardiac shunts or regurgitation from the valves or narrowed or blocked cardiac vessels. If the left side of the heart needs to be examined, then the catheter is advanced up the aorta, across the aortic valve, and into the left ventricle, and abnormalities are visualized, and blood samples obtained as indicated. Follow-up care following this procedure is important to prevent complications of cardiac catheterization. The client is monitored closely after the procedure. The nurse would assess for shortness of breath and monitor the client's mental status, because pulmonary edema, dysrhythmias, PE, MI, cardiac tamponade, and bleeding are all complications of this procedure. VS are monitored every 15 minutes initially, and then every 30 minutes for 2 hours or until the VS are stable, as per agency policy. The affected extremity (not both extremities) needs to be kept straight for a period of 2 to 6 hours after the procedure to prevent bleeding; therefore activity as tolerated would be avoided. A soft knee brace on the affected extremity can help the client to remember to keep the leg straight. Typically the client is placed in a supine position, and the head of bed would not be elevated above 30 degrees as prescribed by the cardiologist. The insertion site is assessed every 15 to 30 minutes to monitor for bloody drainage or hematoma. SCDs are used to improve blood flow to the lower extremities but are not indicated following cardiac catheterization and could potentially increase the risk for bleeding in the insertion site.

Test-Taking Strategy: Note that the question is asking about planning care for the client following cardiac catheterization. Think about the clinical scenario, what is involved with the procedure, and the potential complications of the procedure. Look at each option provided, and think about the potential effect of the intervention and how that relates to promoting safe client care. Organize your thought process as illustrated in the table.

Test-Taking Strategy

Intervention	Potential Effect After Cardiac Catheterization	Promotes/Inhibits Safety or Neither
Assess for shortness of breath.	Helps detect complications of procedure.	Promotes
Keep both extremities straight.	Keeping affected extremity straight is necessary, but it is not necessary to keep both extremities straight.	Promotes for the affected extremity, neither for the other extremity
Encourage activity as tolerated.	Bed rest needs to be maintained to prevent bleeding and to promote hemodynamic stability.	Inhibits
Apply a soft knee brace to the left leg.	May help the client to remember to keep the affected extremity straight.	Promotes
Position the client in a supine position.	Helps to maintain hemodynamic stability, minimizes pain, prevents bleeding at insertion site.	Promotes
Monitor the client for changes in mental status.	Helps detect complications of the procedure.	Promotes
Monitor the VS every 15 minutes initially.	Helps detect complications of the procedure.	Promotes
Assess the insertion site for bloody drainage or hematoma.	Assesses for postprocedural bleeding.	Promotes
Apply SCDs to both lower extremities.	May increase risk for bleeding.	Inhibits
Assess circulation, sensation, and motion of the affected extremity.	Helps detect complications of the procedure.	Promotes

Consider the rationale behind each of the interventions in the context of whether it would promote or inhibit safety, or if the action would not make a difference either way. Assessing for shortness of breath; monitoring the client's mental status; monitoring VS frequently initially; and assessing circulation, sensation, and motion of the affected extremity all help to detect complications of the procedure and therefore promote safety and are correct. Regarding the option that states to keep both extremities straight, note that although it would promote safety to keep the affected extremity straight, it would not make a difference for the unaffected extremity, and therefore this option is incorrect. Remember that for an option to be a correct answer, all aspects or parts of the option need to be correct. Encouraging activity as tolerated may increase the risk for bleeding and hemodynamic instability and therefore inhibits safety and is incorrect. Applying a soft knee brace may help the client to remember to keep the extremity straight and therefore would help prevent bleeding at the insertion site; this promotes safety and is correct. Positioning the client in a supine position helps to promote hemodynamic stability, minimizes pain, and helps to prevent bleeding at the insertion site and therefore promotes safety and is correct. Assessing the insertion site for bloody drainage or hematoma also promotes safety and is correct. Applying SCDs to both lower extremities, although it promotes circulation, may increase the risk for bleeding following this procedure and therefore inhibits safety and is incorrect. All options that promote safety should be selected as correct answers, and all options that inhibit safety or neither promote nor inhibit safety would be incorrect and should not be selected. Remember that in order to *Generate Solutions,* you need think about expected outcomes and use your hypotheses to define a set of interventions that will enable the client to achieve the expected outcomes.

CJ Cognitive Skill: Generate Solutions

Practice Question 10.23   Unfolding Case Study 4

A 70-year-old client was diagnosed with acute MI and post-myocardial heart failure with an ejection fraction of 30%. The nurse is initiating discharge teaching related to medication therapy.

*Which information will the nurse teach the client regarding the discharge medications? Choose the **most likely** option for the missing information in the table below by choosing from the lists of options provided.*

Medication	Dose, Route, Frequency	Drug Class	Indication
Aspirin	81 mg orally daily	Antiplatelet	MI prevention
Carvedilol	6.25 mg orally twice daily	Beta blocker	Heart failure with reduced ejection fraction
Atorvastatin	20 mg orally daily	HMG-CoA reductase inhibitor	Atherosclerotic cardiovascular disease
Lisinopril	5 mg orally daily	Angiotensin converting enzyme inhibitor	Heart failure with reduced ejection fraction
Nitroglycerin	0.4 mg sublingual every 5 minutes as needed up to 3 times	Vasodilator	Acute angina

Options for 1	Options for 2	Options for 3	Options for 4	Options for 5
Aspirin	0.6 mg sublingually every 15 minutes as needed up to 5 times	Fibrate	Acute angina	Hypertension
Ibuprofen	0.4 mg sublingually every 5 minutes as needed up to 3 times	Bile acid sequestrant	Hypertension	Hyperlipidemia
Diclofenac	0.6 mg sublingually × 1 before strenuous activity	HMG-CoA reductase inhibitor	Heart failure with reduced ejection fraction	Heart failure with reduced ejection fraction

Rationale: Aspirin, an antiplatelet medication, in the dose of 81 mg orally daily, is used for MI prevention and is prescribed at discharge following acute MI. Ibuprofen and diclofenac are similar in that they are also NSAIDs, but these medications are not used for MI prevention. Nitroglycerin is a vasodilator and, when prescribed at a dose of 0.3 to 0.6 mg sublingually every 5 minutes as needed up to 3 times, is indicated for acute angina (not every 15 minutes or up to 5 times). For acute angina, clients are also taught that if there is no relief after the first dose, they need to call EMS and then take a second and a third dose if still no relief occurs while waiting for help to arrive. Nitroglycerin may also be prescribed sublingually × 1 before strenuous activity for acute angina prevention, but can be used up to 3 times when being used for an acute angina episode. Atorvastatin is classified as an HMG-CoA reductase inhibitor. One use is for treatment of atherosclerotic cardiovascular disease and lowering cholesterol. Fibrates can be used to lower cholesterol, and fenofibrate and gemfibrozil are examples of fibrates. Bile acid sequestrants are also used to lower cholesterol, and include medications such as cholestyramine and colestipol. Carvedilol is a beta-blocker, is used for post-MI heart failure with reduced ejection fraction, and works by preventing cardiac remodeling and thereby improving contractility of the heart. It can also be used for hypertension, but hypertension is not usually the reason in post-MI management. Carvedilol is not used to manage acute angina. Lisinopril is an angiotensin-converting enzyme inhibitor and also helps with post-MI heart failure with reduced ejection fraction by the same mechanism as with carvedilol. Like carvedilol, lisinopril can also be used for hypertension, but this is not usually the reason in post-MI management. It is not used for hyperlipidemia.

Test-Taking Strategy: Note that this question is asking you about the information you will provide to the client when doing discharge teaching following acute MI with subsequent heart failure. You will need to draw on your knowledge of pharmacology in order to answer this question correctly. Use strategies for answering pharmacology questions, including recognizing common letters, such as the prefix or suffix, to place the medication into a classification, as illustrated in the table. Once you have placed the medication into a classification, then you can think about the indications for use. This strategy will help you with four of the five medications in this question.

Test-Taking Strategy

Medication	Prefix/Suffix	Medication Classification
Carvedilol	-lol	Beta-blocker (e.g., carvedilol, metoprolol, atenolol)
Lisinopril	-pril	Angiotensin-converting enzyme inhibitor (e.g., lisinopril, enalapril, captopril)
Atorvastatin	-statin	HMG-CoA reductase inhibitor (e.g., atorvastatin, simvastatin, rosuvastatin)
Nitroglycerin	Nitro-	Vasodilator

Once you are able to determine the classifications and indications for four medications, think about the last medication, *aspirin,* and recall that it is an antiplatelet agent. In the baby aspirin dose (81 mg), it is used for MI prevention. You will need to rely on your pharmacology knowledge to determine the correct dose for the nitroglycerin. Remember that in order to *Take Action,* you need to think about the solution that addresses the highest priorities. In this scenario the teaching is focused on the discharge medications, and the actions are focused on which information is included.

CJ Cognitive Skill: Take Action

The nurse is caring for a 70-year-old client who had a cardiac catheterization yesterday to confirm an MI and has completed discharge teaching using the teach-back method. This morning the nurse is evaluating the client's understanding of the discharge plan of care.

*For each of the statements made by the client, click or specify with an X whether the statement indicates an **Understanding** or **No Understanding** of the teaching provided.*

Client Statements	Understanding	No Understanding
"I should walk 1 mile at least once a day in the beginning."	☐	☒
"I will be sure to carry my nitroglycerin with me."	☒	☐
"I will check my pulse before, during, and after I do my exercises."	☒	☐
"If I notice my pulse is more than 5 BPM higher than what it usually is, I won't exercise."	☐	☒
"I will exercise indoors as much as possible."	☐	☒
"I will make sure to walk at least 3 times per week."	☒	☐
"I need to avoid straining, so I won't do push-ups or pull-ups."	☒	☐

Rationale: Cardiac rehabilitation is an important part of the recovery process following acute MI. Usually a cardiac rehabilitation specialist will provide direction on an activity and exercise schedule, depending on the specific cardiac condition and the cardiac procedures performed. The client should remain near home during the first week after discharge and should engage in a walking program, light housework, or any activity done while standing that does not cause angina. Then, during the second week, the client can increase social activities and may even be able to return to work part-time depending on the severity of the cardiac event and treatment procedures. By the third week, the client can begin lifting objects and engaging in progressively more intense activity. The client with coronary artery disease and stent placement, as in this scenario, should begin by walking approximately 400 feet 3 times each day. Walking 1 mile is an eventual goal, but not immediately following discharge. Clients should carry their nitroglycerin with them in the event they experience angina. They should check their pulse before, during, and after exercise. If their pulse increases more than 20 BPM above what it usually is, they should not continue with the activity. They should also stop the activity if they experience shortness of breath, angina, or dizziness. They should exercise outdoors when the weather is good and do not necessarily have to exercise indoors all the time. The client should progressively increase activity, with a goal of walking at least 3 times a week and increasing the distance every other week, until the total distance is 1 mile during exercise sessions. The client needs to avoid straining, such as with lifting, push-ups, pull-ups, and straining during bowel movements because of the stress these activities place on the heart.

Test-Taking Strategy

Test-Taking Strategy: This question is asking you to evaluate understanding of discharge teaching for the client following acute MI. Remember that cardiac rehabilitation is a mainstay in long-term treatment, and activity or exercise is integral to health promotion. Think about each of the client statements in the context of safety in the immediate discharge period. If the client statement described a safe action during this period, then you should categorize it as Understanding. If it is potentially unsafe during this time, then you should categorize it as No Understanding. Use a thinking process as illustrated in the table.

Client Statement	Safe/Not Safe/Incorrect in the Immediate Discharge Period
"I should walk 1 mile at least once a day in the beginning."	Not safe
"I will be sure to carry my nitroglycerin with me."	Safe
I will check my pulse before, during, and after I do my exercises."	Safe
"If I notice my pulse is more than 5 BPM higher than what it usually is, I won't exercise."	Incorrect
"I will exercise indoors as much as possible."	Incorrect
"I will make sure to walk at least 3 times per week."	Safe
"I need to avoid straining, so I won't do push-ups or pull-ups."	Safe

Carrying nitroglycerin; checking the pulse before, during, and after exercise; walking at least 3 times per week; and avoiding straining are all safe during the immediate discharge period. Walking at least 1 mile per day in the immediate discharge period is potentially unsafe, and activity needs to be gradually increased. It is safe to exercise unless the pulse rate is greater than 20 BPM higher than what is usually is, and exercising outdoors is also acceptable. Remember that in order to *Evaluate Outcomes,* you need compare observed outcomes against expected outcomes, and look for evidence that the interventions were effective. In this case, you need to determine whether the client statements demonstrate understanding or no understanding with regard to post-MI discharge teaching related to self-care and activity and exercise.

CJ Cognitive Skill: Evaluate Outcomes

Stand-alone Item 1: Trend

Content Area: Medical-Surgical Nursing
Priority Concept: Elimination
Reference(s): Ignatavicius et al., 2021, pp. 1375–1383; Pagana, et al., 2019, pp. 205–206, 269, 295, 299

The nurse is caring for a 56-year-old client admitted 2 days ago from the ED for recurring atrial fibrillation. The client has a history of obesity, heart failure, and hypertension. Today the client reports increasing pitting edema of ankles and is worried about another episode of heart failure. Morning VS are as follows: T = 98°F (36.7°C); HR = 84 BPM; RR = 20 bpm; BP = 158/92. A review of the client's I&O record shows that 24-hour urinary output on hospital day 1 was 750 mL; yesterday urinary output decreased to 535 mL. The nurse reviews the client's lab profile to compare lab results from this morning with those on the day of admission.

Health History	Lab Results	Imaging Studies	Nurses' Notes

Laboratory Test	Laboratory Results on Admission	Laboratory Results Today	Normal Reference Range
Sodium (Na)	141 mEq/L (141 mmol/L)	138 mEq/L (138 mmol/L)	136–145 mEq/L (136–145 mmol/L)
Potassium (K)	5.0 mEq/L (5.0 mmol/L)	5.5 mEq/L (5.5 mmol/L) H	3.5–5.0 mEq/L (3.5–5.0 mmol/L)
Glucose	106 mg/dL (6.0 mmol/L)	100 mg/dL (5.5 mmol/L)	70–110 mg/dL (3.9–6.1 mmol/L)
Calcium (Ca)	9.0 mEq/L (9.0 mmol/L)	8.6 mEq/L (8.6 mmol/L) L	9.0–10.5 mEq/L (9.0–10.5 mmol/L)
Blood urea nitrogen (BUN)	28 mg/dL (10.0 mmol/dL) H	38 mg/dL (13.6 mmol/L) H	8.0–23.0 mg/dL (2.9–8.2 mmol/L)
Creatinine	1.8 mg/dL (157.2 mcmol/L) H	3.1 mg/dL (274.1 mcmol/L) H	0.6–1.2 mg/dL (53–106 mcmol/L)
Hemoglobin (Hgb)	14.2 g/dL (142 g/L)	14.0 g/dL (140 g/L)	14.0–18.0 g/dL (140–180 g/L)
Hematocrit (Hct)	46% (0.46 volume fraction)	44% (0.44 volume fraction)	42%–54% (0.42–0.54 volume fraction)

*Based on the client's laboratory results, which **six physician's orders** would the nurse anticipate?*

- ☒ Prepare client for kidney imaging studies.
- ☐ Administer fluid challenge.
- ☒ Begin diuretic therapy.
- ☒ Maintain strict I&O.
- ☒ Insert indwelling urinary catheter.
- ☒ Record hourly urinary output.
- ☒ Weigh client daily before breakfast.
- ☐ Prepare client for hemodialysis.

Rationale: The clinical scenario indicates that the client is retaining fluid as evidenced by the history of heart failure and worsening ankle edema. The client also has a 24-hour urinary output that totaled 535 mL, which is only about 22 mL/hr. The minimum normal urinary output is 30 mL/hr, which the client produced on the first hospital day. Decreased urinary output may be the result of impaired kidney function, so the nurse would review the client's laboratory results. Today the client has hyperkalemia and hypocalcemia. Although there are a number of causes for these electrolyte imbalances, the rapid increase in serum creatinine indicates possible AKI. An acute impairment of kidney function results in an increased potassium and increased phosphate level. Phosphate and calcium have an inverse relationship in the body; an increased phosphate level causes a decrease in serum calcium. Creatinine is a protein waste product that is normally excreted via the kidneys to keep the serum level of this toxin as low as possible in the body. An increase of 1 to 2 mg/dL of serum creatinine per day accompanied by decreasing urinary output is consistent with AKI. The client's BUN is increased, which could be due to dehydration or AKI; urea is also a protein waste product that is eliminated by the kidneys. Although both BUN and creatinine are associated with kidney function, creatinine is the most reliable and kidney-specific test that when elevated indicates kidney impairment.

   Given that the client is likely beginning to have manifestations of AKI, the nurse would anticipate the need for collaborative interventions. A CT scan, ultrasound, and/or other imaging study would likely be ordered to help determine the cause of the impaired kidney function. Diuretic therapy is used to rid the body of excess fluid, which the client is experiencing. The client's fluid status is best monitored by taking accurate daily weights using the same scale before breakfast. Strict I&O with hourly urinary output measurements helps monitor the effectiveness of diuretic therapy and kidney function. Hourly urine output can be measured accurately if the client has an indwelling urinary catheter. A fluid challenge would not be done in this client's case because he has fluid retention with heart failure. It is too soon to determine if the client will need kidney replacement therapy such as hemodialysis.

Test-Taking Strategy: To answer this test item correctly, you'll need to approach it in a stepwise manner because it measures several cognitive skills. First, review the clinical scenario and the client's laboratory results to identify findings that are currently abnormal. Next, create a table like the one shown here to help determine which of those abnormal client findings are relevant and require immediate attention by the nurse. This step enables you to *Recognize Cues* that you will then need to analyze.

Test-Taking Strategy

Abnormal Client Finding	Abnormal Client Finding That Is Relevant and of Immediate Concern	Abnormal Client Finding That Can Be Addressed at a Later Time or Is Not of Immediate Concern
H/O obesity, heart failure, and hypertension	☐	☒
Increasing pitting ankle edema	☒	☐
Decrease in 24-hour urinary output	☒	☐
BP 158/92 mm Hg	☒	☐
Serum potassium increase	☒	☐
Serum calcium decrease	☒	☐
Blood urea nitrogen increase	☒	☐
Serum creatinine increase	☒	☐

As you can see from the table, most of the abnormal client findings are relevant in this clinical scenario and are of immediate concern to the nurse. *Analyze Cues* to determine what these data mean. The client's increasing ankle edema and increased BP indicate that the client likely has fluid retention (hypervolemia). However, the client's kidneys are not working adequately to rid the body of the excess fluid. Instead the 24-hour urinary output demonstrates that the client is eliminating less than the minimum normal output of at least 30 mL/hr. Given that the client has impaired urinary elimination, you then need to review the laboratory results and compare the previous results with today's values. Four of the eight lab tests show significant changes between admission and today. All of those changes in potassium (increased), calcium (decreased), BUN (increased), and creatinine (increased) are associated with the client's *priority* condition of AKI *(Prioritize Hypotheses)*.

Once you have determined the client's condition supported by abnormal physical and lab findings, you need to answer the test item by thinking about the interventions that are needed for clients with early-stage AKI. Use this table to help you answer the test item to measure *Generate Solutions*.

Potential Physician Order	Indicated for Clients With Early AKI	Not Indicated for Early AKI or Contraindicated for This Client
Prepare client for kidney imaging studies.	☒	☐
Administer fluid challenge.	☐	☒
Begin diuretic therapy.	☒	☐
Maintain strict I&O.	☒	☐
Insert indwelling urinary catheter.	☒	☐
Record hourly urinary output.	☒	☐
Weigh client daily before breakfast.	☒	☐
Prepare client for hemodialysis.	☐	☒

Note that the client has early-stage AKI. Apply your knowledge of pathophysiology to determine the potential interventions for this condition. Also consider the client's coexisting problems and how the interventions may affect those conditions. Use the options checked in the "Indicated" column as the correct responses for this Stand-alone item.

CJ Cognitive Skills: Recognize Cues, Analyze Cues, Prioritize Hypotheses, Generate Solutions

Stand-alone Item 2: Trend

Content Area: Medical-Surgical Nursing
Priority Concept: Gas Exchange
Reference(s): Ignatavicius et al., 2021, pp. 559–562, 608

Practice Question 10.26 | **Stand-alone Item 2: Trend**

The nurse in the surgical unit is caring for a 51-year-old postoperative client with non–small cell lung cancer (NSCLC) of the right lung who had a thoracotomy. The client has a chest tube attached to a stationary closed chest drainage system.

Health History	Physical Assessment	Vital Signs	Nurses' Notes

1300: Arrived from the PACU. Alert and oriented × 3. Resting comfortably in bed, no restlessness. Closed chest tube drainage system intact. Upper tube is near the right front lung apex, occlusive dressing dry and intact. Lower tube on the right side near the base of the lung, occlusive dressing dry and intact. Drainage chamber = 70 mL red fluid. Water seal chamber = fluctuation of fluid, no bubbling. Suction control chamber = gentle bubbling. No subcutaneous emphysema. No shortness of breath or difficulty breathing. Lung sounds clear bilaterally. HOB elevated. Trachea midline. O_2 2 L per NC. Having difficulty with coughing and deep breathing and using incentive spirometer. Pain 4/10.
1400: Alert and oriented × 3. Reports nausea. Restless, states pain is 8/10. Closed chest tube drainage system intact. Occlusive dressings dry and intact. Drainage chamber = 170 mL red fluid. Water seal chamber = fluctuation of fluid with intermittent bubbling. Suction control chamber = gentle bubbling. No subcutaneous emphysema. States difficulty breathing due to pain. Lung sounds clear bilaterally. HOB elevated. Trachea midline. O_2 2 L per NC. Refusing to cough and deep breathe or use incentive spirometer due to pain. Able to tolerate respiratory treatment with assistance of respiratory therapist. Nausea and pain medication administered as prescribed.
1500: Sleepy but arousable. Restless, states nausea subsided, pain 7/10. Closed chest tube drainage system intact. Occlusive dressings dry and intact. Drainage chamber = 170 mL red fluid. Water seal chamber = continuous bubbling. Suction control chamber = gentle bubbling. Small amount subcutaneous emphysema around upper tube near the right front lung apex. States difficulty breathing. Lung sounds = crackles in lower lobes bilaterally. Trachea = slight deviation to the left. O_2 2 L per NC. Refusing to cough and deep breathe.

Health History	Physical Assessment	Vital Signs	Nurses' Notes

	1300	1400	1500
T	99.6°F (37.5°C)	100.4°F (38.0°C)	101.6 F (38.6°C)
HR	88 BPM	96 BPM	110 BPM
RR	18 bpm	22 bpm	26 bpm
BP	100/62 mm Hg	128/88 mm Hg	140/90 mm Hg
SpO$_2$	94% on 2 L O_2 per NC	92% on 2 L O_2 per NC	90% on 2 L O_2 per NC

*Click (or check with an X) to indicate whether each nursing action listed below is either **Anticipated** (appropriate or necessary) or **Contraindicated** (could be harmful)/**Not Helpful** for the client's plan of care at this time.*

Nursing Action	Anticipated	Contraindicated/ Not Helpful
Contact the surgeon.	☒	☐
Clamp the chest tube.	☐	☒
Request an order for a stat chest x-ray.	☒	☐
Monitor the client for continued changes over the next hour.	☐	☒
Request an order for additional pain medication.	☐	☒
Flush the chest drainage tube.	☐	☒
Increase the amount of suction in the suction control.	☐	☒

Rationale: Postoperative care of a client who underwent thoracotomy requires closed-chest drainage to drain air and blood that collect in the pleural space. Stationary chest tube drainage systems, such as the Pleur-evac system, use a water-seal mechanism that acts as a one-way valve to prevent air or liquid from moving back into the chest cavity. The first chamber in the system is the drainage collection chamber, located where the chest tube(s) from the client connects to the system. Drainage from the tube(s) collects in this chamber, which has a series of calibrated columns for measurement of the drainage. The second chamber in the system is the water seal to prevent air from moving back up the tubing system and into the chest. Water oscillates (fluctuates) in this chamber (moves up as the client inhales and moves down as the client exhales). The third chamber is the suction control chamber, which provides suction when attached to a suction device, such as wall suction. The nursing care priorities for a client with a chest tube are to monitor the client closely for changes in status, ensure the integrity of the system, promote comfort, ensure chest tube patency, and prevent complications. Common complications of chest tube placement are malpositioning and empyema. Malpositioning can lead to pneumothorax or tension pneumothorax. A pneumothorax is air in the pleural space, causing a loss in negative pressure in the chest cavity, a rise in chest pressure, and a reduction in vital capacity, which can lead to lung collapse. A tension pneumothorax is a life-threatening complication of pneumothorax in which air continues to enter the pleural space during inspiration and does not exit during expiration. If not promptly detected and treated, tension pneumothorax can quickly be fatal. Empyema is the collection of purulent material in the pleural space, which can develop following lung surgery. The nurse would monitor for complications of chest tubes closely and report any unexpected findings to the surgeon immediately. The amount of drainage from the chest tubes should be no greater than 70 to 100 mL/hr. The surgeon is notified immediately if drainage amounts are greater, if drainage becomes bright red, or if drainage in the tube stops in the first 24 hours postoperatively. According to the Nurses' Notes, the client had no drainage between 1400 and 1500. Continuous bubbling in the water seal drainage is unexpected and could indicate an air leak in the system; the surgeon is notified if continuous bubbling is noted. The nurse would ensure that there is continuous gentle bubbling in the suction control chamber. Thus there are assessment findings that indicate a deterioration in the client's condition. The client has become restless because the reported pain level decreased only from 8/10 to 7/10 after the administration of pain medication. There is continuous bubbling in the water seal chamber, and some subcutaneous emphysema is noted around the upper tube near the right front lung apex. The client also states that she is experiencing difficulty breathing. Crackles are heard on auscultation of the lungs bilaterally, and there is slight deviation of the trachea to the left. In addition, the T, HR, RR, and BP have increased and the SpO_2 has decreased. Contacting the surgeon is the immediate nursing action, along with requesting a stat chest x-ray. The chest x-ray will assist in determining the cause of the deterioration in the client's condition. Clamping the chest tube is contraindicated and may increase pressure and tension in the lungs. Monitoring the client for continued changes over the next hour delays necessary immediate and life-saving interventions. Requesting an order for additional pain medication is *not* a safe action. The client received pain medication 1 hour prior, and administering additional pain medication may make the client sleepier and mask signs of a worsening deterioration. Flushing the chest tube is contraindicated. Disconnecting a chest drainage system can cause a pneumothorax. Increasing the amount of suction in the suction control chamber will not increase the drainage outflow and is not helpful. In fact, increasing the amount of suction could be harmful to lung tissue because too much suction can cause mechanical injury.

Test-Taking Strategy

Test-Taking Strategy: Note that this question is asking you to determine nursing actions based on assessment findings for a client with a chest tube following thoracotomy. Use your nursing knowledge to interpret each finding. Looking at each of the interventions listed in the options, determine whether it will help or not help the client, and also think about the rationale as to why it would help, not help or not be needed or potentially worsen the client's condition.

Intervention	Helps or Does Not Help/Potentially Worsens/Not Needed	Why?
Contact the surgeon.	Helps	Assessment findings suggestive of tension pneumothorax, contacting surgeon for further orders for necessary interventions.
Clamp the chest tube.	Does Not Help/Potentially Worsens	Increased pressure and tension in lungs.
Request an order for a stat chest x-ray.	Helps	Allows visualization of lungs and chest tube placement to determine the possible cause of the deteriorating condition.
Monitor the client for continued changes over the next hour.	Does Not Help/Potentially Worsens	More frequent assessment is needed to monitor symptoms and intervene accordingly.
Request an order for additional pain medication.	Does Not Help/Potentially Worsens/Not Needed	May mask signs of further deterioration; does not address cause of pain.
Flush the chest drainage tube.	Does Not Help/Potentially Worsens	Can cause further respiratory compromise, can cause or worsen pneumothorax.
Increase the amount of suction in the suction control.	Does Not Help/Potentially Worsens	Will not address the problem and could potentially worsen pneumothorax and harm lung tissue.

You need to identify relevant data *(Recognize Cues)*, and analyze those data and interpret their meaning in the clinical scenario *(Analyze Cues)*. Then you need to determine the priority concerns *(Prioritize Hypotheses)* and think about the solutions that address these concerns. Finally, determine the interventions that would promote safe care of the client with a chest tube *(Generate Solutions* and *Take Action)* and result in desired outcomes *(Evaluate Outcomes)*.

CJ Cognitive Skills: Recognize Cues, Analyze Cues, Prioritize Hypotheses, Generate Solutions, Evaluate Outcomes

Stand-alone Item 3: Trend

Content Area: Pediatric Nursing
Priority Concept: Gas Exchange
Reference(s): Hockenberry et al., 2019, pp. 904–905

| Practice Question 10.27 | Stand-alone Item 3: Trend |

A 2-year-old child is seen in the ED, where the ED physician diagnoses moderate acute laryngotracheobronchitis.

| Health History | Nurses' Notes | Vital Signs | Physical Assessment |

Neurologic: Alert and responsive. Resting comfortably in bed, no restlessness. Responsive to verbal and tactile stimuli.
Respiratory: Chest symmetrical. Suprasternal retractions with nasal flaring. Barking cough, labored breathing, use of accessory muscles. Inspiratory wheezes bilaterally.
Cardiovascular: S1 and S2 noted, pulse 110 BPM. No murmurs, rubs, gallops. No cyanosis, edema, clubbing, pulsations. Radial pulses 2+ bilaterally. Pedal pulses 2+ bilaterally.

| Health History | Nurses' Notes | Vital Signs | Physical Assessment |

	1000	1015	1030
Temperature	99.6°F (37.5°C)	99.4°F (37.4°C)	99.6°F (37.5°C)
Apical pulse	110 BPM	112 BPM	112 BPM
RR	34 bpm	36 bpm	34 bpm
BP	100/62 mm Hg	98/60 mm Hg	98/60 mm Hg
SpO$_2$	94% on RA	92% on RA	90% on RA

The nurse is preparing to collaborate with the ED physician about the child's plan of care. Based on the assessment findings, highlight the interventions the nurse anticipates the ED physician to order. Select all that apply.

- ☒ Oral dexamethasone
- ☒ Supplemental oxygen
- ☒ Cool mist via facemask
- ☐ Intubation with ventilation
- ☐ Strict NPO status
- ☒ Nebulized epinephrine every 20 to 30 minutes prn
- ☐ Limited interaction between the parents and child

Rationale: Acute laryngotracheobronchitis (LTB) is a type of croup experienced by children ages 6 to 36 months old. Parainfluenza viruses types 1, 2, and 3; adenoviruses; respiratory syncytial virus; and *Mycoplasma pneumoniae* are common causes. The illness is preceded by an upper respiratory infection, which descends to the lower airway structures. Clinical manifestations include low-grade fever and a barky, brassy cough after awakening, sometimes with inspiratory stridor. Agitation and crying exacerbate the symptoms and are often worse at night. A major concern with acute LTB is inflammation of the larynx and trachea, causing a narrowing of the airway. Inhaling air past the inflammation into the lungs can be difficult. This is the cause of the classic sign, inspiratory stridor. Other common manifestations include hoarseness, nasal flaring, intercostal retractions, tachypnea, and continuous stridor. Hypoxia and decreased oxygen saturation can occur when the obstruction is severe enough, which can lead to respiratory acidosis and respiratory failure. Maintaining airway patency and providing adequate respiratory support are the mainstays in the treatment of acute LTB. Oral dexamethasone is given to decrease subglottic edema. Intravenous or intramuscular dexamethasone may be given if the child is unable to tolerate oral administration. Supplemental oxygen, sometimes with mist, may be needed if hypoxemia is present. Cool mist may be provided via face mask or as blow-by and helps to constrict edematous blood vessels in the airway, thereby reducing narrowing. This child's SpO$_2$ is decreasing; therefore use of supplemental oxygen and cool mist is anticipated. Intubation and ventilation may be required if the airway obstruction is severe. Signs of impending airway obstruction include increased pulse and RR; substernal, suprasternal, and intercostal retractions; nasal flaring; and increased restlessness.

The child is not exhibiting signs of severe airway obstruction. It is important to allow the child to drink beverages of choice if the client can tolerate fluids. IV fluids may be needed if airway obstruction is severe or if the child is intubated. Nebulized epinephrine is administered every 20 to 30 minutes prn for moderate to severe cases and causes mucosal vasoconstriction and subsequent decreased subglottic edema. Children need the security of a parent's presence to minimize crying, as this can worsen the airway obstruction. Parents should be encouraged to use comfort measures such as rocking, holding, singing, and reading books with their child.

Test-Taking Strategy: Note that this question is asking you to anticipate physician orders based on assessment data in the question for the child with moderate acute LTB. Use your nursing knowledge to recall the pathophysiology associated with this condition. Recall that moderate acute LTB can cause severe airway obstruction and hypoxemia. Looking at each of the interventions listed in the options, determine whether it will help or not help this child. Also think about the rationale as to why it would help, not help or potentially worsen the child's condition, or not be needed.

Test-Taking Strategy

Intervention	Helps or Does Not Help/Potentially Worsens/Not Needed	Why?
Oral dexamethasone	Helps	Reduces epiglottic edema.
Supplemental oxygen	Helps	Treats hypoxemia related to airway narrowing.
Cool mist via facemask	Helps	Reduces airway narrowing.
Intubation with ventilation	Not Needed	Not severe enough; pulse and RR are still normal; no restlessness.
Strict NPO status	Does Not Help/ Potentially Worsens	Because airway obstruction is not severe, oral fluids can still be taken in; without adequate hydration, condition could worsen.
Nebulized epinephrine every 20 to 30 minutes prn	Helps	Reduces airway narrowing.
Limited interaction between the parents and child	Does Not Help/ Potentially Worsens	Can cause fear in the child and thus increase crying and worsen airway narrowing.

You need to identify relevant data *(Recognize Cues)*, and analyze those data and interpret their meaning in the clinical scenario *(Analyze Cues)*. Then you need to determine the priority concerns *(Prioritize Hypotheses)*, think about the solutions that address these concerns *(Generate Solutions)*, and determine the interventions that would promote safe care of the child with moderate acute LTB *(Take Action)* and result in expected outcomes *(Evaluate Outcomes)*. Oral dexamethasone will help to reduce airway narrowing. Because the child's airway is still patent as noted through the physical assessment and VS, this medication can safely be given orally; therefore this is a correct answer. Supplemental oxygen is indicated and will treat the hypoxemia as noted by the low SpO_2 level, and this option is correct. Cool mist via facemask may also help to reduce airway narrowing and therefore is a correct option. Signs of impending airway obstruction are not present; therefore intubation and ventilation would not be anticipated at this time. Strict NPO status would be needed if airway obstruction were severe; because it is not severe, the child should be encouraged to continue taking in oral fluids to prevent dehydration, and this is an incorrect option. Nebulized epinephrine every 20 to 30 minutes prn will help to reduce airway narrowing and therefore is a correct answer. Lastly, recall that interaction between the child and parents is important during stressful times and will reduce fear and distress and crying, thereby helping with maintaining a patent airway, making this option incorrect.

CJ Cognitive Skills: Recognize Cues, Analyze Cues, Prioritize Hypotheses, Generate Solutions, Evaluate Outcomes

Stand-alone Item 4: Bow-tie

Content Area: Pharmacology
Priority Concept: Tissue Integrity
Reference(s): Burchum & Rosenthal, 2019, pp. 1039–1042; Ignatavicius et al., 2021, pp. 452–455; Lilley et al., 2020, p. 598

Practice Question 10.28   **Stand-alone Item 4: Bow-tie**

The nurse is assigned to care for a 74-year-old client who was admitted this morning for a spider bite (type unknown) on the left calf that occurred 3 days ago while hiking. Since that time, the leg has become increasingly reddened, hot, swollen, and painful. This morning the bite area started to drain a moderate amount of greenish-yellow exudate, which prompted the client to go to the ED. VS: T = 98.4°F (36.9°C); HR = 85 BPM; RR = 16 bpm; BP = 128/76 mm Hg; SpO$_2$ = 97% on RA. The client's medical history includes type 2 DM, chronic heart failure, and hypertension. The client was admitted for IV drug therapy with ceftriaxone and observation. The nurse is preparing to administer the first dose of ceftriaxone to the client.

Complete the diagram by dragging from the choices below to specify what drug classification ceftriaxone is in, two actions the nurse would take when caring for the client receiving this drug, and two parameters the nurse would monitor to assess the client's progress and the effectiveness of the drug.

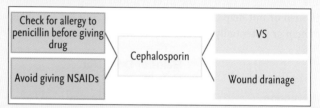

Actions to Take	Drug Classification	Parameters to Monitor
Check for allergy to penicillin before giving drug.	Penicillin	Oxygen saturation
Assess for fluid retention.	Carbapenem	VS
Monitor for seizures.	Cephalosporin	Wound drainage
Avoid giving NSAIDs.	Monobactam	Breath sounds
Assess for dysrhythmias.		Serum potassium

Rationale: The client is started on ceftriaxone, which is a long-acting third-generation cephalosporin (antibiotic), because of a local infection known as cellulitis. The client's infection seems to be localized because the client does not have a fever or other indications of systemic infection. The client was likely hospitalized rather than managed at home because the client is older and has type 2 DM. Because cephalosporins are structurally and pharmacologically similar or related to the penicillin class of antibiotics, some clients who are allergic to penicillins are also allergic to cephalosporins. Therefore before administering the first dose of ceftriaxone, the nurse would check the medical record for allergies and ask the client about any known penicillin allergy. Unlike many of the cephalosporins, ceftriaxone can cause bleeding. The nurse would observe for bleeding or excessive bruising and avoid giving the client any other drug that can cause bleeding such as NSAIDs. In addition, NSAIDs can lead to or worsen AKI. Cephalosporins do not cause fluid retention. This class of drugs is also not associated with development of seizures or dysrhythmias. Antibiotic therapy with a cephalosporin should resolve the client's cellulitis, which is a skin and tissue infection from a spider bite in this clinical scenario. The client currently has *local* signs and symptoms of infection including a moderate amount of greenish-yellow wound drainage. If the infection does not respond to IV antibiotic therapy, the infection may become *systemic,* causing an increase in body temperature, increased white blood cells, and possibly sepsis. Therefore the nurse would want to monitor the client's VS for possible systemic infection, especially the development of a fever. The nurse would also monitor the characteristics and amount of drainage from the wound. If the client's cellulitis resolves, the nurse would expect the drainage to decrease and change from greenish-yellow to clear or tan. Monitoring oxygen saturation and breath sounds would not provide the information that is needed about the client's cellulitis. Ceftriaxone does not affect serum potassium levels.

Test-Taking Strategy: Because this type of NGN test item can measure all clinical judgment cognitive skills, you'll need to use a multistep approach to select the correct responses in each part of the Bow-tie figure. First, you need to *Recognize Cues* to determine relevant abnormal client findings that would be immediately concerning. The client presented to the ED with a spider bite that caused signs and symptoms that worsened at home. These signs and symptoms when grouped together are indicative of skin and tissue infection, a condition called cellulitis. Once you *Analyze Cues* to ascertain the priority and immediate client condition *(Prioritize Hypotheses),* you then need to determine what type of drug would be prescribed. Given that the client has an infection, antibiotic therapy would be the most appropriate drug to be administered. Apply knowledge about ceftriaxone and recall that it is classified as a cephalosporin. Consider each of the options in the test item as to whether the action (in the left well of the Bow-tie) would be appropriate for a client taking ceftriaxone. A table as illustrated here will help you determine which actions are appropriate for a client receiving ceftriaxone.

Potential Nursing Action	Appropriate Nursing Action to Take for Client Receiving Ceftriaxone	Not an Appropriate Nursing Action to Take for Client Receiving Ceftriaxone
Check for allergy to penicillin before giving drug.	☒	☐
Assess for fluid retention.	☐	☒
Monitor for seizures.	☐	☒
Avoid giving NSAIDs.	☒	☐
Assess for dysrhythmias.	☐	☒

The last part of the test item asks you identify the parameters in the right well of the Bow-tie that the nurse would monitor while the client is receiving ceftriaxone to determine if it was effective. The nurse could conclude that drug therapy is effective if the client's condition improves as shown in the table.

Potential Parameter (Client Finding) the Nurse Would Monitor While Client Is Taking Ceftriaxone	Parameter Would Support Client Is Improving and Ceftriaxone Is Effective? Yes or No	Expected Outcome That Would Indicate Client Is Improving
Oxygen saturation	No	N/A
VS	Yes	Temperature and pulse within normal limits
Wound drainage	Yes	Less wound drainage and color change from greenish-yellow to tan or clear
Breath sounds	No	N/A
Serum potassium	No	N/A

N/A, Not applicable.

Consider the client's condition and assessment findings. Two of the parameters (client findings) indicated by a "Yes" should be monitored because they indicate if the wound and cellulitis are improving, the client is progressing, and the drug is effective in managing the local infection. These parameters, VS and wound drainage, are the correct responses to this part of the test item.

CJ Cognitive Skills: Recognize Cues, Analyze Cues, Prioritize Hypotheses, Generate Solutions, Take Action, Evaluate Outcomes

Stand-alone Item 5: Bow-tie

Content Area: Pharmacology
Priority Concept: Clotting
Reference(s): Burchum & Rosenthal, 2019, p. 620; Ignatavicius et al., 2021, pp. 652–653;
Lilley et al., 2020, pp. 404–406

| Practice Question 10.29 | Stand-alone Item 5: Bow-tie |

A 72-year-old client is being prepared for hospital discharge following treatment for a new-onset episode of atrial fibrillation. The client's medical history notes that the client has a long-term history of heart failure that has been treated with diet and medications, including furosemide, lisinopril, and carvedilol. Apixaban 5 mg orally twice daily has been added to the home medication regimen. The nurse plans discharge teaching for the client about the new medication.

Complete the diagram by dragging from the choices below to specify the primary adverse effect of apixaban, two points the nurse would teach the client, and two statements that indicate understanding following teaching.

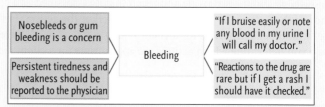

Teaching Points	Primary Adverse Effect	Statements Indicating Understanding
Headaches are a common side effect of the drug and are expected.	Bleeding	"Ibuprofen is best to take if I have a headache."
Right side pain radiating to the shoulder is common.	Hypotension	"I really hope that I don't end up getting gallbladder stones from this drug."
Urinary retention can occur during treatment.	Gallbladder stones	"If I bruise easily or note any blood in my urine I will call my doctor."
Nosebleeds or gum bleeding is a concern.	Renal impairment	"I need to have my blood work checked twice weekly while I am taking this medication."
Persistent tiredness and weakness should be reported to the physician.		"Reactions to the drug are rare but if I get a rash I should have it checked."

Rationale: Heart failure, also called pump failure, is a general term for the inability of the heart to work effectively as a pump. In atrial fibrillation (AF), multiple rapid impulses from many atrial foci depolarize the atria in a totally disorganized manner at a rate of 350 to 600 times a minute; ventricular response is usually 120 to 200 BPM. The result is a chaotic rhythm with no clear P waves, no atrial contractions, loss of atrial kick, and an irregular ventricular response. The atria merely quiver. Often the ventricles beat with a rapid rate in response to the numerous atrial impulses. The rapid and irregular ventricular rate decreases ventricular filling and reduces cardiac output. This alteration in cardiac function allows for blood to pool, placing the client at risk for clotting concerns such as DVT, PE, or stroke. AF is frequently associated with underlying cardiovascular disease because of the atrial fibrosis and loss of muscle mass that occurs. These structural changes are common in heart diseases such as hypertension, heart failure, and coronary artery disease. Because clotting problems is a concern, these clients require long-term anticoagulation to prevent stroke and thrombus formation. Apixaban is an anticoagulant that may be prescribed to prevent these complications of AF. The primary adverse effect of apixaban is bleeding; therefore the client needs to be taught to monitor for any signs of bruising or bleeding such as from the nose or gums. In addition, persistent tiredness and weakness could be a sign of occult bleeding; if indications of bleeding occur, the physician needs to be notified. Headaches are not expected and are not a common side effect of the medication. However, persistent headaches could be an indication of bleeding. Ibuprofen would not be given because it is an NSAID and can increase the risk for bleeding. Hypotension is not an adverse effect of this drug, although the BP would drop if the client was bleeding. Gallbladder stones are not an adverse effect and are not associated with this drug; therefore right side pain radiating to the shoulder is not likely to occur. Renal impairment is not an adverse effect; however, if the client has renal impairment, then the excretion of apixaban can be delayed, increasing the risk of bleeding. Urinary retention is not associated with this drug, although this could be a manifestation of a coexisting renal problem if one existed. The client taking apixaban does not need to have blood work checked twice a week. Laboratory tests, such as hematocrit, hemoglobin, and red blood cell count, and coagulation studies may be performed periodically to monitor progress or check for adverse effects, or they may be done before any invasive procedure is performed to ensure that bleeding is not a risk. Reactions to the drug can occur but are rare. If a reaction does occur, the client is likely to develop a rash and needs to contact the physician for instructions.

Although the client is also on furosemide, lisinopril, and carvedilol, because the apixaban is a new medication, the nurse would be sure to thoroughly conduct teaching and evaluate effectiveness of the teaching related to this medication.

Test-Taking Strategy: Recall that this NGN item type measures multiple clinical judgment cognitive skills. First, you need to *Recognize Cues* to determine relevant data that would be the priority in planning care for this client. The client has new-onset AF and is being discharged to home after starting a new medication. Next, *Analyze Cues* by considering the client's health problems, a long-term history of heart failure, and other prescribed medications. Note that the client is taking furosemide, lisinopril, and carvedilol, and that apixaban is being added as a new medication. *Prioritize Hypotheses* by focusing on apixaban because it is a new medication for this client, and think about the primary adverse effects of this medication. Start to answer this question by selecting the adverse effect from the middle well of the Bow-tie. Use knowledge about apixaban, and recall that it is classified as an anticoagulant, to choose bleeding as the primary adverse effect. Next, consider each of the teaching point options (in the left well of the Bow-tie) and their relation to apixaban as an anticoagulant *(Generate Solutions* and *Take Action)*. Use a thinking process as illustrated in the table to choose the correct teaching points for this question.

Test-Taking Strategy

Teaching Point	Related to Apixaban and Bleeding as an Adverse Effect	Not Related to Apixaban and Bleeding as an Adverse Effect
Headaches are a common side effect of the drug and are expected	☐	☒
Right side pain radiating to the shoulder is common	☐	☒
Urinary retention can occur during treatment	☐	☒
Nosebleeds or gum bleeding is a concern	☒	☐
Persistent tiredness and weakness should be reported to the physician	☒	☐

The last part of the question asks you to identify the evidence of teaching effectiveness, in the right well of the Bow-tie. The nurse would determine that teaching about apixaban is effective based on the client statements *(Evaluate Outcomes)*.

Client Statement	Would Help Prevent or Detect Bleeding or Other Adverse Effects/May Pose Further Risk/Is Not Necessary or Not Related
"Ibuprofen is best to take if I have a headache."	May pose further risk
"I really hope that I don't end up getting gallbladder stones from this drug."	Would not help prevent or detect bleeding Not related
"If I bruise easily or note any blood in my urine I will call my doctor."	Would help detect bleeding
"I need to have my blood work checked twice weekly while I am taking this medication."	Is not necessary
"Reactions to the drug are rare but if I get a rash I should have it checked."	Would help detect an adverse effect

Consider the client's condition and assessment findings, note that apixaban is a new medication, and recall that apixaban is an anticoagulant. Two of the client statements provide evidence of client understanding of the teaching. Bruising or bleeding is evidence of an adverse reaction. Also recall that if a rash presents in a client taking a medication, especially a new medication, an allergic reaction should be suspected.

CJ Cognitive Skills: Recognize Cues, Analyze Cues, Prioritize Hypotheses, Generate Solutions, Take Action, Evaluate Outcomes

Stand-alone Item 6: Bow-tie

Content Area: Maternal-Newborn Nursing
Priority Concept: Gas Exchange
Reference(s): Lowdermilk et al., 2020, pp. 310, 462–463, 492, 714, 757

Practice Question 10.30   **Stand-alone Item 6: Bow-tie**

The nurse in the birthing suite performs an initial assessment on a newborn and documents the following data in the Nurses' Notes.

| Health History | Nurses' Notes | Vital Signs | Lab Results |

0800: Newborn of 43 weeks' gestation born via vaginal delivery. Apgar score at 1 minute = 3. Newborn limp, skin color bluish, RR 80 bpm, grunting during breathing with nasal flaring. Lacks cry with minimal response to gentle slap on soles. Nails and umbilical cord stained a yellow-green color. Blood glucose 40 mg/dL (2.2 mmol/L). Profuse scalp hair. Length 23 inches (58.42 cm), weight 5.5 lb (2500 g). SpO_2 = 90% on RA.

Complete the diagram by dragging (or selecting) from the choices below to specify which potential condition the newborn is most likely experiencing, two assessment findings that support that condition, and two potential interventions to treat the condition.

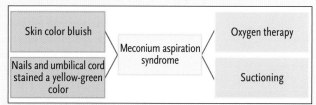

Supportive Assessment Findings	Potential Conditions	Potential Interventions
Skin color bluish	Acrocyanosis	Suctioning
Profuse scalp hair	Meconium aspiration syndrome	Oxygen therapy
Skin dry and cracked without lanugo	Large for gestational age	Early feedings with dextrose
Length 23 inches (58.42 cm), weight 5.5 lb (2500 g)	Transient tachypnea	Phototherapy with a bili-blanket
Nails and umbilical cord stained a yellow-green color		Abdominal decompression with an NG tube

Rationale: Meconium aspiration syndrome is a condition that occurs when a newborn breathes a mixture of meconium and amniotic fluid into the lungs in utero around the time of delivery or during delivery. Meconium is a dark green fecal material that is produced in the intestines of a fetus before birth. Normally the newborn will pass meconium stools after delivery for the first few days of life. If the fetus is stressed before or during birth, meconium stool may be passed while still in the uterus. The meconium stool then mixes with the amniotic fluid that surrounds the fetus. The fetus may then breathe the meconium and amniotic fluid mixture into the lungs shortly before, during, or immediately after birth. Fetal stress often results when the amount of oxygen available to the fetus is reduced. Common causes of fetal stress include a pregnancy that goes past the due date (more than 40 weeks), a difficult or long labor, maternal hypertension, diabetes, or infection. Respiratory distress is the most prominent sign, and the newborn may breathe rapidly or grunt during breathing. Therefore tachypnea, grunting, a bluish skin color (cyanosis), limpness, retractions, nasal flaring, and lung crackles may be present. The newborn's nails, skin, and umbilical cord may be stained a yellow-green color. A diagnosis is made based on the newborn's clinical manifestations and the presence of meconium in the amniotic fluid. Blood gas analysis may be done to evaluate oxygen and carbon dioxide levels, and a chest x-ray may be done to determine if meconium has entered the newborn's lungs. If meconium aspiration occurs, the newborn needs immediate treatment via suctioning to remove the meconium from the airway. After emergency treatment is provided to remove the meconium, additional treatment may be needed to avoid complications. These include oxygen therapy, the use of a radiant warmer to help maintain body temperature, antibiotics to prevent or treat an infection from aspiration, possibly the use of a ventilator to help the newborn breathe, and extracorporeal membrane oxygenation (ECMO) if the newborn is not responding to other treatments or has pulmonary hypertension. Profuse scalp hair, dry and cracked skin without lanugo, and a long and thin body are characteristics of a postterm newborn. Although this newborn is postterm, this fact is not one of the options for a potential condition. Even though a newborn is postterm, it does not necessarily mean that the newborn is large for gestational age. Early feedings may be an intervention for a large-for-gestational-age newborn because of hypoglycemia. However, this would not be an intervention for meconium aspiration syndrome; feedings would not be initiated until the syndrome was treated and stabilized. Phototherapy may be prescribed for a newborn with hyperbilirubinemia. Abdominal decompression is not necessary in meconium aspiration syndrome but may be a necessary intervention in an acute inflammatory disease of the GI tract such as necrotizing enterocolitis, most often seen in preterm newborns. Acrocyanosis is often seen in healthy newborns and refers to the peripheral cyanosis around the mouth and the hands and feet. It is normal in the first few hours after birth and may also be seen intermittently for 7 to 10 days after birth. A large-for-gestational-age newborn is one who is plotted at or above the 90th percentile on the intrauterine growth curve. Assessment findings would include respiratory distress, hypoglycemia, and signs of birth trauma or injury. Interventions include monitoring for and treating any respiratory distress that may occur, monitoring for hypoglycemia, and early feedings. Transient tachypnea of the newborn is a respiratory condition that results from the incomplete reabsorption of the fetal lung fluid in full-term newborns. This condition usually disappears within 24 to 48 hours. Assessment findings include tachypnea, retractions, nasal flaring, fluid breath sounds on auscultation, and cyanosis. Interventions include oxygen administration and supportive care.

Test-Taking Strategy: To begin answering this question, organize your thought process into two parts. This question is asking you to decide on the potential condition by analyzing relevant data provided in the clinical scenario (*Recognize Cues* and *Analyze Cues*). List the potential conditions and then think about each assessment finding to decide if it is consistent with the condition listed, as illustrated in the table.

Potential Conditions

Acrocyanosis
Meconium aspiration syndrome
Large for gestational age
Transient tachypnea

Supportive Assessment Finding[a]	Potential Condition
Skin color bluish	Meconium aspiration syndrome, transient tachypnea
Profuse scalp hair	Postterm (not an option)
Skin dry and cracked without lanugo	Postterm (not an option)
Length 23 inches (58.42 cm), weight 5.5 lb (2500 g)	N/A to any potential condition
Nails and umbilical cord stained a yellow-green color	Meconium aspiration syndrome

[a]No supportive assessment findings for acrocyanosis or large for gestational age.
N/A, Not applicable.

Bluish skin color and nails and umbilical cord stained a yellow-green color are both specific to meconium aspiration syndrome. Profuse scalp hair and dry skin that is cracked without lanugo are both found with postterm newborns, but recall that this does not specifically mean that the infant is large for gestational age. The length and weight identified in the question are not supportive of any of the potential conditions listed, and there are no supportive assessment findings for acrocyanosis or large for gestational age in the clinical scenario. Now that you have identified the most likely potential condition that is the priority problem *(Prioritize Hypotheses)*, the second part of your thought process will be to decide on the most appropriate nursing actions for the care of the newborn with meconium aspiration syndrome *(Generate Solutions)*. To decide on the two interventions the nurse would take or *Take Action*, think about what occurs in meconium aspiration syndrome. Next, determine whether there are data to support performing the listed intervention, as illustrated in the table.

Action to Take	Supporting Data
Suctioning	Yes
Oxygen therapy	Yes
Early feedings	No
Phototherapy with a bili-blanket	No
Abdominal decompression with an NG tube	No

The Apgar score and physical assessment findings including the muscle tone, skin color, RR and other respiratory findings, level of responsiveness, and umbilical cord findings are all supportive findings for suctioning and oxygen therapy. Remember that with meconium aspiration system, the first priority is to stabilize breathing and address potential or existing respiratory failure. There are no data supporting early feedings, which would actually be contraindicated until the newborn is stabilized. There are also no data to support phototherapy with a bili-blanket or abdominal decompression with an NG tube.

CJ Cognitive Skills: Recognize Cues, Analyze Cues, Prioritize Hypotheses, Generate Solutions, Take Action

References and Bibliography

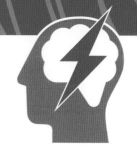

Betts, J., Muntean, W., Kim, D., Jorion, N., & Dickison, P. (2019). Building a method for writing clinical judgment items for entry-level nursing exams. *Journal of Applied Testing Technology, 20*(S2), 21–36.

Burchum, J., & Rosenthal, L. (2022). *Lehne's pharmacology for nursing care* (11th ed.). St. Louis: Elsevier.

Burchum, J., & Rosenthal, L. (2019). *Lehne's pharmacology for nursing care* (10th ed.). St. Louis: Elsevier.

Centers for Disease Control and Prevention (CDC). *Interim clinical guidance for management of patients with confirmed coronavirus disease (COVID-19).* CDC updated February 2021. https://stacks.cdc.gov/view/cdc/89980.

Dickison, P., Haerling, K. A., & Lasater, K. (2019). Integrating the National Council of State Boards of Nursing Clinical Judgment Model into nursing educational frameworks. *Journal of Nursing Education, 58*(2), 72–78.

Halter, M. J. (2022). *Varcarolis' foundations of psychiatric-mental health nursing* (8th ed.). St. Louis: Elsevier.

Hockenberry, M. J., Wilson, D., & Rodgers, C. C. (2019). *Wong's nursing care of infants and children* (11th ed.). St. Louis: Elsevier.

Ignatavicius, D. D. (2022). *Developing clinical judgment for practical/vocational nursing and the Next-Generation NCLEX-PN® Examination.* St. Louis: Elsevier.

Ignatavicius, D. D. (2021). *Developing clinical judgment for professional nursing and the Next-Generation NCLEX-RN® Examination.* St. Louis: Elsevier.

Ignatavicius, D. D., Workman, M. L., Rebar, C., & Heimgartner, N. M. (2021). *Medical-surgical nursing: Concepts for interprofessional collaborative care* (10th ed.). St. Louis: Elsevier.

Lilley, L. L., Collins, S. R., & Snyder, J. S. (2020). *Pharmacology and the nursing process* (9th ed.). St. Louis: Elsevier.

Lowdermilk, D. L., Perry, S. E., Cashion, M. C., Alden, K., & Olshansky, E. (2020). *Maternity and women's health care* (7th ed.). St. Louis: Elsevier.

National Council of State Boards of Nursing (NCSBN). (Winter, 2018). Summary of the strategic practice analysis. *NGN News,* 1–4.

NCSBN. (Spring, 2020). The NGN case study. *NGN News.* 1–5.

National Institutes of Health (NIH). *COVID-19 Treatment guidelines: What's new in the guidelines.* NIH updated June 11 2021. https://www.covid19treatmentguidelines.nih.gov/about-the-guidelines/whats-new/.

Pagana, K., Pagana, T., & Pagana, T. (2021). *Mosby's® Diagnostic and laboratory test reference* (15th ed.). St. Louis: Elsevier.

Pagana, K., Pagana, T., & Pike-MacDonald, S. (2019). *Mosby's Canadian manual of diagnostic and laboratory tests* (2nd ed.). St. Louis: Elsevier.

Petersen, E. K., Betts, J., & Muntean, W. (2020). *Next generation NCLEX® (NGN).* [PowerPoint slides].

Potter, P. A., Perry, A. G., Stockert, P., & Hall, A. (2021). *Fundamentals of nursing* (10th ed.). St. Louis: Elsevier.

Silvestri, L., & Silvestri, A. (2022). *Saunders 2022-2023 Clinical judgment and test-taking strategies* (7th ed.). St. Louis: Elsevier (Saunders).

The Joint Commission. (n.d.). Acute myocardial infarction core measure set. Retrieved from https://www.jointcommission.org/-/media/deprecated-unorganized/imported-assets/tjc/system-folders/assetmanager/acute-myocardial-infarctionpdf.pdf?db=web&hash=73B2DBC4D5656B6FEF8AB20B71D57EB8.

Varcarolis, E. M., & Fosbre, C. D. (2021). *Essentials of psychiatric-mental health nursing: A communication approach to evidence-based care* (4th ed.). St. Louis: Elsevier.